Arts in Healthy Aging

Exploring Research, Policy, and Professional Practice

Patricia Dewey Lambert,
Doug Blandy, and
Margaret J. Wyszomirski

OXFORD
UNIVERSITY PRESS

OXFORD
UNIVERSITY PRESS

Great Clarendon Street, Oxford, OX2 6DP,
United Kingdom

Oxford University Press is a department of the University of Oxford.
It furthers the University's objective of excellence in research, scholarship,
and education by publishing worldwide. Oxford is a registered trade mark of
Oxford University Press in the UK and in certain other countries

© Oxford University Press 2024

The moral rights of the authors have been asserted

All rights reserved. No part of this publication may be reproduced, stored in
a retrieval system, or transmitted, in any form or by any means, without the
prior permission in writing of Oxford University Press, or as expressly permitted
by law, by licence or under terms agreed with the appropriate reprographics
rights organization. Enquiries concerning reproduction outside the scope of the
above should be sent to the Rights Department, Oxford University Press, at the
address above

You must not circulate this work in any other form
and you must impose this same condition on any acquirer

Published in the United States of America by Oxford University Press
198 Madison Avenue, New York, NY 10016, United States of America

British Library Cataloguing in Publication Data
Data available

Library of Congress Control Number: 2023942341

ISBN 978-0-19-284760-7

DOI: 10.1093/oso/9780192847607.001.0001

Printed in the UK by
Ashford Colour Press Ltd, Gosport, Hampshire

Links to third party websites are provided by Oxford in good faith and
for information only. Oxford disclaims any responsibility for the materials
contained in any third party website referenced in this work.

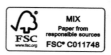

*For our aging family members,
friends, and colleagues
who love the arts.*

Contents

List of Figures — xi
List of Tables — xiii
List of Boxes — xv
Acknowledgments — xvii
About the Authors — xix

1. **Introducing *Arts in Healthy Aging* Policy and Practice** — 1
   - Introducing *Arts in Healthy Aging* — 1
   - A Profile of Older Adults in America — 2
   - Healthy Aging — 6
   - The Need for Research and Resources to Support the *Arts in Healthy Aging* Movement — 11
   - America's Arts and Culture Sector — 13
   - The Interdisciplinary Fields of *Creative Aging* — 20
   - Introducing the Chapters of this Book — 24

2. **Foundational Concepts in Creative Aging** — 28
   - Introduction — 28
   - Creative Aging in the Arts in Health Field — 29
   - Understanding the Needs of Older Adults — 33
   - Engaging in Arts and Culture: A Basic Human Need — 38
   - Choice-Based Arts Participation — 39
   - Public Purposes of the Arts — 43
   - Introducing the *8Ps Framework for Arts in Healthy Aging* — 45
   - Conclusion — 47

3. **Four Strategies to Advance Arts and Aging Policy** — 49
   - Introduction — 49
   - Aging as a Special Constituency: An Advocacy Movement, 1973–1995 — 51
   - The Arts Aim for a Place on the Aging Policy Agenda, 1981–2015 — 56
   - A Change in Frame and Leadership: Creative Aging and the National Center for Creative Aging, 2001–2018 — 62
   - Decentralizing Creative Aging Policy and Diffusing the Arts into Healthy Aging, 2013 to Present — 66
   - Conclusion — 69

4. **How the Arts Support Health and Well-Being Outcomes in Older Adults** — 71
   - Introduction — 71
   - The Sociocultural Context of Older Adults' Health and Well-Being — 71
   - Human Development in Late Life — 72
   - Motivations of Older Adults to Participate in Creative Aging Programs and Activities — 75
   - Healthy Aging in All Phases of the Natural Aging Process — 77
   - Arts Participation and Healthy Aging — 84

Subjective Well-Being in Older Adults — 89
Basic Design Elements of *Arts in Healthy Aging* Programs — 93
Conclusion — 99

5. Centering the Learner in Arts Education for Older Adults — 101
Introduction — 101
Examples of Motivating Factors for Older Adults' Arts Participation — 103
Creativity, Culture, and Folk Groups — 105
The Arts, Making Special, and Expressive Culture — 107
The Arts and the Life Course — 108
Folklore and Creative Aging — 113
The Arts, Education, and Folklore — 114
Conclusion — 116

6. Creating a Learner-Centered Transformative Arts Education Environment for Older Adults — 119
Introduction — 119
Lifelong Learning — 121
Transformative Learning Theory — 123
Transformative Learning, the Extrarational, and the Arts — 128
Transformative Learning and the Role of the Arts Educator — 131
Conclusion — 134

7. Older Adults, Community Arts Participation, and Age-Friendliness — 137
Introduction — 137
Community Resources Available to Older Adults — 138
Health and Well-Being Outcomes Associated with Community Arts — 145
Ageism and Ableism as Barriers to Participation — 149
Age-Friendly Communities and Participation in Arts and Culture — 152
Conclusion — 158

8. Arts Programs for Older Adults in Residential and Clinical Care Settings — 159
Introduction — 159
Overview of America's Eldercare and Healthcare System — 159
Healthcare Quality and Healthcare Consumerism — 162
Medicare, Medicaid, and Long-Term Care — 164
Age-Friendly and Person-Centered Care — 168
Introduction to Settings of Care for Older Adults in America — 173
Independent Living — 173
Independent Living to Assisted Living — 175
Assisted Living — 178
Clinical Care — 181
Conclusion — 183

9. Arts Programs in Hospice and End-of-Life Care — 184
Introduction — 184
A "Good Death" in America — 184
The American Hospice System — 189
Arts in Spiritual Care — 194
Arts for Reminiscence, Legacy, and Ritual — 196
Conclusion — 200

10. Advancing Public Policy and Professional Practice for the	
Arts in Healthy Aging	201
Introduction	201
Findings on the Current State of *Creative Aging* Policy and Practice in America	204
Activating the *Arts in Healthy Aging* Ecosystem	212
Activating the *8Ps Framework for Arts in Healthy Aging*	219
Conclusion	222
Appendix A: America's Arts in Healthy Aging Timeline	225
Appendix B: National Organizations Advancing the Fields of Arts, Health, Aging,	
and Lifelong Learning	231
Notes	237
References	243
Index	259

Figures

1.1	America's aging population	3
1.2	Americans' increasing educational attainment	8
1.3	The creative sector	19
1.4	Fields of knowledge framing creative aging policy and professional practice	21
2.1	The arts in health field in America	32
2.2	Illustrative patterns of functional ability throughout the lifespan	36
2.3	The NEA's *How Art Works* System Map	44
2.4	The *8Ps Framework for Arts in Healthy Aging*	46
4.1	Whole-person health and well-being	78
4.2	Examples of older adults' motivations to participate in creative aging activities that support the health and well-being of the body, mind, and spirit	79
4.3	The sociocultural context of healthy aging	83
4.4	Example of a logic model framework for how creative aging programs contribute to older adults' health outcomes	87
4.5	Domains of subjective well-being in older adults	92
4.6	Creative aging programs in support of program outputs and outcomes of the National Council on Aging's *Aging Mastery Program*	94
4.7	A continuum of creative aging program approaches and outcomes	95
4.8	Representative types of creative aging programs	96
4.9	Creative aging program design by program goals along the natural aging process	98
4.10	Program design by nature of participation and level of autonomy	99
6.1	Phases of transformative learning and extrarational transformative learning through the arts	130
8.1	Senior housing and healthcare settings	161
10.1	America's creative aging institutional infrastructure in 2018	213
10.2	Activating the *8Ps Framework for Arts in Healthy Aging*	220

Tables

1.1	Time spent on leisure activities by older adults	10
1.2	Commonly used terms for describing America's arts and culture sector	16
2.1	Individual choice categories for arts participation	42
4.1	Erikson's eight stages of life development	73
4.2	Cohen's phases of late life	75
8.1	Common chronic physical impairments in older adults	170
8.2	Common chronic cognitive impairments in older adults	171
9.1	Developmental landmarks and task work for the end of life	187
9.2	Ten characteristics of hospice programs in America	191
9.3	Different types of care provided in end-of-life settings	192

Boxes

1.1	*The arts* as defined by the National Endowment for the Arts	14
6.1	Ten phases of transformative learning	125
6.2	Aims within the transformative learning environment leading toward transformative experiences	132
6.3	Prerequisite competencies for working with older adults within the transformative arts education learning environment	134
6.4	Examples of lifelong learning programs for older adults	135
7.1	Examples of community-based arts programs for older adults	142
7.2	Examples of community-wide arts programs for older adults	153
7.3	Questions for community-based arts programs for older adults	156
8.1	Examples of creative aging programs intended to support older adults in long-term care settings	179
8.2	Example of a comprehensive hospital arts program	183
9.1	Uses and benefits of psychosocial support programs in hospice and end-of-life care	198
9.2	Example of an arts program intended for end-of-life care	199
10.1	Findings from the 2015 Summit on Creativity and Aging in America	211
10.2	Our ideas for specific action steps that might be taken by national organizations to move toward building an advocacy coalition for the *arts in healthy aging*	217

Acknowledgments

It is with great appreciation that we take this opportunity to acknowledge several individuals who helped to make this book project possible. We would like to begin with thanking Gay Hanna, one of America's leading scholars in the creative aging field, for her enthusiastic encouragement when we first started this research project. Our research assistant, Rosemarie Oakman, provided extraordinary support in the first two years of developing this project, and we are deeply grateful for her talents in collecting, organizing, and summarizing English-language publications from around the world that informed our study. We thank our additional research assistants for their valuable support of this project: at The Ohio State University, Lizzie Howald and Kuo Guo, for summarizing pertinent documents from the United States and the United Kingdom; and doctoral students Ahyoung Yoon and Nakyung Rhee for sharing their insights about United States and South Korean arts and aging policies. Thank you also to our graduate and undergraduate students who responded to this research within our classes. Several expert reviewers provided valuable feedback on specific chapter drafts in development, and we thank Judy Rollins and Jenny Lee, in particular, for their thoughtful chapter reviews. Heartfelt gratitude goes to Dianne Dewey for her eagle-eyed manuscript review. We are very grateful to our talented digital illustrator, Stephanie McCarthy, for her extraordinary ability to take our complex ideas and our amateur hand drawings and transform them into beautiful visuals for publication. We extend special thanks to the wonderful staff of Oxford University Press, especially to our editor, Martin Baum, for facilitating an excellent book publication process. Finally, we acknowledge financial support for this project that came from the University of Oregon's School of Planning, Public Policy and Management and from a University of Oregon Faculty Research Award.

About the Authors

Patricia Dewey Lambert, PhD, is Professor at the University of Oregon's School of Planning, Public Policy and Management. Her research and teaching specialize in arts administration, arts in health, cultural policy, nonprofit management, and international public policy. Her employment experience in Europe and the United States comprises positions as a professional classical singer, opera administrator, foundation programs administrator, English (ESL) instructor, marketing communications consultant, research fellow, and college teacher. Her numerous academic fellowships, grants, and awards include a Fulbright European Union Affairs Research Program Grant, grant support from the Canadian Embassy and Canadian Consulate in Seattle, and a Rotary Ambassadorial Scholarship. Prof. Lambert has published articles in *Higher Education*, the *International Journal of Arts Management*, the *International Journal of Cultural Policy*, the *Journal of Arts Management, Law and Society*, and *Studies in Art Education*, among others. She serves on the editorial board of the *Journal of Arts Management, Law and Society*. Her recent book publications include *Managing Arts Programs in Healthcare* (Routledge 2016) and *Performing Arts Center Management* (Routledge 2017). She served as lead author and editor of a major national white paper, titled *Arts, Health & Well-Being in America*, published by the National Organization for Arts in Health (NOAH) in 2017. From 2021 to 2024, she served as a board member of the NOAH, for which she oversaw national professionalization initiatives for advancing the field. Prof. Lambert contributed to this book project research her expertise in arts in healthcare leadership, performing arts management, and cultural policy.

Doug Blandy, PhD, is Professor Emeritus in the School of Planning, Public Policy and Management and in the Folklore Program at the University of Oregon. His research and teaching address arts educational experiences in community-based settings that meet the needs of all students within a lifelong learning context. Prof. Blandy's research has been published in *Studies in Art Education*, *Art Education*, *Visual Arts Research*, the *Journal of Multicultural and Cross-Cultural Research in Art Education*, and the *Visual Sociology Review*, among other journals. His book publications comprise *Art in a Democracy* (1987), *Pluralistic Approaches to Art Criticism* (1991), *Remembering Others: Making Invisible Histories of Art Education Visible* (2000), *Histories of Community-Based Art Education* (2001), *Matter Matters* (2011), *Happy Clouds, Happy Trees: The Bob Ross Phenomenon* (2014), and *Learning Things: Material Culture Studies in Art Education* (2018). Prof. Blandy has served on the editorial boards of *Studies in Art Education*, the *Journal of Cultural Research in Art Education*, and the *Journal of Social Theory and Art Education*. From 2007 to

2009, he was senior editor of *Studies in Art Education*. Prof. Blandy's contributions to the field of arts education have been recognized by the National Art Education Association (NAEA)'s *Manuel Barkan Award* for scholarly publication, the *NAEA Art Educator of the Year* (2010), the NAEA *Beverly Levett Gerber Special Needs Lifetime Achievement Award* (2014), and the United States Society for Education's *Art Edwin Ziegfeld Award* (2015). Prof. Blandy is a member of the NAEA Distinguished Fellows. He is past chair of the board of Local Learning: The National Network of Folk Arts in Education. Prof. Blandy contributed to this book project his expertise in visual arts education, lifelong learning, community cultural development, material culture studies, folklore, and disability studies.

Margaret J. Wyszomirski, PhD, is Professor Emerita at The Ohio State University's Department of Art Administration, Education and Policy, where she directed the graduate Arts Policy and Administration Program from 1998 to 2014. Her research and teaching have focused on American arts policy and arts administration, comparative cultural policy, arts entrepreneurship, and cultural diplomacy. An internationally known scholar, she served as staff director for the bipartisan Independent Commission on the National Endowment for the Arts (1990) and as director of the Office of Policy Planning, Research and Budget at the National Endowment for the Arts (1991–1994). She was a founding member of the Research Advisory Committee of the American Council for the Arts (now Americans for the Arts) and was chairman of the Research Task Force for the Center for Arts and Culture in Washington, DC. She was a member of three American Assembly steering committees, including the 1997 American Assembly on *The Arts and the Public Purpose*. Her arts and cultural policy research has been funded by the Ford Foundation, the Pew Charitable Trusts, and The Aspen Institute, among others. She has published a number of books and monographs, including *Arts, Ideology and Politics* (1985); *America's Commitment to Culture: Public Policy and the Arts* (1995); *The Public Life of the Arts in America* (1999); *Going Global: Negotiating the Maze of Cultural Interactions* (2000); *Understanding the Arts and Creative Sector in the United States* (2008); *International Cultural Connections: The Times, They Are A-Changing* (2011); and *Professionalism in the Creative Sector* (2023). Prof. Wyszomirski contributed to this book project her expertise in cultural policy and arts administration.

1
Introducing *Arts in Healthy Aging* Policy and Practice

Introducing *Arts in Healthy Aging*

Arts in Healthy Aging is about why and how the arts can support the health and well-being of older adults in America. We investigate the intentional design of arts-based lifelong learning and arts participation programs to achieve health and well-being outcomes in older adults.

This field is commonly called *creative aging*, which is viewed as a set of theoretical approaches and practices that "leverages the benefits of making, sharing or otherwise engaging in the arts to foster the mental, emotional and physical health and well-being of older adults" (National Assembly of State Arts Agencies 2019a, 1). In creative aging, creativity is celebrated as an inherent human trait that can be nurtured throughout the lifespan. Creative expression does not diminish with age; indeed, tapping into one's creativity can awaken human potential in the second half of life (Cohen 2005).

Although there are many different forms of creativity and creative expression, this book is focused on the arts. "Art is the transformation of the tangible (bodies, instruments, paper, ink, clay, fabric) and intangible (words, sounds, memories, emotions, ideas) into something new, such as sculpture, living history theater, musical performances, stories, paintings, dance, quilts, or poems. The process of creating, as well as the art that is created, transforms the participants and the people around them" (Boyer 2007, 15). In this book, we emphasize examples of arts-based educational programs and participatory visual and performing arts programs for older adults, which are provided in both community settings and eldercare facilities.

Older adults everywhere want a high quality of life in their senior years. In the United States and around the world, there are ever-increasing demands for *arts in health* programs for older adults. Many older adults—defined in this book as people over the age of 60—engage regularly in the arts for educational, enrichment, spiritual, and therapeutic purposes. However, very few resources exist that can help cultural organizations, artists, educators, and healthcare facilities in designing and implementing arts in health and arts for wellness programs for older adults. Similarly, there are very few resources that inform *arts-based lifelong learning* for older adults. In addition, although we know the dramatically growing cohort of people over the age of 60 are active participants in arts and cultural programs in their communities, very little scholarship focuses on this larger demographic group and the intersectional subgroups associated with race, ethnicity, gender, sexual orientation, and socioeconomic status as arts participants.

The time is right for a robust study that contributes to developing the theory and practice of lifelong learning in the arts and to developing a public policy agenda and strategies for arts engagement that support the *creative aging* movement and field. In this book, we refer to *arts in healthy aging* and *creative aging* interchangeably.

Arts in Healthy Aging specifically investigates why and how arts-based lifelong learning and participation in the arts can contribute to the health and well-being of older adults in America. This first chapter clarifies key concepts and introduces the fields of knowledge that inform the present-day creative aging field of public policy and professional practice. The chapter concludes with summarizing the scope of our study on *arts in healthy aging* and introducing the subsequent chapters of this book.

A Profile of Older Adults in America

A profound demographic transformation is taking place around the world because people are having fewer children and are also living longer. Disproportionate growth of older age groups varies among countries and regions. Many of the oldest countries are in Europe, with an expected increase in the percentage of older adults to 27.6% of the total population by 2050. In both Asia and Latin America, the percentage of people aged over 65 will be more than double (to about 19% in these two regions). In contrast, Africa's percentage of older adults in 2050 will be comparatively very low, i.e., 6.6%. The continent of North America anticipates growth in the population of those aged 65 and older from 15.1% in 2015 to 22.5% in 2050 (Federal Interagency Forum on Aging-Related Statistics [FIFARS] 2021). The world's population of older adults will increase to 1 billion by 2030 and will reach an estimated 1.6 billion by 2050 (Coughlin 2017, 5), comprising 16.7% of the world's total population by the middle of the twenty-first century (FIFARS 2021).

Although the entire world's population is growing older due to lower birth rates, it is important to recognize that gains in healthy life expectancy are enjoyed mainly by wealthy societies and often by high-education and high-income populations within those societies. This is certainly the case in the United States, where wealthier and better-educated people both live longer and enjoy better health in their old age (Coughlin 2017, 21). Life expectancy of Americans rose by roughly 30 years from 1900 to the present. "Longevity is creating [a] new age between middle age and old age. What this stage of life will include or even be named is still in the formative phase" (Hanna 2013, 1).

Since 1900, the percentage of Americans aged 65 and older nearly quadrupled (from 4.1% in 1900 to 16% in 2019—the most recent year for which data are available at the time of writing this book), and the number increased more than 17 times (from 3.1 million to 54.1 million). By 2030, when the entire baby boom generation

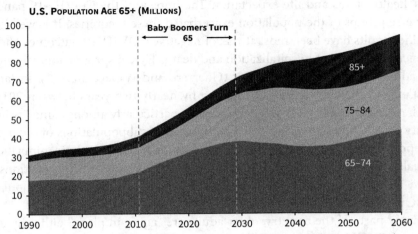

Figure 1.1 America's aging population
Source: Peter G. Peterson Foundation (pgpf.org)

(those born from 1945 to 1965) will be over the age of 65, the nation's percentage of older adults will rise to 21%. The older population in 2030 is projected to be more than twice as large as it was in 2000, growing from 35 million to 73 million. By 2035, the number of people aged over 65 will surpass the number of those under the age of 18 for the first time in the country's history. The over-65 population group in the United States is projected to reach 80.8 million by 2040 and 94.7 million by 2060 (see Figure 1.1).

The older population itself is also becoming increasingly older, with worrisome trends indicating that the number of working-age adults per retired adult is falling dramatically. In 2019, people reaching the age of 65 had an average life expectancy of 19.6 more years (20.8 years for women and 18.2 years for men). In 2019, the 65–74 age group was more than 14 times larger than this group was in 1900; the 75–84 age group was 20 times larger; and the 85+ age group was more than 53 times larger. The 85-and-older age group is now the fastest-growing segment of the US population, and a child born today has a high probability of living to 100 years (Administration for Community Living 2021; FIFARS 2020; Population Reference Bureau 2019).

In general, older adults in America are now better educated and more ethnically diverse than they were in previous generations, and they are also working longer past the age of 65. The gender gap in life expectancy is narrowing, and the poverty rate for older Americans has dropped sharply over the past 50 years (FIFARS 2021).

However, wide economic and health disparities are evident across different population subgroups. Even before the COVID-19 pandemic, a range of factors—such as income inequality, an inadequate social safety net, racial inequality, and some population groups' limited access to healthcare—led to stark differences among older adults' health status and life expectancy. The impact of the COVID-19 pandemic on diverse groups of the population exacerbated these inequities. It is well known that older adults have been most at risk of negative COVID-19 outcomes and consequences, and rates of hospitalization and deaths have disproportionately affected older adults in communities of color (Guerrero and Wallace 2021, 1). In fact, life expectancy in the United States decreased by nearly two years between 2018 and 2020, largely due to the COVID-19 pandemic, particularly among minority groups (Bukaty 2021, 1). Public health research shows that subpopulations of older adults disproportionately impacted by COVID-19 include racial and ethnic minorities, individuals with disabilities, rural populations, tribal populations, populations with limited English proficiency, and socioeconomically disadvantaged populations (NORC at the University of Chicago 2021, 3).

In many parts of the country, older adults are "aging in place," either by choice or because it is the only choice that they have. About 95% of Americans aged over 65 live independently in traditional communities. Significant risk of social isolation exists among older adults, especially for women. Among women aged 85 and over, 70% of women are widowed. Roughly one-fourth of women aged 65–74 currently live alone. This share jumps to 39% among women aged 75–84 and to 55% among women aged 85 and older. The aging population is also fueling a rapid increase in the number of older adults requiring nursing home care. In 2019, a relatively small number of people (1.2 million) aged 65 and older lived in nursing homes. The percentage of older adults in nursing homes increases with age, i.e., from 2% for people aged 75–84 to 8% for people aged over 85 (Administration for Community Living 2021, 7; FIFARS 2020; Population Reference Bureau 2021).

Despite wide disparity among diverse groups of older Americans (as well as internationally), those aged over 65 are generally enjoying higher levels of educational attainment and economic well-being than ever before. In 2019, 86% of the older population were high school graduates or more, and 29% had a bachelor's degree or more (FIFARS 2020, 79). People in the high-income group (roughly 40% of older adults) now make up the largest single share of older people by income category. In the United States, consumers over the age of 50 now control 83% of household wealth (Coughlin 2017, 8), and "wealthy and highly educated Americans are reaping the bulk of our continued longevity gains" (21). Coughlin notes that the enormous cohort of aging baby boomers controls vast personal wealth, is fluent in the use of technology, and is "accustomed to shaping the economic and physical world around it" (89–90). This consumer cohort is driving what he refers to as the *longevity economy*, which offers enormous economic potential to businesses and organizations able to tap into this group's demands for high-quality products and experiences in their retirement years.

No universally applied framework for categorizing and describing older adults in America exists, although data captured nationally and internationally usually reference age 65 and above. In the United States, around age 65 is when people usually cease or scale back work and enter into retirement with the expectation that they will be able to pursue leisure activities thereafter, health and wealth permitting. Age 65 is also when Americans are currently eligible to join Medicare, the federal health insurance program for older adults. Social Security, pensions, and disbursals from individual retirement accounts also usually begin in one's 60s. Once the idea of the "golden years" was promulgated in the 1950s and 1960s, "a happy retirement became something that consumers would pay for and, in funds provided by Social Security and Medicare, voters would demand. Within decades, it would become hard to even think of following up one's primary career with anything other than the pursuit of leisure" (Coughlin 2017, 53). In addition, many retirees are now rethinking retirement in their quest to be "*more* active, *more* engaged, and *more* stimulated" due to "a natural outgrowth of inner desires we all have for learning, social relationships, a sense of meaning, and giving something back to society" (Cohen 2005, 138).

Americans' popular conceptualization of retirement as "golden years" to consume leisure activities as an entitlement—that is, as a reward to be eagerly anticipated after the working years—reflects a growing *age consciousness*. By the middle of the twentieth century, there was an increased sensitivity to the role of age and generation on behavior. "Today, age consciousness has so penetrated our society that one's membership in a particular generation or *birth cohort* is often offered to explain a variety of behaviors—from consumption decisions to political preferences" (Stern 2011, 15). For studying older adults in America at the time of writing this book, there are three birth cohorts that are commonly referenced. The *silent generation*—sometimes referred to as the *World War II generation*, or the *1935 cohort*—is the demographic cohort defined as people born from 1928 to 1945. The *baby boom* generation has the birth years 1945 to 1965, often divided in half by demographers as *early baby boom* (1945) and *late baby boom* (1955) cohorts. *Generation X*, with birth years from 1965 to 1980, is a smaller cohort currently just beginning to enter the preretirement or early retirement years.

For Americans entering retirement, planning for a single retirement lifestyle to potentially extend from one's 60s well into one's 90s is unrealistic. Many retirement planners and advisers refer to the three stages of retirement as the *go-go years*, the *slow-go years*, and the *no-go years*, first popularized by Stein (1998) in his book titled *The Prosperous Retirement*. As the terminology suggests, the first phase of retirement, until the early to mid-70s if one is healthy, involves the pursuit of desired leisure activities, such as travel, volunteering, and other activities. In the slow-go years, typically from the mid-70s to the mid-80s, some physical and cognitive limitations may begin to affect the high levels of activity enjoyed previously. The slow-go years become the no-go years at some point, typically around age 85 or so, after which retirement spending tends to be allocated more to healthcare needs than to travel and entertainment.

Retirement planning for the three stages of a retirement lifestyle aligns with mainstream studies on adult development. Erikson (1982), who defines *late adulthood* as extending from age 65 to death, developed the most commonly applied theory of adult psychosocial development that is used to explain changes as people age. Other scholars divide late adulthood into three stages: early (65–75, to some still considered middle life), middle (75–85), and old (85+) (Rollins 2013, 33–34). In addition, many people retire in their early 60s or even in their 50s, offering a similar lifestyle at that age to those in the 65–75 age bracket. Everyone over the age of 50 is eligible to join the American Association of Retired Persons (AARP).

> Depending when you decide old age begins, the group can be said to account for people found anywhere along a 50-plus span of life, with every imaginable level of physiological health, cognitive ability, and wealth represented, along with every type of personalities; ideologies of every stripe; and every race, nationality, creed, gender, and sexual identity to be found on this blue Earth. Yes, many things become harder with age, and biological reality eventually limits what we can achieve as we grow older. But aging unfolds differently for everyone. We all enter the process at unique starting points and then proceed through a wild variety of physiological experiences at rates that vary from person to person. The idea that there exists one single state of older being that kicks in at age 50, 65, or at any other single age, defies all logic. So does the idea that there is one, single normal way to live a later life. (Coughlin 2017, 15–16)

We decided to study the role of the *arts in healthy aging* for Americans aged 60 and over. While recognizing that the experience of aging varies dramatically from person to person, for purposes of this study, we chose to use the three stages of late adulthood for analysis. We consider the early stage of aging to comprise ages 60–75, an age bracket currently being filled by the baby boom cohort. The middle stage of aging represents ages 75–85, comprised of the baby boom cohort and the silent generation. The late stage of aging, from age 85 to 100+, currently includes only members of the silent generation birth cohort. The last of the baby boom generation will reach the age of 60 in 2025, at which time the Generation X cohort will also begin to enter the first stage of late adulthood.

Healthy Aging

It is a reasonable assumption that everyone wants to be as healthy and happy as possible as long as possible in their lives. A metric for measuring how long a person can expect to live without frailty and disability is referred to as *healthy life expectancy* (Coughlin 2017, 21) or *healthspan* (Population Reference Bureau 2016, 1). Most people hope for a long life with as short a period of terminal sickness as possible, a concept known as *compression of mortality* (Coughlin 2017, 198). As people reach their 80s, 90s, and beyond, they experience higher risk of age-related health problems and disability. Extensive research is underway that seeks to unravel the determinants of health and well-being in longer lifespans (Population Reference Bureau 2016).

Understanding the health and well-being of older adults is so essential that *healthy aging* has become the focus of the World Health Organization (WHO)'s work on aging from 2015 to 2030, replacing its previous focus on *active aging*. As explained by WHO documents, "healthy aging is about creating the environments and opportunities that enable people to be and do what they value throughout their lives. Everybody can experience healthy aging. Being free of disease or infirmity is not a requirement for healthy aging, as many older adults have one or more health conditions that, when well controlled, have little influence on their well-being" (WHO 2020, 1). On December 14, 2020, the United Nations General Assembly proclaimed 2021–2030 to be the "Decade of Healthy Aging," announcing efforts to promote research and practices that would help "improve the lives of older people, their families, and the communities in which they live" (WHO 2021).

The determinants of healthy aging are a mixture of genetic, biological, environmental, psychological, cultural, and social factors, which vary from person to person and across societies. In America, the opportunities that any individual may have for healthy aging tend to be discussed in terms of inherited physiological factors (inherited medical risks), socioeconomic status (education and income), and individual lifestyle choices (such as diet, exercise, and social activities).

> While there is no one simple explanation, aging is affected by intrinsic factors, such as heredity and age-related changes, and extrinsic factors, such as environment, disease, and lifestyle . . . . In the absence of disease, many limiting effects of normal aging are often not even felt until sometime after age 75. Even then, an older adult can adapt his or her normal routine to accommodate these physical-biological and social-emotional changes. (Boyer 2007, 3)

The Federal Interagency Forum on Aging-Related Statistics publishes periodic reports on the condition of older adults in the United States, tracking forty indicators in the areas of population, economics, health status, health risks and behaviors, healthcare, and the environment (FIFARS 2020). For purposes of this book, the most relevant indicators of the well-being of older adults include educational attainment, functional limitations, and use of time.

As illustrated in Figure 1.2, educational attainment among Americans has continuously increased over the past century. Most recent data indicate that approximately one-third (33%) of older adults have a bachelor's degree or higher, although the education level of older adults varies considerably by race and ethnic origin (Administration on Aging 2021, 16). As argued in the *Older Americans 2020* report, "educational attainment has effects throughout the life course and plays an important role in well-being at older ages. Higher levels of education are usually associated with higher incomes, higher standards of living, and above-average health and life expectancy" (FIFARS 2020, 79).

The WHO defines healthy aging as "the process of developing and maintaining the functional ability that enables well-being in older age" (WHO 2020, 2). *Functional*

8 Arts in Healthy Aging

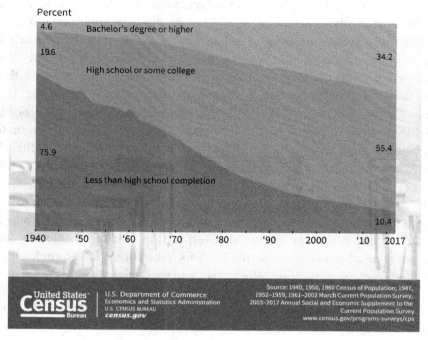

Figure 1.2 Americans' increasing educational attainment
Source: Infographic prepared by the US Census.

ability is explained by the WHO to consist of "the intrinsic capacity of the individual, relevant environmental characteristics, and the interaction between them" (2). In more general terms, the WHO clarifies, functional ability is about older adults having the ability to meet their basic needs; learn, grow, and make decisions; be mobile; build and maintain relationships; and contribute to society (2).

> Intrinsic capacity comprises all the mental and physical capacities that a person can draw on and includes their ability to walk, think, see, hear and remember. The level of intrinsic capacity is influenced by several factors such as the presence of diseases, injuries and age-related changes.
>
> Environments include the home, community and broader society, and all the factors within them such as the built environment, people and their relationships, attitudes and values, health and social policies, the systems that support them and the services that they implement. Being able to live in environments that support and maintain one's intrinsic capacity and functional ability is key to healthy aging. (WHO 2020, 2)

Two significant frameworks for analyzing environmental factors that support functional ability are the *social determinants of health* and the *age-friendly ecosystem*.

These terms are introduced in subsequent chapters of this book. Of equal importance to environmental influences on healthy aging are the individual behavioral decisions of older adults. Intrinsic capacity mainly has to do with the individual health of the person, but it also involves lifestyle choices.

Most older adults have at least one chronic health condition that may affect their functional ability; the prevalence of functional limitations increases with age. The leading chronic health conditions among older adults are currently arthritis (48%); diabetes (29%); cancer (25%); coronary heart disease (14%); COPD, emphysema, or chronic bronchitis (10%); myocardial infarction (9%); stroke (9%); and angina (4%) (Administration on Aging 2021, 17). Of particular concern to many older Americans and their families is the potential to experience severe cognitive limitations due to various forms of dementia, including Alzheimer's disease. One-third of all older adults die with Alzheimer's disease or another form of dementia (Alzheimer's Association 2021). It is also noteworthy that falls are the leading cause of fatal and nonfatal injuries among older adults, and roughly one in four older adults falls each year (NCOA 2021b, 2). Illness or injury of all kinds may result in functional limitations among older adults, which affect their well-being and ability to fully and independently participate in society.

> In 2018, 22 percent of the population age 65 and over reported having a disability as defined by having a lot of difficulty or being unable to do at least one of the following functioning domains: vision, hearing, mobility, communication, cognition, or self-care.
>
> ... Disability increases with age. In 2018, 46 percent of people age 85 and over reported any disability, compared with 16 percent of people ages 65-74. People age 85 and over also had higher levels of disability than people ages 65-74 in all the individual domains of functioning. (FIFARS 2020, 107)

The population's educational attainment and functional limitations are both crucial factors to understand when considering the topic of this book. Even more important, however, are social and behavioral factors, which can be assessed by examining how older adults choose to spend their time. It is noteworthy that, despite much longer and healthier lifespans, societal expectations of older adults have changed very little over the past century. The FIFARS report titled *Older Americans 2020: Key Indicators of Well-Being* presents particularly valuable data on leisure activities (see Table 1.1). "Leisure activities are those done when free from duties such as working, shopping, doing household chores, or caring for others. During these times, individuals have flexibility in choosing what to do" (133). True to the societal expectation that Americans' retirement years are meant for leisure activities, people aged 65–74 report allocating 30% of their time to such activities, and this figure increases to 32% in the 75+ age group.

When delving more deeply into these data, one quickly discovers that very little time is spent doing things that proactively contribute to older adults' well-being and that of others. Watching TV is the activity that occupies the most leisure activity

10 Arts in Healthy Aging

Table 1.1 Time spent on leisure activities by older adults

	55 and over Average hours per day	55 and over Percent of leisure time	55–64 Average hours per day	55–64 Percent of leisure time	65–74 Average hours per day	65–74 Percent of leisure time	75 and over Average hours per day	75 and over Percent of leisure time
Socializing and communicating	0.60	9.2	0.59	10.7	0.67	9.3	0.53	6.8
Watching TV	4.00	61.1	3.36	61.3	4.34	60.6	4.78	61.7
Participation in sports, exercise, and recreation	0.24	3.7	0.23	4.2	0.28	3.9	0.21	2.7
Relaxing and thinking	0.44	6.7	0.37	6.8	0.42	5.9	0.59	7.7
Reading	0.50	7.7	0.27	5.0	0.61	8.6	0.80	10.3
Other leisure activities	0.76	11.6	0.67	12.1	0.84	11.7	0.84	10.8

Note: "Other leisure activities" includes activities, such as playing games, using the computer for leisure, doing arts and crafts as a hobby, experiencing arts and entertainment (other than sports), and engaging in related travel.

Reference population: These data refer to the civilian noninstitutionalized population. Source: Bureau of Labor Statistics, American Time Use Survey.

Source: FIFARS (2020, 133)

time—more than 60% of this time—for adults aged over 65 (see Table 1.1). Older adults in all age brackets report 11%–12% of their leisure time to include "activities such as playing games, using the computer for leisure, doing arts and crafts as a hobby, experiencing arts and entertainment (other than sports), and engaging in related travel" (FIFARS 2020, 134).

Older adults now have the most leisure time available to them of any population group in history. However, as the data on leisure time activities indicate, most people are generally unprepared for what to actually "do" with their longevity. Twenty-first century retirement is being reinvented in social and psychological ways as an ever-increasing number of older adults pursue rich, active, and engaged lifestyles. "More and more people are realizing that this time of life, far from being the downside of the 'hill,' is full of potential for improving life, expanding skills, and fulfilling dreams and expectations" (Cohen 2005, 163).

At the forefront of national initiatives to encourage social and behavioral decisions that will improve the health and well-being of older adults is the National Council on Aging (NCOA)'s *Aging Mastery Program*, which was launched in 2013. The program assumes that older Americans are, to some extent, responsible for their own healthy lifespans through individual decisions and actions that they take. The *Aging Mastery Program* is an educational program designed "to change societal expectations about the roles and responsibilities of baby boomers and older adults and to create fun and easy-to-follow pathways for getting more out of life" (NCOA 2021a, 1). The program's guidebook, titled the *Aging Mastery Playbook*, notes the urgent need for resources to help older adults individually set goals for aging well. Quality of life is emphasized throughout the educational program's materials, and participants are guided in "developing sustainable behaviors across many dimensions that will lead to improved health, stronger financial security, enhanced well-being, and increased connectedness to communities" (NCOA 2021a, 1).

The *Aging Mastery Playbook* is built on the six interconnected dimensions of aging well that have been identified by the NCOA:

- Gratitude and Mindfulness
- Health and Well-Being
- Finances and Future Planning
- Connections and Community
- Creativity and Learning
- Legacy and Purpose

The educational program and an array of related program activities have been designed to guide individuals in developing positive behavior changes in these six dimensions in order to be more aware and intentional about how they spend their time, and to encourage them to share their talents with others to strengthen their communities (Firman and Stiles 2018, 11–15). The *Aging Mastery Program* is currently one of the few resources available to older Americans that is purposively designed to support individual decision-making for healthy aging.

The emphasis on individual behavioral choices as essential to healthy aging underpins new thinking about what makes life worth living in the last 30–40 years of one's lifespan. Programs and services that support this stage of life will only increase in importance as this population segment continues to grow. The *longevity revolution* now underway is essentially a new paradigm for aging, which is focused on health and wellness, lifelong learning, and community engagement based on aging in place (Hanna and Perlstein 2008, 15; Hanna 2016, 193). The term *retirement*, with all its negative connotations, and even the sappy phrase *the golden years* are increasing obsolete as more and more older adults discover that "the second half of life can be more rewarding, stimulating, enjoyable, and rich than the first half" (Cohen 2005, 140).

The Need for Research and Resources to Support the *Arts in Healthy Aging* Movement

The academic and professional field focused on the *arts in healthy aging* is growing dramatically as the aging population around the world demands a high quality of life in their senior years. Despite the enormous potential of the arts to engage older adults in educational, enrichment, and therapeutic programs, few resources exist to support cultural organizations, artists, and healthcare institutions in designing and implementing *arts in health* and *lifelong learning* programs for this population group. A robust array of arts education concepts, theories, and practices has evolved over many decades for K-12 education; however, scant scholarship exists for arts education in lifelong learning for older adults. Similarly, the lack of research on arts participation and cultural engagement for people over the age of 60 is striking, given the size and economic/political power of this demographic group.

Another large gap in the field stems from the dearth of information available to seniors about the kinds of programming, activities, and services that relevant organizations offer in the field of creative aging. In addition, although aging populations may be the direct concern of creative aging policies and programs, they are not the only group that can benefit from widespread information on policy and practice in this field. Many individuals—including professional medical staff and family caregivers—are intimately involved in what kinds of activities "work" for specific aging demographics and in specific circumstances. Furthermore, everyone regardless of their current age will age over time. Healthy aging is an issue with the potential to affect every citizen directly or indirectly—no matter whether they are young or old.

The broad issue of how arts and cultural participation and engagement of all kinds can help define the social goals of healthy aging for an increasing population cohort has begun to attract policy discussion and the attention of national and local governments in many industrialized countries. The first decade of the twenty-first century saw many countries begin to explore these issues primarily through research, professional development, and program development to develop a community of practice that is research and experience based. Concerned academics and professionals undertook definitional efforts that framed the arts and cultural response to the general widespread growth in an aging population with regard to other policy agendas, especially health, well-being, lifelong education, and intergenerational relations. During the next decade, efforts to build program delivery capacity, advocacy networks, interagency collaborations, and public–private partnerships took on momentum throughout the policy infrastructure. As discussion began to frame public discourse and thinking, interested advocates, researchers, practitioners, and policymakers began to develop the necessary components of a policymaking system, as well as mechanisms to share ideas, information, and implementation tools across nations.

This book addresses the specific ways in which advancing the *arts in healthy aging* will involve rethinking arts education, which has historically been focused on the education of children and youth. *Lifelong learning* is one area for such rethinking, along with a deeper understanding of the subgroups that are likely to be segmented within a broad aging population. These subgroups will be divided by various dimensions. One dimension is age itself, since not all people over 60 share a similar condition of activity. For example, young retirees may not face access and participation barriers while the "older old" may experience limiting physical and/or mental conditions. Another relevant dimension is health and socioeconomic status, which pertains to older adults with certain disease-specific or condition-specific health issues (Alzheimer's disease, depression, physical disabilities, etc.), as well as certain access and social-specific conditions (such as social isolation or limited financial means).

Each targeted group of older adults raises its own set of needs and may give rise to a different set of program design and implementation choices. The personal histories of individuals regarding their lifetime engagement and participation in the arts and culture are another key factor. Some older adults will be building on and extending long-standing engagement with the art and culture and finding new time and opportunities to expand and/or diversify that pattern. Others may be engaging with cultural activities and the arts for the first time. Institutions, such as hospitals, assisted living and retirement communities, senior centers, colleges, universities, community-based adult education organizations, arts and cultural institutions, and the tourism industry, are all focusing on the aging population as a market and reimagining their role as service providers and caregivers for these individuals. Families, communities, and government agencies are also grappling with understanding their relevant roles, resources, and capabilities. Addressing creative aging in all this diversity requires cross-institutional and cross-sectoral collaborations, partnerships, and coalitions.

America's Arts and Culture Sector

No single framework for describing the arts and culture sector exists because the composition of this sector is determined by its social and economic context, its location, and the nature of the community. Although there is no common analytical framework for this sector, the definition of *culture* articulated by the United Nations Educational, Scientific and Cultural Organization (UNESCO) is widely accepted around the world. UNESCO (2001, 1) frames *culture* broadly, as "the set of distinctive spiritual, material, intellectual and emotional features of society or a social group that encompasses, not only art and literatures, but lifestyles, ways of living together, value systems, traditions and beliefs." The arts are a core element of this anthropological definition of culture and take shape in nations around the world as both a societal sector and an economic sector. The arts manifest as expressive culture, as well as cultural goods and services, which possess both a cultural value that reflects the representation of diverse values, meanings, and beliefs and an economic value that can commodify the good or service when it is bought or sold (Throsby 2001).

In order to understand how the arts can be used in programs to intentionally support health and well-being outcomes for older Americans, it is useful to briefly explain the overall structure of the arts and culture sector. In the United States, the specification of what is included in "the arts" may be best understood by examining the establishing legislation of the National Endowment for the Arts (NEA). As

> **Box 1.1 *The arts* as defined by the National Endowment for the Arts**
>
> (b) The term "the arts" includes, but is not limited to, music (instrumental and vocal), dance, drama, folk art, creative writing, architecture and allied fields, painting, sculpture, photography, graphic and craft arts, industrial design, costume and fashion design, motion pictures, television, radio, film, video, tape and sound recording, the arts related to the presentation, performance, execution, and exhibition of such major art forms, all those traditional arts practiced by the diverse peoples of this country[,] and the study and application of the arts to the human environment.
>
> (c) The term "production" means plays (with or without music), ballet, dance and choral performances, concerts, recitals, operas, exhibitions, readings, motion pictures, television, radio, film, video, and tape and sound recordings, and any other activities involving the execution or rendition of the arts and meeting such standards as may be approved by the National Endowment for the Arts established by section 954 of this title.
>
> *Source:* National Foundation on the Arts and the Humanities, U.S. Code 20 (1965), § 952

quoted in Box 1.1, a comprehensive list of arts activities can be defined by discipline and/or genre.

Unlike many other countries, the United States does not have a Department or Ministry of Cultural Affairs. Rather, it has a core quartet of federal cultural agencies, as well as a cluster of independent cultural institutions (such as the Library of Congress, the Smithsonian Institution, and the John F. Kennedy Center for the Performing Arts). These federal institutions are complemented by an array of arts, heritage, and cultural programs in numerous other federal agencies and departments. Both the NEA and the National Endowment for the Humanities were established in 1965 as part of the National Foundation on the Arts and the Humanities Act (NFAH Act). Two years later, the Corporation for Public Broadcasting was created. In 1976, the Institute of Museum Services (IMS) was added to the NFAH Act. In 1996, the IMS was consolidated with the Library Programs Office of the United States Department of Education to become the Institute of Museum and Library Services. Each of these four core agencies is focused on a particular set of cultural interests. Each receives annual appropriations from Congress and is subject to periodic reauthorization by Congress.

As the lead federal agency concerned with the arts and arts policy, the NEA is dedicated to advancing Americans' access to and excellence in the arts. Its enabling legislation explained further that it was "to help create and sustain not only a climate encouraging freedom of thought, imagination, and inquiry but also the material conditions facilitating the release of this creative talent" (U.S. Code 20 (1965), § 20, Sec. 2 (7)). To address this mission, the chairperson was authorized to support projects to maintain and encourage professional excellence, emphasize American creativity and cultural diversity, support wider distribution of the arts, and encourage public knowledge, education, understanding, and appreciation of the arts (U.S. Code 20 (1965) § 954 (c)). The NEA is structured into over a dozen program divisions that address the needs of major arts fields, such as music, dance, literature, folk and traditional arts, visual arts, design, theater, opera/musical theater, media arts, and museums. It also has divisions focused on arts education, expansion arts (i.e., arts in culturally specific communities), state arts agencies, and local arts agencies. Each field has organized a set of professional interest groups that bring issues of concern to the NEA and lobby Congress regarding agency policies, resources, and regulations. The NEA formulates arts policy both at the general agency level and within each program through consultations with its field and solicits the advice of peer panels on both policy and grant-making (Wyszomirski 2013).

In fiscal year 2022, the NEA awarded 3,474 grants for a total of $227.45 million (usaspending.gov). The NEA is headed by a chairperson who is nominated by the president and confirmed by the Senate. In addition, a National Council advises the chair and is composed of esteemed individual artists and other professionals knowledgeable about and supportive of the arts. Members of this network also include relevant members of Congress, congressional committees, and their staff. This governance network is further extended by a set of similarly structured, officially designated arts agencies in all fifty states plus six special jurisdictions, and a complement of over 3,000 local arts agencies. The arts policy community is comprised of most of these governmental actors and is augmented by the many nonprofit arts organizations who are NEA grantees, arts-related professional associations, a group of private foundations concerned with cultural philanthropy, and the many citizens who are arts donors and members of the arts audience.

In the United States, when we refer to public policy focused on the arts, we turn to the field of *cultural policy*. At the time of the founding of the NEA, cultural policy was largely understood as government arts funding policy. Since the mid-twentieth century, however, cultural policy has come to encompass many more aspects of the ever-evolving artistic creativity that occurs across the nonprofit, for-profit, public (government), and unincorporated organizational forms. It involves the activities of many individuals (professionals, semi-professionals, volunteers, board members, technicians, administrators, audiences, and so on). It engages many types of organizations operating in the visual, performing, popular, and digital arts, as well as in folk arts and crafts, humanities, and copyright industries, among others.

Table 1.2 describes the ever-evolving array of arts segments commonly understood to be associated with cultural policy. This table is suggestive of the complexity and breadth of the sector and the terminological profusion that exists. The main operating rationales, predominant organizational forms, types of engagement, and examples are provided for each arts segment. It is important to note that, as an ever-evolving sector, the boundaries between the types of arts are highly permeable. For example, video games are largely commercial but are also considered to be a type

Table 1.2 Commonly used terms for describing America's arts and culture sector

Arts Segment	Main Economic Sector	Main Operating Rationale	Participation Examples of how people engage in these art forms	Examples of organizations and activities
Visual, Performing, and Literary Arts *Terminology associated with this segment includes:* "Community Arts" "High Arts" "Fine Arts" "Traditional Arts" "Folk Arts" "Creative Industries" *(this is the creative economy term for this segment)*	Nonprofit Public sector	Art for art's sake Public purposes of the arts Arts in social practice	*Individuals can choose to . . .* curate, create, collect, compose, choreograph, dance, sing, play, act, document, write, critique, exhibit, perform, record, interpret, visit, view, read, teach, etc.	museums and galleries symphony orchestras dance companies opera companies theater companies performing arts centers cultural centers creative writing narrative critique memoirs mural making and graffiti
Commercial Arts *Also known as:* "Entertainment" "Cultural Industries" *(this is the creative economy term for this segment)*	For profit	Arts for profit	*Representative categories:* shareholders, consumers, subscribers, fans, collectors, producers, distributors, marketers, teachers	media video games galleries commercial film television and streaming services commercial galleries popular music and dance publishing
Applied Arts *Also known as:* "Instrumental Arts" Any of the arts segments listed in this table when they relate to nonarts utility	For profit Public sector	Arts for the potential to enhance profit Arts used in support of multiple professional purposes	*Representative categories:* clients, manufacturers, producers, patients, customers, marketers, therapists, teachers	architecture product design graphic design fashion design creative and expressive arts therapies arts education

Attached Arts *This is a political label for this segment, which is also known as:* "Instrumental Arts"	Public sector Nonprofit For profit	Arts attached to other larger policy arenas to advance the arts' agenda, acquire advocacy resources, and broaden political and public support	*Representative categories:* advocates, lobbyists, civil servants, public officials, educators, planners, contributors — arts in cultural diplomacy arts in urban planning arts in healthcare policy and advocacy arts in education policy and advocacy
DIY Arts *Also known as:* "Amateur Arts" "Community Arts" "Hobbies" "Unincorporated Arts"	Voluntary Unincorporated Informal	Arts for self-actualization Arts for building community	*Individuals can choose to…* curate, create, collect, compose, choreograph, dance, sing, play, act, document, write, critique, exhibit, perform, record, interpret, visit, view, read, teach, etc. — church choirs and community choral groups community theater, orchestras, and bands quilting circles book groups self-published books, comics, and zines square dancing
Heritage Arts *Also known as:* "Traditional Arts" "Folk Arts" "Historic Preservation"	Nonprofit Public sector For profit Voluntary	Public purposes of the arts Commodification of heritage Respect for authenticity Respect for items of natural, historical, and cultural significance	*Organizations and individuals can engage in…* preservation, curation, restoration, collecting, touring, documenting, interpreting, teaching, exhibiting, performing, visiting, viewing, reading, etc. — cultural heritage celebrations heritage site tourism archaeological sites antiques collecting festivals and fairs historic landscapes and buildings

of visual art and are being added to museum collections. The work of some do-it-yourself (DIY) artists, such as traditional or folk artists, will also manifest as visual arts collected by museums or heritage sites. Similarly, church choirs may be invited to perform at major performing arts centers.

As Table 1.2 suggests, when we discuss *the arts* throughout the pages of this book, we are referring to the multiple ways that people participate in self-defined arts activities coupled with theoretical perspectives and organizational structures supporting that participation. The participatory arts programs that we profile in the chapters that follow primarily emphasize participation associated with the visual and performing arts. We focus on *two-dimensional arts*, such as painting, drawing, printmaking, still photography, and fiber arts; *three-dimensional arts*, such as ceramics and sculpture; *time-based arts*, such as film and video; *literary arts*; *theater*; *dance*; and *music*. Organizations that offer participation in the arts are structured as nonprofit organizations, public sector (government) entities, for-profit businesses, unincorporated entities, and hybrid organizational forms combining one or more of the preceding organizational structures. While we recognize the plethora of categorizations of the arts that exist—such as "fine arts," "heritage arts," "expressive culture," "making special," and so on—our position is consistent with that of the American Assembly (1997)'s *Art and the Public Purpose* in that we resist "calling up the conventional dichotomies that have separated the arts into high and low, fine and folk, professional and amateur . . ." (10–11). We do not privilege one form of art over another or believe that one form of art ranks higher or lower. Our model of arts participation is introduced in Chapter 2; however, it is important to understand at this point that arts participation by older adults, as is accurate to all people, takes place across and within all the possibilities implied in the above. Ultimately, as is emphasized by NEA (2012, 12), we understand *art* to be "an act of creative expression done within the confines of a set of known or emerging practices and precedence that is intended to communicate richly to others." In this regard, the chapters in this book will delineate arts participation practices that are advantageous to healthy aging outcomes.

With blurring boundaries between various arts fields and an ever-widening public understanding and interest in diverse forms of the arts, the American arts and culture sector has gradually become more clearly structured by applying a concentric circles model. This visual conceptualization of the cultural sector, which is in wide use internationally, generally positions *core creative arts* (such as the creation and expression of the visual arts and performing arts) at the center, surrounded by a next layer of *core cultural sector industries* (museums, galleries, theaters, etc.). The next concentric circle outward consists of wider cultural industries, such as media, publishing, and so on. The outermost concentric circle contains creative industries where the applied commercial output is emphasized, such as fashion and design.

America's enormous arts and culture sector, also commonly referred to as the *creative sector*, is effectively depicted in Figure 1.3. This illustration may be best understood as a variation of a concentric circles model of the creative economy, wherein the core arts and cultural industries are positioned in the center, surrounded by support

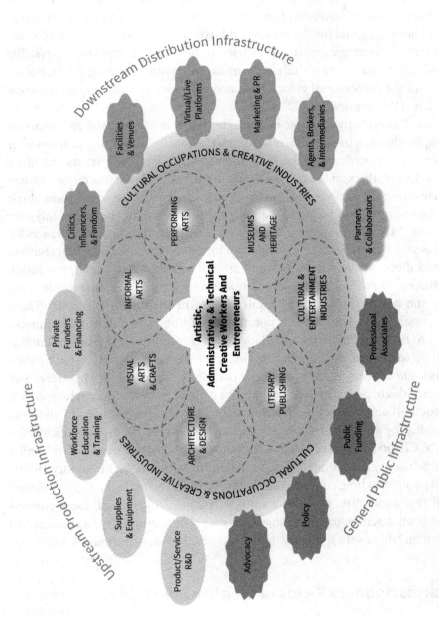

Figure 1.3 The creative sector
Source: Adapted from Wyszomirski (2008, 209).
Illustration by Stephanie McCarthy.

systems and infrastructure. The schematic is particularly useful for analyzing the complex industrial structure of the creative sector in terms of the *upstream production infrastructure*, the *downstream distribution infrastructure*, and the *general public infrastructure* as the support system for the sector as a whole. To briefly clarify, the upstream production infrastructure provides equipment, services, private monetary capital, and human capital for the creative industries. The downstream distribution infrastructure connects the cultural industries to their markets and consumers. The general public infrastructure includes an emphasis on public funding, public policy, advocacy, and the professional associations across the sector that support the creative industries (Wyszomirski 2008).

Figure 1.3 illustrates the creative sector as both a social sector and an economic sector. People who seek to use the arts to support health and well-being outcomes for older adults are able to draw on the skills and services of teaching artists and other types of creative workers and entrepreneurs noted at the center of this model. Unlike many other economic sectors, the creative sector locates its core in the individuals who often work independently or in small groups rather than clusters of industry organizations. Many types of arts activities are created at the center of this model, such as drawing, painting, singing, playing an instrument, acting, dancing, reading, writing, and more. When similar types of artistic activities are created, produced, and distributed by mid-sized and large organizations, these cluster into the array of creative and cultural industries illustrated in the middle ring of the model. These industries manifest in a wide array of nonprofit, for-profit, and public (government) organizations that differ in their constellation in every community across the county.

In addition to this breadth of organizational partners that can be accessed for program design and delivery, many prospective partners exist on both the upstream and downstream sides of program distribution. The general public infrastructure, which is largely focused on advocacy, policy, public funding, and partnerships, is also crucial in establishing a societal framework that supports arts programs specifically for older adults. Chapter 3 of this book provides a more detailed discussion of the public policy and advocacy components of the public infrastructure that influence the allocation of public funding, conduct advocacy activities, and policymaking processes and mobilize communities of practice into professions. Together, all these components have been essential to efforts that the arts policy community has pursued to cultivate partnerships with the aging policy and health policy communities.

The Interdisciplinary Fields of *Creative Aging*

Arts in Healthy Aging studies a research field and arena of professional practice that currently lies at the intersection of *arts policy and management, health policy and management,* and *aging policy and management* (see Figure 1.4). In this book, we use *the arts in healthy aging* (our preferred term) interchangeably with *creative aging* (the current term for the field that is often used in publications and professional practice).

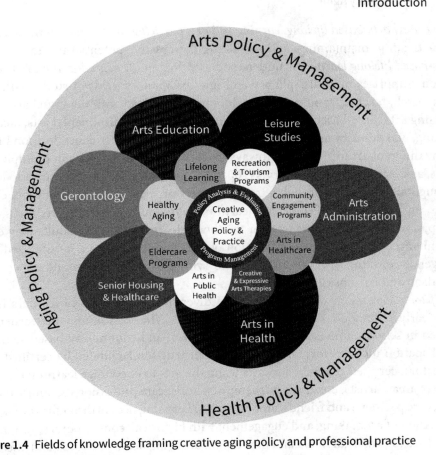

Figure 1.4 Fields of knowledge framing creative aging policy and professional practice
Illustration by Stephanie McCarthy.

Chapter 2 of this book provides insight into foundational concepts, theories, and scholarly fields that have come to shape the field of *creative aging* as it currently exists. We take as a given that the human being is inherently creative, and that this creative potential continues to grow throughout the lifetime. Creativity is a tremendous resource to all older adults throughout what is hoped to be many decades of a healthy aging process (Cohen 2000).

Creative aging is a term that has come to embrace this overarching idea. Herein, *creative* can be understood both in terms of artistic content and processes of creativity, and *aging* can be understood as the natural aging process beginning at age 60. Creative aging is a field of scholarship and professional practice that is focused on engaging creativity, the arts, and the humanities in supporting the health and well-being of older adults in a diverse array of community settings, as well as in healthcare facilities. In creative aging, the arts are seen as an effective tool to address the wellness needs of older Americans who are living longer and healthier lives than ever before. Creative aging has to do with a set of public policies and professional practices that leverage the benefits of engaging in creativity to foster mental, emotional, and physical health and well-being of older adults.

We view *arts-based lifelong learning* and *arts participation* to be essential avenues for activating, maintaining, and sustaining the creative potential in older adults. *Arts-based lifelong learning* is understood as a domain of *arts education*. Arts education comprises multidisciplinary and interdisciplinary fields of study dedicated to research, teaching, and policy development associated with the visual arts, performing arts, time-based arts (such as film and video), environmental arts, creative writing, and culinary arts, among others. In other words, arts education comprises many different art forms and pathways of learning and takes place in multiple settings, as described below. As Jarvis (2008, 20) emphasizes, people continue to learn throughout their lives through a transformative process involving cognition, emotions, and application. People can learn *in*, *with*, and *through* the arts across the lifespan. As argued in Chapter 6 of this book, learning by older adults may even be enhanced through the accumulation of life experiences and a "crystallized" intelligence resulting in a greater ability to synthesize information and experience (Findson and Formosa 2011, 75).

Lifelong learning in the arts assumes a diversified continuum of learners from very early childhood through older adulthood. This continuum of learners is served in schools, universities, arts organizations, and community-based settings. Participation includes formal and informal instruction facilitated by certified arts educators, certified general educators using the arts to encourage learning in other subject areas, artists, creative arts therapists, healthcare professionals, family members, care partners, and friends, among others. Learning occurs through art making, discussion of art making, and engagement with historical, contemporary, and traditional arts. Formal curricula and instruction are informed by research and effective practices, such as Gardner (1983)'s theory of multiple intelligence, particularly associated with the visual–spatial, linguistic–verbal, bodily–kinesthetic, musical, and existential intelligences. Learning is also informed by developmental factors associated with age, life course, ethics, gender, race, ethnicity, and culture.

People engage in lifelong learning in the arts individually and collectively through a wide array of classroom and community-based opportunities. Education in the arts occurs formally and informally in multiple face-to-face and online settings associated with schools, community arts centers, performing arts centers, colleges and universities, museums, healthcare settings, religious institutions, arts supply businesses, and within unincorporated affinity groups associated with one or more art forms. Participation may occur within intergenerational groups or groups based on age. Arts organizations across the country are becoming increasingly responsible for serving the educational needs of their larger communities, with programs focused on children, youth, adults, and families.

Our research has also emphasized understanding older adults' individual choices regarding *arts participation*. Although our research has emphasized the ways in which older adults participate in the visual arts (such as painting, drawing, sculpture, glasswork, and ceramics, or visiting a museum) and performing arts (such as playing an instrument; dancing, singing, and acting; or attending a performance), we are mindful of the much broader array of active and receptive cultural engagement opportunities that are available to older adults. After all, arts participation goes far beyond buying a ticket to a theater performance or visiting a museum. Older adults everywhere are active participants in choirs, knitting circles, dance groups, book clubs, and so much more. Older adults are also a prime target market for cultural tourism around the world.

The intended outcome of creative aging programs and initiatives is the health and well-being of people aged over 60. We ascribe to a broad understanding of *health* as "a state of complete physical mental, or social well-being and not merely the absence of disease or infirmity" (WHO 2022) and that of *well-being* as "the state of being comfortable, healthy, or happy" (Oxford Dictionary). In this sense, creative aging can perhaps be understood as either closely aligned with or even a subfield of arts in health. *Arts in health* is defined as "a broad and growing academic discipline and field of practice dedicated to using the power of the arts to enhance human health and well-being in diverse institutional and community contexts" (NOAH 2017, 9).

In this book, we clearly specify a focus on the arts within a broader framework of creativity. The illustration provided as Figure 1.4 positions the academic and professional field of *creative aging* policy and practice to be at the center of a flower. This flower is located at the intersection of arts policy and management, health policy and management, and aging policy and management. The first ring of petals encircling the creative aging center represents the specific types of programs that creative aging practice comes from. The larger outer ring of petals shows the domains of knowledge and professional expertise that contribute to this field. These fields of expertise are introduced and discussed throughout the pages of this book.

On the health side of the field, there is the large arts in health field, which includes subfields in the creative and expressive arts therapies, arts in healthcare (which refers to programs in formal healthcare facilities), and arts in community health or in public health programs. This field adjoins the eldercare world of senior living and healthcare facilities, which often feature arts programs of various kinds for their residents and caregivers. A focus on health and aging are jointly represented by the large gerontology field with its smaller petal focusing on healthy aging programs.

Blurred boundaries then lead to the arts side of the program, where one finds arts education with the specific focus on lifelong learning. Arts administration is also located here, which refers to the management of arts organizations, such as museums, symphony orchestras, and dance companies—and the full array of community engagement programs that community-based arts organizations can offer to older adults.

There is also the field of leisure studies, which also contains a broad array of arts-based programs for older adults, as well as the enormous fields of recreation and cultural tourism. Due to the health and well-being benefits associated with the leisure time available to older adults as discussed in Chapter 7, the field of leisure studies is relevant and necessary to any discussion of creative aging. Carpenter (2008, 15) succinctly defines *leisure* as "a person's free, unobligated time." The availability of leisure time, according to Carpenter, will vary across the lifespan, which for many people will be most available in "childhood and later adulthood" (15). Limitations to leisure time are associated with "income and physical and social psychological challenges" (15). Within the field of leisure studies, *serious leisure*, in contrast to *casual leisure*, requires "perseverance, personal effort to obtain special knowledge and skill" and "commitment to regular participation" (21). For older adults engaging with the arts, engagement may be serious or casual, or both. Leisure studies is also where relevant factors for creative aging research can be found, such as frameworks for thinking about longer lifespans and the economic support that is needed for an active retirement.

Introducing the Chapters of this Book

This book addresses a large gap in extant scholarship on *creative aging* to meet the needs of a wide array of students and professionals around the world. Although grounded in an international comparative analysis of relevant public policy and exemplar programs, this reference book focuses primarily on opportunities for arts engagement to support health and well-being of older adults in the United States. This book project sought to address an urgent need for resources on this topic and will contribute to a new interdisciplinary research trajectory taking shape across the fields of medicine, public health, gerontology, healthcare administration, social work, creative and expressive arts therapy, arts management, and arts education.

The three co-authors of this book are qualitative researchers working at the intersection of the arts, humanities, and social sciences. All three of us are engaged as educators in the broad academic field of arts administration, education, and policy. The specialized areas of research expertise brought to this book project are arts education (Blandy), arts in health (Lambert), and arts and cultural policy (Wyszomirski). The specific focus of this book is an investigation into why and how arts-based lifelong learning and participation in the visual, performing, and literary arts can contribute to the health and well-being of older adults in America. As mentioned previously, the research team has concentrated on studying how creative aging programs can be designed and implemented so that their participants receive the maximum health benefit. The overarching goals of this book project were twofold: (1) to develop recommendations for a national public policy infrastructure to advance the *arts in healthy aging* ecosystem in America and (2) to articulate smart practices in *arts in healthy aging* program design and professional practice.

Given the interdisciplinary and exploratory nature of this study, qualitative research methodologies were emphasized. Research methods and data collection tools were comprised of literature review, document analysis, key informant interviews, and case studies. Secondary analysis of statistical data and major findings from relevant publications discussing the physiological and psychological benefits of arts engagement also contributed to our findings. Throughout our multi-year study, we pursued two main objectives. We wanted to develop the "why" of the creative aging movement in order to ground this field of public policy and professional practice in research. We also wanted to offer a set of best practices on the "how" of creative aging program design, implementation, and evaluation.

The result of our study is a book divided into two main sections. The first part of the book (Chapters 2–6) offers a deep dive into conceptual and theoretical material that explains key concepts in creative aging, creative aging policy analysis, and the institutional infrastructure that supports creative aging. Although we have focused primarily on creative aging in America, these chapters will also integrate some information from other nations to help place the creative aging movement in its global context. The first section of the book concludes with a chapter that addresses the ways that arts education needs to be reimagined to address the lifelong learning interests of older adults.

In Chapter 2, we begin by developing theoretical frames for conceptualizing *aging*, and we argue that the contemporary field of *creative aging* would be more effectively framed as *the arts in healthy aging*. Building on introductory material from Chapter 1 on the arts as both a social sector and an economic sector in America, Chapter 2 develops an understanding of the *public purposes of the arts, cultural engagement,* and *choice-based arts participation*. Significant in Chapter 2 is also a more thorough introduction to America's *arts in health* field, within which the *arts in healthy aging* can be understood as a subfield. Chapter 2 concludes with our articulation of the *8Ps Framework for Arts in Healthy Aging* that we will be referencing throughout the book.

Chapter 3 turns to a descriptive analysis of the evolution of *arts in healthy aging* policy strategies in the United States. This chapter outlines four overlapping phases of the creative aging movement over the past 50 years. The first three phases are identified as *arts advocacy for older adults as a special constituency* (1973–1995), *the arts seeking a place on the aging policy agenda* (1981–2015), and *creative aging as a program asset for health policy* (2000–2015). The chapter critically discusses the opportunities and challenges presented throughout these three movements, all of which provide important context for our current stage of policy evolution in the field, *decentralization of creative aging policy* (2015 to the present).

Chapter 4 presents a set of conceptual tools that can be used to understand how the arts support specific health and well-being outcomes in older adults. The chapter begins with essential information regarding the sociocultural context of older adults' health and well-being and then develops frameworks for understanding how human development manifests in late life. A detailed examination of the motivations of older adults to choose to participate in creative aging programs and activities leads to material that clarifies the mechanics of why and how arts programs can contribute to healthy aging. Finally, the chapter turns to an analysis of basic design elements that must be considered when developing arts programs for older adults.

Chapters 5 and 6 serve as two chapters that systematically formulate why and how the field of arts education needs to be reconceptualized for older adults and provide theoretical modeling for developing arts-based lifelong learning programs for older adults. These chapters address head-on the fact that the field of lifelong learning, specific to arts-based education programs for older adults, is largely undertheorized in comparison with, for example, such programs for children and youth. Drawing on scholarship in relevant fields, such as gerontology, folklore, and arts education—and by developing concrete recommendations for using transformative learning theory in arts-based lifelong learning—these two chapters present a robust resource for creative aging programs designed to achieve educational outcomes.

The second section of the book (Chapters 7–9) then follows how the *arts in healthy aging* can support every step of the natural aging process. We begin by looking at active lifelong learning by individuals living independently in community settings. The chapters gradually turn their focus to programming that takes place in healthcare institutions and in end-of-life care. Illustrative program examples are included throughout these chapters.

Chapter 7 investigates arts programs and services for older adults that are provided as either a primary or a secondary focus of community-based organizations of various kinds. This chapter includes specific content on older adults' choices to engage in arts and culture activities in their leisure time and discusses barriers to participation that arise from *ageism, ableism,* and the recent challenges of COVID-19. The global movement toward *age-friendly communities* is discussed in detail. The chapter culminates in a robust set of questions that advocates for *arts in healthy aging* can ask to support the design, planning, implementation, and evaluation of arts-based programs for older adults that are provided in America's communities.

Chapter 8 moves the reader from a focus on community-based programs that older adults are able to access independently to understanding how *arts in healthy aging* programs can be provided in senior living settings and healthcare facilities. The landscape of eldercare facilities is complex and is essential to understand for those interested in developing arts programs for older adults. This chapter provides a concise overview of America's eldercare and healthcare system, matters pertaining to healthcare quality and healthcare consumerism, and basic information pertaining to Medicare, Medicaid, and long-term care. Key concepts in *age-friendly healthcare* and *person-centered care* are introduced. The chapter then shifts to a descriptive analysis of pathways for arts programs to be developed to serve patient groups across the care continuum ranging from *independent living,* to *assisted living,* to *clinical care.*

Chapter 9 extends the care continuum even further, with a focus on arts programs for older adults and their caregivers in hospice and end-of-life care. This chapter describes important human development tasks that take place at the end of life and also describes how the arts can assist older adults and their loved ones with attending to these final tasks. *Hospice* is introduced in depth, with a particular focus on the use of the arts in supporting spiritual care within hospice services. The chapter then profiles how the arts can be used specifically to support activities of reminiscence, legacy, and ritual at the end of life.

Chapter 10—the final chapter in the book—builds on all the material provided in Chapters 1–9 to develop concrete recommendations for advancing public policy and professional practice for the *arts in healthy aging* field. After summarizing the major arguments made throughout the book, the chapter articulates four main research findings from our research on the current state of *creative aging* policy and practice in America. The chapter then turns to specific recommendations for activating the *arts in healthy aging* ecosystem and recommendations for activating our *8Ps Framework for Arts in Healthy Aging*.

To support the work of researchers, students, and practitioners in this field, the back pages of the book include an appendix titled *America's Arts in Healthy Aging Timeline* and an appendix that lists federal agencies and nationally focused organizations across the fields of arts, health, aging, and adult education.

2
Foundational Concepts in Creative Aging

Introduction

We encourage readers of this book to imagine all the ways in which they might want to participate in the arts as older adults. Individual activities at home might be as simple as reading, listening to music, knitting, watching movies, playing video games, and so on. Many people wish to have social connections and a sense of community, which can be fostered through group participation in community choirs, bands, and orchestras; by attending museum and gallery exhibits; by attending pre-concert lectures before orchestral performances; by participating in discussion sessions after theater performances; by engaging in faith-based arts activities; by joining group heritage international tours; by taking painting classes in a local arts center; and so much more. Opportunities to engage in arts and culture through community-based organizations are plentiful. Most arts organizations in America's communities seek to be as accessible as possible through intergenerational programs and services.

Throughout the natural aging process, however, older adults will likely have changing interests and needs that lead to different choices regarding arts participation. Medical conditions can be supported through specific arts programs that support physical and cognitive health, such as memory care programs offered by museums. Arts programs can be provided in many different types of community-based organizations—such as educational institutions, craft centers, gyms, senior centers, performing arts organizations, and churches—and these arts programs can be purposefully designed to support physical, cognitive, social, emotional, and spiritual well-being. Internationally, a strong body of quantitative, qualitative, and arts-based evidence exists regarding the health benefits derived from the arts. In recent decades, arts programs intended to support health and well-being have grown rapidly in healthcare facilities and in community contexts. Older adults can benefit, for example, from arts programs designed to support specific needs of residents in long-term care and in healthcare settings.

Chapter 1 argued that there is tremendous potential for the power of the arts to be harnessed to support health and well-being among older adults. Now, Chapter 2 lays a conceptual foundation for how *creative aging* "works" to provide healthy aging outcomes.

Chapter 1 of this book offered a profile of the changing demographics and leisure activity patterns of older adults in America, pointing to the urgent need for expanded programs and services that support all stages of the aging process. *Healthy aging* was first introduced, and supporting an individual's *functional ability* was identified as being essential for everyone over the age of 60. America's arts and culture sector was introduced as both a social sector and an economic sector. We clarified that we understand categorizations of *the arts* to be very broad, and that older adults engage in creative activity across all the arts segments identified in Table 1.2; however, this book emphasizes the visual and performing arts as "tools" that can support healthy aging processes and goals. Then, Chapter 1 introduced the interdisciplinary fields of knowledge and professional practice engaged by creative aging policy and practice, across the domains of the arts, health, aging, and education.

Building on this introduction to the book, Chapter 2 introduces approaches to systems thinking and the use of logic models to activate the arts in pursuit of healthy aging goals. This field of research and practice has come to be known as *creative aging*—a term that is in common use at present when referring primarily to opportunities for the arts participation (as opposed to a much wider concept of creative practice) for older adults. Throughout this book, the terms *creative aging* and *arts in healthy aging* are used interchangeably. However, as we argue consistently throughout the chapters, the time is right to reframe research, policy, and practice in the field to more strategically link the arts, health, aging, and education communities depicted in Figure 1.4. Shifting to an *arts in healthy aging* re-conceptualization of the field may enhance opportunities for developing systems of policy and practice that can more effectively build the field across the nation and, by extension, internationally as is contextually appropriate.

Chapter 2 begins with positioning the current *creative aging* field within its closest cognate field, *arts in health*. Similar to other distinct population groups served by arts in health programs, older adults have specific needs. We discuss these needs by further developing the concept of *functional ability*, and we also introduce the *age-friendly ecosystem* and barriers to older adults' well-being that result from *ageism* and *social justice issues*. This discussion of older adults' needs then shifts to explaining how engaging in arts and culture is understood globally to be a basic human need. From this wide discussion of the human need for cultural engagement, we turn to a detailed analysis and modeling of choice-based arts participation. Our discussion of arts participation leads into introducing systems thinking and logic model elements for operationalizing the arts as an instrument to achieve individual and community benefits. Ultimately, building arts participation is viewed as resulting in societal benefits, which can be best understood as the public purposes of arts participation that can be fostered through effective policy development. The chapter concludes with introducing our *8Ps Framework for Arts in Healthy Aging*, an analytical model can be applied to any arts program purposefully designed to benefit older adults.

Creative Aging in the Arts in Health Field

The field of *arts in healthy aging*, also called *creative aging*, may be usefully conceptualized within the much larger field of *arts in health*, first introduced in Chapter 1 of this book. *Arts in healthy aging* encompasses many other domains of study and practice, including arts education, arts administration, policy analysis, leisure studies, and gerontology, and others (see Figure 1.4); however, the field of arts in health provides considerable insight into the intentional design of arts programs intended to support health and well-being outcomes. In short, *arts in healthy aging* is inherently embedded within the *arts in health* field for the purposes of policy analysis, research, and professional practice.

Internationally, the terminology used to describe the field that engages the arts in support of health and well-being is *arts, health, and well-being* (see, for example, All-Party Parliamentary Group on Arts, Health and Wellbeing 2017). In the United States, there is not agreement on a term to be used to describe the field as a whole. In this chapter, we use the term *arts in health* to refer to this broad field, although we recognize that there will be disagreement in the field with regard to our use of this descriptor. Regardless of the term used, "the primary purpose of [this field] is to use creative activities to lessen human suffering and to promote health, in the broadest sense of the word" (Sonke et al. 2009, 107). The former Society for the Arts in Healthcare described this field as "a diverse, multidisciplinary field dedicated to transforming the healthcare experience by connecting people with the power of the arts at key moments in their lives. This rapidly growing field integrates the arts, including literary, performing, and visual arts and design, into a wide variety of healthcare and community settings for therapeutic, educational, and expressive purposes" (quoted in Lambert et al. 2016, 4).

In the United States, the arts, humanities, architecture, and design are being used to enhance healthcare and patient experience, to provide essential clinical care, to buttress caregiver wellness, and to strengthen public health. This broad field of practice includes several distinct and related disciplines of particular relevance to our study, including the creative arts therapies (art therapy, music therapy, dance/movement therapy, drama therapy, poetry therapy, and psychodrama), expressive arts therapies, and arts in health. In America, the broad field of *arts in health* has evolved over the past 40 years, in contrast with the creative arts therapies that have been recognized as professional disciplines since the 1940s.

There are several core professional domains that engage the arts in support of health and well-being. Several definitions provided in the National Organization for Arts in Health (2017, 9) white paper on *Arts, Health, and Well-Being in America* may assist in clarifying scope of practice. The overarching term used for this field in this book is *arts in health*, which refers to "a broad and growing academic discipline and field of practice dedicated to using the power of the arts to enhance human health and well-being in diverse institutional and community contexts." This field has two major subfields that refer to clinical facilities and community settings. *Arts in healthcare* (also referred to as *arts in medicine*) is the domain of arts in health that engages the arts in clinical settings. *Arts in public health* (also referred to as *arts in community health*) is the domain of arts in health that uses the arts in community health or public health settings. Whereas these areas of engagement are very broad, professional creative and expressive arts therapists require board certification, registration, and/or licensure to provide clinical services to patients. The *creative arts therapies* define their field as "six well-established health professions that 'use distinct arts-based methods and creative processes for the purpose of ameliorating disability and illness and optimizing health and wellness. Treatment outcomes include, for example, improving communication and expression, and increasing physical, emotional, cognitive, and/or social functioning' (www.nccata.org)" (NOAH 2017, 9). The term *expressive arts therapy* officially refers to "a professional field that 'combine(s) the visual arts, movement, drama, music, writing, and other creative processes to foster deep personal growth and community development' (www.ieata.org)" (NOAH 2017, 9). In practice, the work of all these professionals can look quite similar. However, it is only credentialed creative arts therapists and expressive arts therapists that are able to offer individualized patient clinical care focused on a medical diagnosis and treatment plan.

The National Organization for Arts in Health (NOAH 2017), established in 2016, promotes five arenas in which the arts generally support Americans' health and well-being: healthcare environments, patient care, caring for caregivers, health sciences education, and community health and well-being. Professionals working in the domains listed in the prior paragraph concentrate on one or more of these arenas. For example, clinical services in hospitals include arts programs that are provided by expressive arts therapists or certified creative arts therapists. In hospitals, artists in healthcare focus more generally on enhancing the patient experience by improving the environment of care. Artists and administrators working in arts in health engage in a continuum of care ranging from a clinical focus at one end of the spectrum to a broad public health focus at the other end. It is noteworthy that there are also many other healthcare professionals—such as child life specialists, recreational therapists, occupational therapists, and nurses—who frequently use the arts in their professional practice. Moreover, many artists focus their individual creative work on health and well-being in their communities.

For understanding how the American *arts in health* field has come into being, it is useful to think of the field as a 100-year-old tree with five main branches (see Figure 2.1). The first branch of the tree is that of the creative arts therapies, which includes the related field of expressive arts therapy. This first branch has been growing steadily since the 1940s; however, the other branches of the tree (i.e., the arts in health branches) have experienced their own rapid growth over the past 40 years. The three *arts in healthcare* branches have allowed the flourishing of *environmental arts, participatory arts*, and *arts for caregivers* in healthcare facilities. Whereas the creative arts therapies involve a clinical diagnosis and treatment plan for a specific patient, the purpose of the arts in healthcare branches is to promote the general well-being of patients, patients' families and friends, and medical staff and other caregivers, as well as including the arts and humanities in health sciences education (Lambert et al. 2016, 6–11).

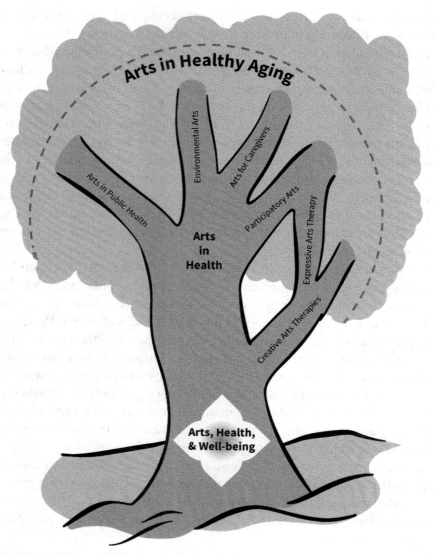

Figure 2.1 The arts in health field in America
Illustration by Stephanie McCarthy.

A new branch has recently grown on this tree, *arts in public health* or *arts in community health and well-being*, which includes programs that engage the arts in support of public health and community health goals (Sonke et al. 2019). Recent programs branching from this limb include a focus on the use of the arts in caring for military and veteran populations, the use of the arts in promoting public health, and engaging the arts in addressing long-term and preventive healthcare needs. The field of arts in public health, which is much more well established in other regions of the world (for example, see the chapters in Clift and Camic 2016), suggests great potential for rapid development in the United States.

This book investigates arts programs specifically designed to achieve health and well-being outcomes in older adults. Similar to other distinct population groups—such as children or veterans or people with a cancer diagnosis—older adults comprise a targeted participation group that intersects with all branches of the *arts in health* tree. In arts programs for older adults, specific arts in health subfields will include the work of clinical creative and expressive arts therapists, and the environmental arts, participatory arts, and arts for caregivers found throughout America's formal healthcare facilities. The field is even larger when we consider the arts in community health and well-being, which includes a dizzying array of community-based artists, arts organizations, community organizations, senior centers, and lifelong learning opportunities. Representative arts programs offered in community-based organizations, senior living communities, and healthcare facilities are introduced throughout the chapters of this book.

Understanding the Needs of Older Adults

Over the past two decades, organizations such as the World Health Organization and the American Association of Retired Persons have developed designations for "age-friendly" cities and communities. The focus on age-friendliness began with ensuring that a community's physical environment, transportation options, housing, and community services were accessible to people of all ages. The scope of age-friendliness has gradually expanded beyond the municipal level to also include healthcare systems, public health systems, colleges and universities, businesses, and entire states. Together, this comprehensive approach to providing community-wide support for older adults is referred to as *the age-friendly ecosystem*. Each domain of the age-friendly ecosystem has its own set of guiding principles and characteristics. For example, age-friendly health systems refer to their "4Ms" of what matters, medication, mentation, and mobility (see Chapter 8); age-friendly public health refers to its "5Cs" system; and age-friendly universities refer to "six pillars" and "ten principles" (Fulmer et al. 2020). Although age-friendly principles and practices may be distinct to each domain—whether cities and communities, businesses, universities, or health systems—the policies and practices prescribed in each arena of policy and practice also support age-friendly principles in the other domains. The most developed arena of age-friendly practices is that of "livable communities," which is addressed in more detail in Chapter 7 of this book.

The essence of being "age-friendly"—regardless of the institutional context of age-friendly policies and practices—is to understand and proactively respond to the diverse needs of older adults. Understanding the specific needs of older adults throughout the aging process and retirement must be the first step in developing policies and programs to serve this population group (and all of its subgroups).

The field of *gerontology* studies aging and older adults. Two subfields—*social gerontology* and *critical gerontology*—provide particularly relevant concepts for research on the *arts in healthy aging*, and theories developed in these fields are presented in depth in Chapter 5 of this book. Key concepts from social gerontology explain how the experience of aging will differ across and within cultures, and how these social contexts influence social expectations associated with older adults (Elder and Glen 1994; Quadagno 2005). Deep patterns of culture structure how Americans think about the aging process and how they view the needs of older adults (Lindland et al. 2016). Within this sociocultural construct, critical gerontology offers "an important critique of prevailing social policies and practices around aging, while promoting the rise of new retirement cultures and positive identities in later life" (Katz 2005, 85). Experts in the field of gerontology provide valuable insight into understanding aging as a normal and natural stage of life.

> [Aging] is a part of our biological design and is distinct from disease and decline. This means that older adults can remain healthy and maintain high levels of independence and functionality—even while experiencing natural changes in vision, hearing, mobility, and muscle strength . . . . [The] process and experience of aging are grounded in, and shaped by, the complex interaction between social, cultural, economic, and other contextual factors. (Lindland et al. 2016, 216).

The aging experience is popularly understood as an element of the retirement years. The need to better understand current retirement cultures of older Americans led to a national study conducted jointly by Edward Jones, Age Wave, and The Harris Poll and published in 2022 as *Longevity and the New Journey of Retirement*. This report argues that four major forces are reshaping the national landscape for Americans' experience: greater longevity; the *baby boom* retirement wave; the need to match healthy life expectancy with total life expectancy; and the "demise of the three-legged stool for funding retirement" (3). These forces, as well as the recent major disruption of the COVID-19 pandemic, are changing the expectations, attitudes, and preparations of Americans for this extended stage of life. The report emphasizes that the experience of aging has changed significantly in recent decades.

> Retirement is now a longer and more important stage of life—and today's retirees increasingly want to make the most of it. The expectations and hopes about retirement and its character have shifted. For the parents of today's retirees and pre-retirees, the focus of retirement was mostly on "rest and relaxation." Now the majority of retirees and pre-retirees view retirement as "a new chapter in life." (9)

Of the three population cohorts either entering into their retirement years or in any stage of retirement (i.e., the *silent generation, baby boom generation,* and *Generation X*), it is the enormous *baby boom* generation of roughly 70 million Americans that is largely reshaping the experience of older adulthood. With reference to Figure 1.1, however, it is crucial to understand that the impact of lifestyle demands of large groups of retirees now and in the future will continue throughout the twenty-first century. In 2022, *Generation X* (born between 1965 and 1980) comprised around 65.8 million Americans, *millennials* (born between 1981 and 1996) stood at 72.19 million, and *Generation Z* (born between 1997 and 2012) totaled 68.6 million. In contrast, older adults born before 1946 accounted for only around 20 million Americans in total (statista.com/statistics/797321/us-population-by-generation/). The large retirement swells of the baby boom generation and the generations to come are fundamentally redefining what it means to be an older adult in America.

> As Baby Boomers become the majority of retirees, their attitudes prevail—more experimental and iconoclastic, less conservative and frugal than the previous generation of retirees. Women Baby Boomers have literally changed the mix in the workplace, on the home front, and now in retirement. Today's new retirees want a very different, more active and engaged retirement than their parents had. (Edward Jones 2022, 5)

The report team concludes that the new experience of the retirement years evolves in four distinct stages that differ for everyone in priorities, dreams, timing, financial circumstances, and experiences. These stages are named *anticipation* (10–0 years before retirement), *liberation / disorientation* (0–2 years after retirement), *reinvention* (3–14 years after retirement), and *reflection / resolution* (15+ years after retirement) (Edward Jones 2022, 12). Of these four stages, effective arts programs for older adults will most likely be designed specifically for the reinvention and reflection/resolution stages. In the reinvention phase, retirees exhibit a great variety of activities and experiences as they redefine their post-work identities and lifestyles. In the fourth stage, retirees continue to lead active and satisfying lives, but they also shift their focus toward "preparing the legacies they'd like to leave behind, including what life lessons they want to pass along to their loved ones" (20).

No matter what the stage of retirement is, it is the capacity of older adults to define for themselves their desired lifestyle that will drive their individual sense of purpose and well-being throughout the aging process. The term *functional ability*, first introduced in Chapter 1, is an essential concept discussed throughout this book. It is the functional ability that largely enables an individual perception of well-being for older adults (WHO 2020a, 2). Functional ability has to do with the "attributes that enable people to be and to do what they have reason to value" (WHO 2015, 28), which means that functional ability can be activated as either an asset that an individual possesses or an output of a carefully designed program that can lead to desired outcomes.

For analyzing the creative aging field, a useful definition of *functional ability* is the motivation and capacity of older adults to do the things that they value. How this translates into specific program design elements is presented in detail in Chapter 4 of this book. As a foundational concept in the creative aging field, however, functional ability may best be understood simply as each person's goal to live a happy and healthy life as long as possible.

People everywhere hope for a long life without frailty and disability, and with as short a period of terminal illness as possible. These are concepts that are discussed by Coughlin (2017) as *healthy life expectancy* (21) and *compression of mortality* (198). Whereas *longevity* or *lifespan* refers merely to the length of one's life, the term *healthspan* is increasingly used to address the difference between healthy life expectancy and total life expectancy. Research shows that the average American "spends the last 12+ years of life with their activities at least partially—and often seriously—curtailed by illness, injury, or cognitive impairment" (Edward Jones 2022, 6). As the 2022 report titled *Longevity and the New Journey of Retirement* argues, "closing the gap between healthspan and lifespan is one of the greatest medical and social challenges we face" (6).

The *longevity revolution* that engages a focus on health and wellness, lifelong learning, and community engagement based on aging in place (Hanna 2016) assumes that older adults will continue to benefit from a healthy life expectancy. In healthy longevity, older adults will be able to do the things that are important to them individually. However, a wide array of health patterns in older age is possible, as depicted in Figure 2.2. An older adult may exhibit any one of these patterns of

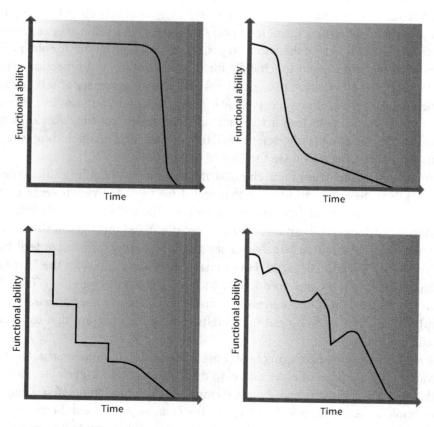

Figure 2.2 Illustrative patterns of functional ability throughout the lifespan
Illustration by Stephanie McCarthy.

increased or decreased functional ability over time or any combination of these patterns throughout late adulthood. Each illustrative pattern of changes in functional ability over time—no matter whether the period of time is short or long—implies the need for different supports and services to support individual health and well-being. At any given time, an arts program designed to support an older adult's functional ability may emphasize lifelong learning, skills development, social engagement, emotional and spiritual well-being, or specific physical and cognitive health benefits. The chapters of this book demonstrate how *arts in healthy aging* programs can support this full spectrum of older adults' needs. Intended outcomes of these programs may involve any combination of goals concerning older adults' functional ability, such as changing, modifying, building, enhancing, expanding, or maintaining their capacity to do the things that they value. Supporting functional ability can also include support that older adults may receive from caregivers and medical/health adaptive devices. It can also include interventions associated with environmental adaptations (such as universal design) that support the changing needs of older adults.

However, not all older adults are able to access the support programs that they need to support their individual health and well-being throughout their aging process. Health inequity is well documented in the literature and is often associated with underrepresented minority groups. Mehrotra and Wagner (2019) argue for the importance of considering diversity among older populations when recognizing the connection that exists between providing services and the needs of people from diverse backgrounds. The urgency of doing so is based on the growing racial and ethnic diversity within the current population of older adults and that is increasing exponentially among younger age groups. *Health inequality* is definable as "inequity or injustice because the difference in a health outcome is considered preventable" (Ferraro, Kemp, and Williams cited in Mehrotra and Wagner 2019, 220). The indisputability of health inequities among people generally and among older adults specifically, is resulting in "lost lives, lost potential, and lost resources" (Weinstein et al. cited in Mehrotra and Wagner 2019, 221). A 2017 National Academies of Sciences report identifies a number of factors supporting health equity, including recognizing good health as being "crucial for the well-being and vibrancy of communities." The report recognizes health to be "a product of multiple determinants" emerging out of "social, economic, environmental, and structural factors, and their unequal distribution matter more than health care in shaping health disparities." Health inequities are also associated with "poverty, structural racism, and discrimination," and the report argues that the "collaboration and engagement of new and diverse (multisector) partners is essential to promoting health equity" (Weinstein et al. cited in Mehrotra and Wagner 2019, 221).

There is a continuing urgent need to address the health inequities among all people. For older adults, such inequity will be a matter of life and death and, if not addressed, will undermine members of underrepresented groups to benefit from engagement with the arts as introduced in Chapter 4 and throughout this book. Arts and cultural organizations must be one of the partners promoting health equity. *Not* doing so will undermine any arts and cultural programming promoted as serving the public interest.

In addition to health inequity, barriers to participation by older adults in the arts include ageism and ableism. Age should be considered as a part of reaching diverse audiences as is race and ethnicity. First referenced in 1969, *ageism*, as a social construct, was defined "as a combination of prejudicial attitudes toward older people, old age, and aging itself; discriminatory practices against olders; and institutional practices and policies that perpetuate stereotypes about them" (Applewhite 2016, 13). The consequences of ageism include shame, fear of the future, and abuse (Applewhite 2016). As with health equity, arts and cultural organizations should partner with other organizations and continually evaluate their own practices to promote a non-ageist society.

Aligned with ageism, another significant barrier is "ableism." *Ableism*, like ageism, is a social construct, defined as "prejudice and discrimination aimed at disabled people, often with a patronizing desire to 'cure' their disability and make them 'normal.' Ableism, either subtly or directly, portrays individuals who are being defined by their disabilities as inherently inferior to nondisabled people" (Dunn 2021, 1). Again, arts and cultural organizations must partner with other organizations, and examine their own practices, to confront ableist attitudes. In this regard, it will be important to not see any disability an older adult is experiencing as definitive of who they are. Strategies for serving older adults experiencing disabilities are discussed in Chapters 5–7.

Engaging in Arts and Culture: A Basic Human Need

Throughout our lifetimes, we are all programmed to seek out larger cultural meaning, cultural connections, and cultural expression (Dissanayake 1988). This very broad concept of *culture* reflects the widely cited UNESCO (2001, 1) framing of the field, with its definition of *culture* articulated as "the set of distinctive spiritual, material, intellectual and emotional features of society or a social group that encompasses, not only art and literatures, but lifestyles, ways of living together, value systems, traditions and beliefs." This is an anthropological framing of culture that positions cultural engagement as a basic human need. Indeed, the right to participate in cultural life is a universal human right enshrined in the *Universal Declaration of Human Rights* as Article 27, which states that "Everyone has the right to freely participate in the cultural life of the community, to enjoy the arts and to share its scientific advancement and its benefits" (United Nations 1948). The *International Covenant on Economic, Social and Cultural Rights*, in Article 15.1.a, similarly calls on states to recognize the right of everyone to participate in cultural life (as cited in UNESCO 2014, 83).

> Culture plays a central role in sustaining and enhancing individuals' and communities' quality of life and well-being. Cultural practices, assets and expressions are also key

vehicles for the creation, transmission and reinterpretation of values, aptitudes and convictions through which individuals and communities express meanings they give to their lives and their own development. Those values, aptitudes and convictions shape the nature and quality of social relationships, have a direct impact on a sense of integration, empowerment, trust, tolerance of diversity, and cooperation. (UNESCO 2014, 82)

The term *culture*, therefore, refers to a whole way of life, including material, intellectual, and spiritual dimensions. Culture is recognized in shared values, attitudes, beliefs, and behaviors. Culture is learned, evolves over time, and is collective in nature. Culture is expressed through tangible and intangible performing, literary, time-based, environmental, culinary, and heritage arts, among other expressive forms. Very basic and essential human needs connect all of us to the values expressed in these various forms of culture.

Cultural engagement similarly refers to all of the ways in which people of all ages can engage with arts, culture, heritage, and the humanities throughout their lifetimes. Engaging in culture can also refer to relevant activities in the fields of leisure, recreation, and tourism. People participate both formally and informally in cultural programs and activities at home, work, museums, performing arts centers, festivals, community arts centers, tours, and heritage site visits, among others. "Cultural [engagement] includes cultural practices that may involve consumption as well as activities that are undertaken within the community, reflecting quality of life, traditions and beliefs" (UNESCO 2014, 85).

One meaning of culture refers to the general body of the arts as a whole; it is the arts in this sense that offer the focus of this book's study. We understand *arts participation* to be a subset of cultural engagement (see Table 1.2). Research conducted for this book project emphasized the ways in which older adults participate in the visual arts (such as painting, drawing, sculpture, glasswork, and ceramics, or visiting a museum), literary arts (such as poetry, storytelling, and writing), and performing arts (such as playing an instrument; dancing, singing, or acting; or attending a performance). In this sense, our study has embraced a basic definition of *the arts* as "painting, sculpture, music, theater, etc., considered as a group of activities done by people with skill and imagination" (merriam-webster.com). As discussed in Chapter 1, we do not privilege one type of the arts over another, and we recognize that individuals will decide for themselves what kind of arts participation they prefer.

Choice-Based Arts Participation

Around the world and throughout history, people of all ages have chosen to participate in the arts for a variety of reasons and in manifold ways. However, in the United States, the twentieth century brought about a deeply entrenched consumption model of measuring arts participation as public attendance at specific types of arts events. As Bill Ivey (2008, 5) writes, "by the early 1960s . . . the concept of participation had already been reshaped to be about audiences and consumption through attendance at nonprofit events." This primary focus on measuring arts consumption meant that in the late twentieth century, "the arts community (i.e., scholars, policymakers, managers) [had] made institutional engagement, or attendance at institutionally sponsored events, its primary area of concern with regard to participation" (Tepper and Gao 2008, 35).

Since 1982, the National Endowment for the Arts (NEA) has regularly tracked arts participation in its *Survey of Public Participation in the Arts*. In recent decades, national discourse about public participation in the arts has expanded beyond the initial concept of participation as passive arts attendance. The NEA's measures of arts participation now also include a concern for geographic availability, access to the arts in light of possible barriers or obstacles to participation, and a diverse array of active engagement in arts and culture. The NEA now contends that Americans participate in the arts by attending live events, by art making and art sharing, by using electronic media, and by arts learning.

Understanding why and how Americans choose to participate in arts and culture is a daunting topic for study. These choices can have significant outcomes at both the individual level and societal level.

> Choice-based cultural participation plays a formative role in building up individual capabilities through exposure to and production of a rich and diversified range of cultural expressions and resources. Indeed, it contributes to the development of critical thinking as well as to a continuous learning process about creativity and cultural diversity. Moreover, cultural participation offers experiences of what is meaningful for each person, and therefore leads to the constant constructions and transmission of individual and collective values influencing how individuals express themselves....
>
> Choice-based cultural participation is also a vector of enhanced well-being and mutual understanding. Indeed, it provides opportunities for individuals to experience positive social connections with their community as well as cultural diversity, which fosters feelings of integration, inclusion and mutual respect. (UNESCO 2014, 83)

The field of cultural economics argues that we consume things that we value, and there are many reasons that people value, engage in, and consume arts and culture. David Throsby (2001; 2010) offers *cultural value* as a multifaceted concept to help clarify a range of qualities possessed by arts programs, products, and activities. Throsby (2001, 28–29) suggests that important characteristics of the arts may be considered as aesthetic value, spiritual value, social value, historical value, symbolic value, and authenticity value. Legacy value may be an additional quality of the arts to consider, and a characteristic of particular importance to some older adults.

Another framework for considering why people choose to engage in the arts has to do with the intrinsic and instrumental benefits that people derive from arts participation. When researching creative aging programs, we found that many programs are designed to achieve specific instrumental benefits, such as measurable knowledge and skills, improved biometric health measures, or improved subjective measures of life satisfaction. In other words, the arts are used as an instrument for achieving specific health and well-being metrics. In this sense, the arts are "attached" to other, larger areas of policy and practice that are the *health* and *aging* fields. In contrast, the intrinsic benefits of arts participation have traditionally been understood as emphasizing a deeply held private or personal value.

A seminal study on benefits associated with arts participation, titled *Gifts of the Muse*, was published in 2004. This publication, and the many publications that built upon this study, sought to reframe Americans' understanding of the relationship between intrinsic and instrumental benefits of the arts. This new framework successfully argues for a strong relationship between intrinsic and instrumental benefits, as they influence and accrue to both the private sphere and the public sphere. Understanding intrinsic benefits of arts participation may be particularly useful for describing the reasons that older adults choose to engage in the arts. The *Gifts of the Muse* report notes that three types of intrinsic benefits exist. Older adults may derive immediate benefits, such as pleasure, from engaging in arts experiences. They may experience growth in individual capacities, such as knowledge and understanding of the world, enhance empathy for other cultures, and so on. And they may create and develop social bonds with other people through sharing arts experiences, revealing a shared sense of community identity, communicating across differences, and expressing common values (McCarthy et al. 2004).

Older adults may be heavily influenced by particular cultural values and by the intrinsic or instrumental benefit that they are seeking through arts participation. Additional motivations and developmental drives that lead to arts participation are discussed throughout this book. All of these factors influence an individual's specific preferences for cultural engagement and ultimately lead to specific choices that older adults make in this arena.

Table 2.1 provides a set of choice categories and a spectrum of choices that can be made within each category for arts participation. These choices can be combined in any way. In existing publications, the spectrum of choice is often set up as a dichotomy (e.g., folk arts vs. fine arts or amateur vs. professional), even if there is no consensus on these dichotomies. We consider these to be false dichotomies and suggest that a full spectrum of choices exists, which should not include any value judgments. Table 2.1 should also be considered as an illustrative—but not exhaustive—menu of individual arts participation choices.

The choices that older adults make for participating in the arts reflect all of the categories provided in Table 2.1. These individual choices are likely not consistent for each person, since people often have wide-ranging interests in the arts and interests may change and evolve over time. The relative weighting of the choice category also varies as interests change and the motivation, goal, or purpose of arts participation shifts.

The first choice category in Table 2.1—the nature or mode of the arts participation activity—offers a particularly strong unit of analysis for creative aging program

Table 2.1 Individual choice categories for arts participation

Choice Category		Illustrative Spectrum of Individual Arts Participation Choices
Mode	The nature or mode of the arts participation activity	Active—Receptive Part of daily life—Going out to special event Arts practice—Arts attendance Creativity—Consumption
Purpose	The goal or purpose of arts engagement	Learning about the arts—Making/doing the arts Entertainment/escape—Meaning/purpose/spirituality Private consumption—Social role/contribution Intrinsic benefit sought—Instrumental benefit sought Acquiring economic value—Acquiring cultural value Chosen by self—Chosen by others Seeking educational outcome—Seeking health outcome
Place	The place or location of arts participation	At home—Not at home Individual participation—Collective participation Live/in-person—Online/digital/virtual/media Synchronous—Asynchronous
Skill	The requisite level or depth of skill, knowledge, or expertise involved in creating or consuming the arts activity	Amateur—Professional Ambient appreciation—Informed appreciation Short-term engagement—Long-term engagement Participating to explore an interest—Participating to develop skills, knowledge, or ability in the art form
Content	The arts field, genre, or type	Popular culture—Public/nonprofit professional arts Folk arts—Fine arts Indigenous arts—Community arts Sacred orientation—Secular orientation

design. This choice category is referenced extensively throughout this book. A range of arts participation modalities can exist along the spectrum from active to receptive participation, from making and doing art to attending a performance or visiting a museum.

Over the past 20 years, an arts researcher and consultant named Alan Brown and his colleagues have been at the forefront of conceptualizing a broader approach to arts participation. This research team's model of arts participation extends from total control over the creative process to one's exposure to the arts with no individual choice or control over the experience. Five modes of participation are clarified as follows:

1. **Inventive Participation** engages the mind, body, and spirit in an act of artistic creation that is unique and idiosyncratic, regardless of skill level (e.g., composing music, writing original poetry, and painting).
2. **Interpretive Participation** is a creative act of self-expression that brings alive and adds value to preexisting works of art, either individually or collaboratively, or engages one in arts learning (e.g., playing in a band and learning to dance).

3. **Curatorial Participation** is a creative act of purposefully selecting, organizing, and collecting art to the satisfaction of one's own artistic sensibility (e.g., collecting arts, downloading music, and burning CDs).
4. **Observational Participation** occurs when one sees or hears arts programs or works of art created, curated, or performed by other people (e.g., attending live performances or visiting art museums). We define two subtypes of observational participation: 1) live event participation and 2) electronic-media-based participation.
5. **Ambient Participation** includes encounters with art that the participant does not select (e.g., seeing architecture and public art or hearing music in a store). (Novak-Leonard and Brown 2011, 32)

Since the development of this model, professional practice in diverse modes of arts participation has continued to evolve. For example, inventive participation can be expanded to include collective participation, as is often seen in the traditional and folk arts. Also, with the COVID-19 epidemic closing arts organizations for a long time, the technological and experiential dimensions of arts participation have flourished in virtual and digital programs of all kinds. That said, all five of these modes of arts participation are highly relevant to our study, and all five of these modes are discussed in the examples of arts participation provided throughout this book.

In sum, the research focus of this book is on diverse forms of arts participation within a broader understanding of cultural engagement as a basic human need. Older adults exhibit individual preferences in choosing specific arts activities in which to engage. They select activities that align with distinct sociocultural values and experiences. These adults also seek a wide array of intrinsic and instrumental benefits through arts participation. Ultimately, when older adults choose to participate in an arts program or activity, this choice represents a full array of decisions made by those individuals in relationship to the availability of opportunities to them. This menu of individual choices is provided as Table 2.1. As the forthcoming chapters of this book argue, organizations should strategically consider the provision of arts experiences for older adults across all of these choice categories.

Public Purposes of the Arts

A full spectrum of arts participation choices is central to understanding the role of arts and culture in society. As explained in the section above, both intrinsic and instrumental benefits can be acquired by the person engaging in the arts. These benefits accrue to the community, resulting in a broader societal impact. For example, if many older adults participate in an arts-based program designed to improve cognitive health, the collective outcome may be distinct measures of improved public health.

The logic connecting the ways that individual arts engagement benefits society as a whole is most clearly explained in the NEA (2012) publication titled *How Arts Work*. This report "proposes a way for the nation's cultural researchers, arts practitioners, policymakers, and the general public to view, analyze, and discuss the arts as a dynamic, complex system" (6) by articulating an "entire system and its implications for the quality of life for all Americans" (7). Figure 2.3 is the oft-cited illustration that depicts the mechanics of the entire arts system by referring to standard elements of a logic model. *Logic models* are used in several chapters of this book to graphically depict hypothesized causes and effects that lead to desired individual and societal outcomes. Logic models are particularly useful as a tool for effective program design, implementation, and evaluation.

In Figure 2.3, the human impulse to create and express is positioned as the primary driver of the system; this is congruent with our assertion that cultural engagement is a basic human need. However, as NEA (2012, 12) argues, "this impulse is a necessary but insufficient condition for arts engagement. Arts engagement requires opportunity." Opportunities to participate in the arts are facilitated by the *arts infrastructure* and *education and training*, both of which serve as inputs in this logic model illustration. The term *inputs* refers to the resources of all kinds that

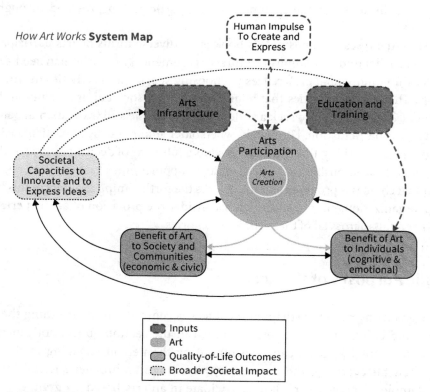

Figure 2.3 The NEA's *How Art Works* System Map
Source: Graphic from the National Endowment for the Arts' publication How Art Works: The National Endowment for the Arts' Five-Year Research Agenda with a System Map and Measurement Model (2012).

are required for effective program design and implementation. By using a systemic approach in our research on arts programs for older adults, we have emphasized identifying essential elements of both these inputs for purposes of successful program design. The arts infrastructure refers to the "institutions, places, spaces, and formal and informal social support systems that facilitate the creation and consumption of art" (NEA 2012, 12). Researching education and training focuses on both formal and informal instruction, and it "refers to the standards, best practices, knowledge models, and skills that inform artistic expression on the one hand, and consumption of [the arts] on the other" (12).

The *How Art Works* logic model illustration positions arts participation as leading to two arenas of interconnected quality-of-life outcomes, which are *benefits to individuals* and *benefits to communities*. As illustrated, this system is mutually reinforcing and cyclical. The ultimate impact lies at the societal level.

If arts participation leads to significant societal impacts, it is important to better understand the public purposes of the arts.[1] Extensive scholarship is available on this topic, including *Gifts of the Muse* (McCarthy et al. 2004) referenced previously, and a book chapter titled "Raison d'Etat, Raisons des Arts: Thinking about Public Purposes" (Wyszomirski 2000). A foundational resource on this topic is the American Assembly (1997, 6) publication titled *The Arts and the Public Purpose*, which identifies four public mandates addressed by the arts:

1. The arts help to define what it is to be an American—by building a sense of the nation's identity, by reinforcing the reality of American pluralism, by advancing democratic values at home, and by advancing democratic values and peace abroad.
2. The arts contribute to quality of life and economic growth—by making America's communities more livable and more prosperous and by increasing the nation's prosperity at home and abroad.
3. The arts help to form an educated and aware citizenry—by promoting understanding in this diverse society, by developing competencies in school and at work, and by advancing freedom of inquiry and the open exchange of ideas and values.
4. The arts enhance individual life—by encouraging individual creativity, spirit, and potential and by providing release, relaxation, and entertainment.

Introducing the *8Ps Framework for Arts in Healthy Aging*

Throughout the chapters of this book, we seek to systematically frame what is needed across the United States for the *arts in healthy aging* movement to advance as a field of research and professional practice. Although it is generally understood that participating in arts activities is inherently a good thing for older adults to do, we specifically focus on the design and implementation of professionally led arts programs intended to achieve explicit health and well-being outcomes. That is, this study concentrates on identifying concrete elements of successful program design.

A strong *arts in healthy aging* program will include a proactive response to external influences and the careful design of internal components, as illustrated in Figure 2.4. The program is designed within the context of public policy and partnerships, which are the first two "Ps" of the *8Ps Framework for Arts in Healthy Aging*. The outermost *policy* sphere attends to the public and governmental context within which arts programs for older adults can be developed, which is discussed in detail in Chapter 3 of this book. The policy domain is paired with *partnerships*, which refers to the institutional infrastructure and potential for cross-sector public, nonprofit, and for-profit funding streams and personnel partnerships that can be harnessed for program development and delivery. This national institutional infrastructure is also introduced in Chapter 3 of this book. Together, the policy and partnerships domains can be thought of as the external ecosystem for creative aging, providing both opportunities and resources to the field as a whole.

Program design, the actual design of the program itself, must carefully address this external ecosystem while manipulating four key program elements: *purpose, people, place,* and *participation*. The first of these internal elements is *purpose*, which refers to the specific intended outcome of the *arts in healthy aging* program. In this book, we discuss this intended program output as a short-term outcome focused on some aspect of the individual's functional ability. Supporting, maintaining, or improving this functional ability will lead to concrete outcomes in health and well-being, as explained in detail in Chapter 4 of this book. The term *purpose* is also understood

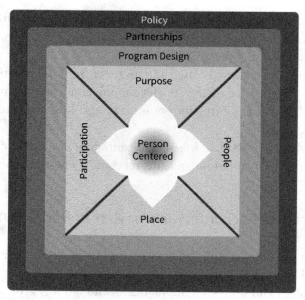

Figure 2.4 The *8Ps Framework for Arts in Healthy Aging*
Illustration by Stephanie McCarthy.

as one aspect of individual choice for arts participation, as listed in Table 2.1. And indeed, *participation* is the second internal program element to consider. When designing arts programs for healthy aging outcomes, program facilitators and participants will need to make decisions on the specific form and nature of arts participation provided by the program. Again, an array of choice categories in the arena of arts participation is listed in Table 2.1, and the mode of arts participation can extend from very active creative engagement to ambient participation.

Decisions regarding purpose and participation will greatly influence the program elements of *people* and *place*. The term *people* refers to the program providers and participants, which may include any combination of artists, facilitators, educators, older adults, family members, and other caregivers. The *place* variable refers to the setting, or site, of program delivery. Also included in Table 2.1, place can refer to a wide array of options for arts engagement, including participation at home or in a community setting, individual or group participation, and in-person or online/remote participation.

At the very center of the 8Ps framework is the final "P": *person-centered*. Our research strongly supports placing a person-centered (or *patient-centered, learner-centered*, or *family-centered*) approach to creative aging program design as the cornerstone of all successful programs. This essential element implies the need for a highly individualized program that takes the goals, motivations, and capacity of the participants into account. It implies the need expressed by older adults for determining their own desired program outcomes, choosing various forms of arts-based learning and arts participation, and creatively co-curating the program itself.

Together, then, the *8Ps Framework for Arts in Healthy Aging* consists of policy, partnerships, program design, purpose, participation, people, and place, and is person-centered at its core. These eight elements of successful *arts in healthy aging* program design are discussed from various perspectives throughout the pages of this book. In the final chapter of this book, we develop recommendations for how to activate this 8Ps framework.

Conclusion

This chapter has built on the introductory material offered in Chapter 1 by providing important foundational concepts that have led to the current generally accepted "framing" of the field of *creative aging* policy and practice. Chapter 2 has explained how the *arts in healthy aging* can be positioned within its closest cognate field, *arts in health*. Indeed, the creative aging field can be understood as seeking to design and implement *arts in health* programs and services to support the specific needs of older adults. This chapter has discussed these specific needs by developing the concept of *functional ability*, by introducing the *age-friendly ecosystem*, and by introducing barriers to older adults' well-being that result from *ageism* and *social justice issues*. This discussion of older adults' needs led to explaining how engaging in arts and culture is a basic human need. From this perspective of understanding the human need for cultural engagement, the chapter turned to a detailed analysis and modeling of choice-based arts participation. This discussion of arts participation led into introducing systems thinking and logic model elements for operationalizing the arts as an instrument to achieve individual benefits and community benefits, specifically through referencing the NEA "How Arts Works" systems model. The chapter explained how arts participation results in both individual and societal benefits. The chapter concluded with introducing the *8Ps Framework for Arts in Healthy Aging*.

Building on the conceptual introduction to the field provided in Chapters 1 and 2, *Arts in Healthy Aging* now turns to an analysis of the evolution of *arts and aging* policy strategies in the United States over the past 50 years.

3
Four Strategies to Advance Arts and Aging Policy

Introduction

Creative aging policy and programming is the current and most recent incarnation of how three policy arenas have interacted in efforts to formulate a meaningful, effective, and, ultimately, sustainable policymaking effort that "leverages the benefits of making, sharing, or otherwise engaging in the arts to foster the mental, emotional, and physical health and well-being of older adults" (National Assembly of State Arts Agencies 2019a, 1). As a policy issue over the past half century, the *arts and aging* has lain at the intersection of arts policy, aging policy, and health policy. This chapter focuses on this trio of policy arenas; however, going forward, it is crucial to add adult education policy to this group of policy domains (see Chapters 5–7 and 10 for a detailed discussion). Historically, both the aging and health policy communities have been older, larger, and higher on the national policy agenda than is arts and cultural policy. Given this asymmetry of political influence, the arts policy community has sought to build alliances with the aging and health policy communities through a series of changing policy images and instrumental utilities.

Policymaking is a multiphase process that involves many possible actors both from within government and outside it. At the national level, inside-government actors include the president, Congress, bureaucratic departments and agencies, and the judicial system. Outside-government policy influencers include interest groups, the media, elections and political parties, public opinion, and independent policy experts (i.e., academics, researchers, consultants, and think tanks). Policy actors participate in various policymaking phases, including issue identification, solution formulation, agenda-setting, enactment, implementation and tool choice, evaluation, and feedback. Similar types of policy actors, processes, and forms also operate at subnational levels, i.e., within states and local policymaking systems, as well as regarding intergovernmental efforts to link federal, state, and local collaboration. The study of policymaking and policy analysis focuses on the dynamics among key actors and how these take on various configurations around particular types of policy (e.g., distributive, regulatory, redistributive, or constituent) or in different policy arenas (e.g., education, economic, defense, housing, health, or arts).

Various policymaking frameworks have noted that competition for priority on the national agenda, which in turn attracts the attention, time, and resources of policymakers, is both intense and limited. It is also influenced by how policy images are framed and how policy problems and solutions are identified and converge (Baumgartner and Jones 1993; Kingdon 1984). The outcomes of such jockeying, plus a consideration of the political circumstances and leadership, play key roles in shaping how policies rise (or fall) on both the priority agendas of specific policy subsystems and on the national policy agenda. These dynamics also influence the design of programs and tools employed in implementing policies and the character of values and standards used to evaluate policy effectiveness. Each policy arena involved in the *arts and aging* policy community encompasses multiple issues competing for priority within their own arena. Policymaking processes are even more complex when they involve an issue that arises at the intersection of multiple policy communities, such as the arts and aging. Each policy domain has developed its own system of values, constituencies, and priorities that, while they may overlap or converge, are likely to differ in significant ways. The aging and the health policy subsystems are larger and more influential than the arts policy subsystem. The arts domain has borne much the challenge of exploring how it might adapt to and accommodate the two larger policy subsystems in hopes of "attaching" the arts to the advocacy and influence "coat-tails" of policy arenas that have higher priority on the national policy agenda.[1]

This chapter has two major concerns: first, to analyze how aging and older adults have been framed, addressed, and positioned within the arts policy agenda as led by the National Endowment for the Arts (NEA) and second, to understand how the NEA has pursued four attempts to reframe arts and aging policy, to more effectively build alliances with the aging and health policy subsystems and to respond to changes, challenges, and opportunities presented by the political environment at a given time. This review focuses on arts and cultural policy at the national level and especially as practiced by the NEA. The NEA is the public policy flagship for formulating and implementing arts policy, as well as an active partner in working with other sectors on subjects of shared interest (e.g., arts education, arts and community development, and cultural diplomacy).

Although *creative aging* is a relatively recent manifestation of NEA action concerning the arts and older adults, it is not the first or only policy approach the agency has explored on this topic.[2] To fully understand how creative aging policy currently fits into the arts (and arts education) policy agenda, we must consider how arts policy has historically addressed the interests, needs, and values of aging people. This longitudinal analysis can be envisioned as four overlapping and quasi-sequential policy formulation strategies that will be discussed in following sections of this chapter. Each of these streams is characterized by a different policy image of *arts and aging* and by variations in the associated policy communities and advocacy coalitions called upon to support and advance relevant policymaking. The detailed timeline provided in Appendix A of this book augments the historical analysis provided in this chapter.

Historically, the first policy strategy viewed aging people as a "special constituency" and was pursued between 1975 and 1995. A second policy strategy sought to reframe the arts as a resource for solutions and services to the aging population and thereby open a policy window for the arts to secure a place on the aging agenda as represented by the White House Conferences on Aging (WHCoAs) that were periodically convened between 1981 and 2015. The first and second strategies overlapped and ran in parallel between 1981 and 1995. "Creative aging" is actually the name for the third policy strategy that redefined aging as a creative stage of the lifespan and repositioned the arts as a vital part of a healthy aging policy agenda. This strategy was marked by the tenure of the National Center for Creative Aging (NCCA) between 2001 and 2018. The final strategy discusses how changes in the national political environment created obstacles to continuing NEA leadership of arts and aging policy formulations. It tracks a consequent devolution of *creative aging* activities and leadership to state and local government actors and private foundations and the emergence of a diffused network policy model. This historical analysis of the evolution of arts and aging policy lays a foundation for our recommendations for advancing the emergent *arts in healthy aging* ecosystem, which we present in Chapter 10 of this book.

Aging as a Special Constituency: An Advocacy Movement, 1973–1995

During the first four decades of the NEA's existence, the most focused arts and aging policy activity was located in the Office of Special Constituencies (OSC) at the NEA and concerned its partnership with the National Council on Aging (NCOA) in an effort to develop an advocacy campaign. This effort aimed to raise awareness about the possible benefits that both the arts and the aging constituencies might secure through a collaborative advocacy movement that could better serve the interests, needs, and quality of life for older adults. However, before turning to the OSC and NCOA partnership, it is useful to discuss three contextual factors that are important to the framing and potential priority of arts and aging policy.

Three Indicators of the Policy Environment for Arts and Aging Policy Development

At this early stage of possible arts and aging policy development, the political environment surrounding major actors was a particularly important variable. Three indicators of this environment concern the character of the crowded arts policy agenda at the NEA, the contested attitudes of arts administrators concerning older adults, and the congressional testimony of NEA leaders about their limited views of what NEA arts policy should attempt. Brief discussions of each indicator follow.

A Crowded Arts Policy Agenda

At the beginning of this stream, the NEA was a young, small agency that was primarily concerned with justifying its main mission: public funding for the arts. Core values of this effort focused on assuring the funding of excellent art; a belief in the arts for art's sake idea; a commitment to broadening the availability of the arts, especially geographically; building and strengthening the institutional infrastructure of the arts sector; developing an arms-length procedural system for grant-making; and promoting the development of a network of professional associations and advocacy groups. Pursuit of this agenda involved a variety of policy tools, including matching grants and encouraging increased philanthropic support for the arts; cultivating a network of state, local, and regional arts agencies across the nation; and funding the growth and proliferation of nonprofit arts organizations, as well as strengthening their finances and supporting audience growth. Writing in 1991, Milton Cummings observed that "a remarkable system of government aid for the arts has been fashioned over the last thirty years" (Cummings 1991, 7). Managing this considerable policy agenda left little attention for older adults and aging issues.

Perceptions of Older Adults in the Arts Policy Community

Even within the arts community, there was little agreement on whether attention to older adults should be on the arts policy agenda. In 1975, the National Research Center of the Arts conducted a public opinion poll with 677 arts administrators. It found that older Americans "... would seem a natural addition to an arts audience..." but that they were "less than a third as likely to attend arts events as those in the early 30s age bracket" (cited in Johnson and Prieve 1976, ii). This prompted the Administration on Aging (AoA) at the United States (US) Department of Health, Education, and Welfare to commission a second survey from the Center for Arts Administration of the Graduate School of Business at the University of Wisconsin Madison to "explore and develop an awareness among arts administrators of the potential for audience development among senior citizens" (Johnson and Prieve 1976, ii). This Wisconsin study[3] found that senior citizens represented less than 10% of the audiences in nearly 80% of the over 200 nonprofit arts organizations across a variety of disciplines that were surveyed. Furthermore, many arts administrators (nearly half) voiced a desire to increase the proportion of their younger audience, but only 7.7% were interested in increasing the senior citizen audience (Johnson and Prieve 1976, 25–26). Clearly, this second survey revealed that arts administrators of the time were divided as to their interest in older adults as a priority audience segment.

Together, these two surveys raise questions regarding what might have been meant when the NEA created an Office of Special Constituencies. Did "special" focus on the initial demographics that older adults were only a small part of the arts audience? Did "special" suggest that older adults faced particular barriers to arts participation as did people who were disabled, institutionalized, or incarcerated? Did it mean "special" in the sense that older adults might need accommodations in pricing, physical venue access, or targeted marketing for regular programming? Or, did "special" imply that older adults were in search of lifelong learning opportunities that were more participatory and tailored to adult learning approaches and scheduling preferences?

Testimony of Agency Leaders Sets Limits on Arts and Aging Attention at the NEA

Another indicator of the contested arts policy image of older adults was visibly displayed in the testimony of NEA leaders at a hearing of the House Select Committee on Aging focused on "The Arts and the Older American," held on February 7, 1981 (U.S. Congress 1981). NEA Chairman, Livingston Biddle made five points:

1. A "major goal" of the agency was to make the arts available to as many people as possible, regardless of age . . . in order to enhance the "quality of life" (9);
2. The Office of Special Constituencies mission was centered on advocacy within the Endowments programs, technical assistance to those seeking to develop arts and aging programming, and cooperative efforts with other federal agencies (9);
3. Advocacy efforts were also to be directed toward "sensitizing" cultural institutions and arts administrators to modify "long-held attitudes about the aged" (10);
4. The arts were more than a form of recreational activities. Rather they were ". . . elements essential to the general physical and mental well-being of older adults" (10); and
5. Speaking as Chair of the NEA, he did not support the idea of creating "line item" status or a budgetary earmark for the Endowment's funding of aging projects. Rather, he saw arts policy at the NEA supporting small demonstration projects, encouraging state arts agencies to do more, and directing funding for elderly artists (12–13).

This last position was reinforced by the Deputy Chair of Programs, Mary Ann Tighe, in her testimony where she states ". . . we have emphatically rejected the notion that special or different arts programs should be developed for the elderly . . ." (15). Biddle's and Tighe's asserted opposition to special programming for older Americans was notably different from the agency's historic commitment to support customized programming for the arts education of children or to establish line-itemed program status to support arts activities of cultural communities of color through the Expansion Arts and Advancement Programs.

Taken together, these three factors indicate that the arts policy community did not have a clear consensus on the priority it was willing to give arts and older adults on its crowded arts policy agenda.

An Arts and Aging Advocacy Partnership: The NEA Office of Special Constituencies and the National Council on Aging

A key characteristic of effective advocacy alliances is that partners arrive at a consensus on core values, issue definitions, and goal priorities. The environmental constraints noted above may have subtly induced tensions into the first strategy to foster an advocacy alliance to convince others of the value of arts-based programs for older Americans. Indeed, the impetus for this alliance may have come from the NCOA.

The NCOA, established in 1950, was the first national charitable organization to advocate with service providers and policymakers the issues concerning older adults. It had played an important role in the passage of landmark legislation, such as the Older Americans Act, and the creation of Medicare and the evolution of Social Security programs. The NCOA's initial priorities focused on a strategy of policy advocacy for congressional mandates focused on the economic status and health of older Americans. In the 1970s, the NCOA began to explore how older adult might more "dynamically express themselves through direct involvement in the creative process" (Sunderland 1982, 195).

The John F. Kennedy Center for the Performing Arts and NCOA formed a distinguished advisory council to explore past and current cultural programs for and by older people in an effort to "bring the elderly into a stimulating environment of creativity . . . thus enriching their lives" (Sunderland 1973, 5). The NCOA received a grant from the AoA to undertake this project with a declared mission ". . . to not only answer the aged's need for essential income and services, but to also find ways to make their [older people's] lives more meaningful and personally gratifying" (10). The resultant report, which included many program examples, was published in the monograph, *Older Americans and the Arts: A Human Equation* (Sunderland 1973). Soon thereafter, the NCOA established the National Center on Arts and the Aging to propel a broad-based advocacy and awareness effort promoting the importance of the arts and creative activities as key support service programs for older persons. These activities included an extensive publication effort, as well as information gathering and awareness building through more than 300 arts and aging workshops and seminars throughout the United States (Sunderland 1982, 195–197). Also starting in 1973, the NEA began awarding a 20-year-long series of annual grants to the NCOA ranging from $10,000 to $35,000 to support their public–private advocacy building activities.

Internally, the NEA started preparing the ground for the creation of an administrative mechanism that would identify and address the artistic interests of a constituency of older adults. The National Council on the Arts passed a resolution at its November 1973 meeting that called for "pilot programs showing how the arts can reach special constituencies" (NEA 1978, 12). In 1976, the NEA created an OSC to oversee and advocate for such targeted activities on an interdisciplinary basis both within NEA program divisions and with other federal agencies. Such interagency partnerships were a priority of the NEA Chair, Livingston Biddle, throughout his 1977–1981 term. Paula Terry was appointed its coordinator and would continue in this role until 2010. The NCOA called the OSC a "benchmark in NEA history" and heralded its efforts to expand access to quality arts activities to as many people as possible. The NCOA also saw the creation of the OSC as an "alert [to] the arts field that older Americans were on the agenda" (Sunderland 1982, 198). The November 1978 Council meeting reaffirmed the agency's interest in reaching "special constituencies" and specifically identified three groups: "handicapped children and adults; the aging; and those institutionalized in hospitals, nursing homes, or prisons" (NEA 1978, 12). By 1979, veterans had been added to the list.

Throughout the 1980s, the NEA continued to work in partnership with major aging organizations. In 1981, the agency signed an interagency memorandum with the AoA to engage in cooperative activities and efforts to put issues of cultural policy and aging on a formal level of discussion for the future (Moody 1988, 247). Additionally, the partnership between the NEA OSC and the NCOA continued. Each year, the NEA provided a funding grant to the NCOA to continue publication[4] and convening activities. Writing in 1988, Moody asserted that ". . . over the last decade, government funding [at both state and local levels] and private initiatives . . . have already created a broad pattern of support for cultural policy on behalf of the elderly" (247). He also argued that arts and aging was a quality-of-life issue (i.e., having to do with personal states of fulfillment), which made it both invisible and hard to measure, and therefore at a disadvantage for agenda status when compared to more measurable issues, such as medical care, financial security, and housing (Moody 1988, 77–103).

The early 1990s coincided with a serious political threat to the existence of the NEA itself, as conservative critics fought to defund or abolish the agency. In the wake of the 1994 congressional elections that won Republican partisan control of the House of Representatives, the elimination of the NEA, the National Endowment for the Humanities (NEH), and the Corporation for Public Broadcasting was high on their agenda. Although these draconian propositions did not succeed, they did prompt the halving of the NEA's budget that, in turn, led to significant staff layoffs, a major reorganization of the agency's programs, and serious losses of grant funding for many of the agency's grantees (Wyszomirski 1995).

In the face of such disruption, the OSC virtually disappeared and the Special Constituencies policy image of older adults in arts policy faded away. The last grant the NEA awarded to the NCOA was in 1990. Between 1991 and 1994, the OSC was absorbed into the Office of Policy Planning, Research, and Budget. It had few projects and made no grants to the NCOA. In 1995, the OSC emerged reframed as the Office of AccessAbility, declaring that its "major focus" for the year was "lifelong learning" and announced an interagency partnership with the WHCoA, the AoA, and the NEH to make "quality arts and humanities opportunities more widely available to older adults" and ". . . to increase the sensitivity of professionals in the aging field to the potential of arts and humanities programs for, by and with older persons . . ." (NEA 1995, 176). The centerpiece of this agreement was to be a conference convened by the NCOA to focus on the "need, demand, and character of arts and humanities involving older and disabled adults" (NEA 1995, 176). This conference fed its recommendations into the 1995 WHCoA.

Ultimately, the NEA OSC's alliance with the NCOA was a temporary relationship joined in pursuit of building constituency awareness within each of their communities about the benefits of working together. Interactions between the two organizations and their constituencies allowed them to become more familiar with each other and to better understand the challenges of positioning arts programming as an issue of aging policy. Twenty years of the experience and knowledge in the artistic practice of providing programming for older adults did lay a foundation for addressing the needs of a rapidly growing population of older Americans—the *baby boom* generation.

The Arts Aim for a Place on the Aging Policy Agenda, 1981–2015

A second policy strategy hoped to "attach" (Gray 2002) the arts to the aging policy agenda as a solution that could be used to address aging issues. Given the size and diversity of issues and interests competing for attention on the national aging agenda, it was unlikely that a lack of arts programming for older adults could come to be seen as a major aging problem. A more likely possibility was that the arts could gain feasibility as a mechanism for addressing aging policy problems. Indeed, one aging policy analyst observed that the experiences of the 1960s and 1970s seemed to demonstrate that ". . . just about every issue or problem affecting some older people . . . could be identified by advocates for the elderly as a governmental responsibility" (Binstock 2005a, 73). Thus, in furthering the goals of the "stronger" aging policy community, the "weaker" policy sector of the arts might gain more political importance and therefore gain allies, generate new work opportunities for artists, and perhaps attract new resources from outside the arts community.

The process of attaching the arts as a mechanism for implementing aging policy focused on building a potential "policy window of opportunity" (Kingdon 1984) that linked arts programming and expertise as a possible and partial "solution" to an assortment of aging policy problems. The tactic chosen to advance this strategy involved participating in the periodic WHCoAs—a device that, historically, drew on the potential influence of a presidential invitation and congressional funding (Cohen 1990, 30). For the arts community, the WHCoA provided an opportunity to build network connections and credibility within the aging policy community, with the hope of eventually securing the endorsement of conference recommendations to accept the arts as a viable provider of aging services. This strategic campaign was waged through participation at national conferences convened in 1981, 1995, 2005, and 2015.

WHCoAs were designed to be a nationwide citizens' forum that engaged in two years of preparatory study and analysis developed through state assemblies formulating recommendations that were ultimately considered by the national conference.[5] The first WHCoA was attended by more than 3,000 people representing fifty-three states and territories as well as 300 national voluntary organizations and saw the coalescing of numerous aging advocacy groups, including the National Council of Senior Citizens and the American Association of Retired Persons (AARP). It produced 947 recommendations on twenty aging policy issue areas. The 1961 WHCoA had a major influence on later policy decisions and was a major reference point for executive branch and legislative policymakers throughout the 1960s (Bechill 1990; WHCoA 1996, 138–140). The 1971 WHCoA was a large grassroots mobilization that took as its theme "Toward a National Policy on Aging," thus signaling that it saw itself as a "focusing event" (Kingdon 1984) for assembling the aging agenda, identifying and advocating for priority issues for designing implementation programs and regulations, as well as cultivating the aging policy community. For the NEA and arts advocates for arts and aging programs, WHCoAs presented another opportunity to advance the development of arts and aging policy.

WHCoA 1981 and 1995: Advocating for Arts Services for Older Americans

The first WHCoA that the arts participated in was held in 1981 and engaged in the usual lengthy citizens' participation activities. Convening in December 1981 meant the conference would be meeting at the end of the first year of the Reagan presidency. Reagan was a president who was both less supportive of aging policies and had waged an "extraordinarily successful effort to win major reductions in domestic programs for the federal FY1982 budget," including arts programs and aging programs (Bechill 1990, 20–23; Lebowitz et al. 1983). These circumstances presented a challenging policy environment[6] for the NEA to attempt to win a place on the national aging agenda through the WHCoA in 1981. Examples of priority recommendations continued to defend financial security, quality healthcare, affordable housing, and long-term care. New priorities focused on mental health and a call for more research to better support policymaking and medical practice (Lebowitz et al. 1983). The NEA, in collaboration with the NCOA and the NEH, organized the first arts-related, WHCoA-sanctioned "Mini-Conference on Arts and Humanities" (Sutherland 1982, 200). Perhaps most noteworthy was the NCOA's call for inclusion of cultural services within the definition of social and community services authorized by the Older Americans Act (WHCoA 1981). Although not included in the final recommendations of the National Conference, this suggestion had the potential to put the arts and humanities on the same statutorily sanctioned footing as other community and social services for older adults. Such a status would have granted arts and humanities aging programs access to authorized funds, instead of treating them as optional, discretionary programs. It would continue to be a policy "prize" that the NCOA and the NEA would continue to pursue for many years.

Although the next WHCoA was congressionally authorized for 1991, it was delayed until 1995 (Binstock 2005b, 9). Throughout the 1980s and 1990s, the NEA and the arts community continued to have a full arts policy agenda.[7] Throughout this period, both the NEA and its arts constituency partners regarded strengthening their lobbying position to be another major priority. A noteworthy milestone in arts advocacy was the first Arts Advocacy Day organized by Americans for the Arts (AFTA). This event brought together a coalition of national arts service organizations, citizen advocates, and local arts agency proponents to visit Washington and urge their members of Congress to support yearly appropriations for cultural agencies, as well as other arts and cultural policy issues as they arose. Eventually, this event became an opportunity to articulate an evolving cultural policy agenda and a mechanism for mobilizing the arts policy advocacy alliance. The strength and cohesion of arts advocacy was tested by the conservative threats to abolish the NEA as part of the so-called "culture wars" that culminated in the largest budget cut in the NEA's history, which triggered its first major reorganization since its founding[8] (Blancato 2004, 66; Wyszomirski 1995).

Despite this political turmoil and existential threat, the NEA OSC worked in partnership with the HHS' AoA and the NEH to collaborate with the NCOA to convene its second pre-WHCoA mini-conference[9] on April 10–11, 1995. The most visible presence of the arts at the 1995 WHCoA was NEA Chair, Jane Alexander's presentation as one of twelve featured dinner speakers at the Delegates Banquet. She focused on the twin goals of creating more opportunities in the arts and humanities for older adults and increasing the sensitivity of aging professionals and practitioners to the possible benefits of arts to quality-of-life issues. She also emphasized the arts as a bridge across generations, as a way out of isolation, and as activities knowing no age limits. Meanwhile, the NEA's partner in promoting *arts and aging* policy, the NCOA, advocated for public support for the arts, as well as for programs in the humanities, adult education, lifelong learning, and museum and library services (Beisgen and Kraitchman 2003). The conference eventually voted to forward forty-five suggested policy issues and implementation strategies endorsed by the entire membership. The arts were only mentioned as part of a recommendation to "emphasize the importance of physical fitness, recreation, the arts and humanities, leisure activities, and education as elements of health promotion for all older persons" (WHCoA 1996, 306).

WHCoA 2005: Baby Boomers, Arts, and Creativity

NEA participation in the 2005 WHCoA was marked by a new partnership and by a new approach. For the first time since 1981, the arts did not partner with the NCOA but rather took the lead in organizing the preliminary mini-conference in partnership with the NCCA, the National Association of Music Merchants (NAMM), and a new representative of the aging community, the AARP. The touchstone of the mini-conference was Dr. Gene Cohen's presentation of the preliminary findings of his NEA-commissioned[10] research project: *Creativity and Aging Study: The Impact of Professionally Conducted Cultural Programs on Older Adults* (Cohen 2006). The theme of the arts mini-conference was "Creativity and Aging in America" and was "focused on the importance and value of professional arts programming for, by, and with Older Americans as a quality of life issue" (Americans for the Arts 2005, 1). The arts mini-conference concentrated on three issues of importance to older Americans: lifelong learning and building community through the arts, designing for the lifespan, and the arts in healthcare (Hanna, Noelker, and Bienvenu 2015, 272). In her mini-conference presentation, Susan Perlstein, the founder and executive director of the NCCA, expressed her hope that the gathering would mobilize support for the inclusion of the arts in the list of social and community services covered in the reauthorization of the Older Americans Act (NEA, NCCA, NAMM, and AARP 2005, 7). For this discussion, it is noteworthy that Cohen's study could be seen as a response to the 1995 WHCoA call for more, and more rigorous, research on aging to inform both policy and practice. Cohen noted that, when published, his study would be the first ever constructed using an experimental design and a control group in the arts and aging field (Americans for the Arts 2005, 12).

The theme of the 2005 national WHCoA was "The Booming Dynamics of Aging: From Awareness to Action." With the first *baby boomers* turning 60 in 2006 and 65 in 2011, everyone at the conference was well aware that the growing constituency of aging baby boomers would make new and different demands on the aging policy support system. However, conference sponsor President George W. Bush and many of the individuals and interests participating in the conference had differing visions of that future. The president was promoting reform of Social Security to avoid the future bankruptcy of the program, asserting that "there is no trust fund" underwriting the system (Binstock 2005b, 9). Hoping to avoid a hostile reception, President Bush became the first president in 50 years who failed to make an appearance at a WHCoA.

Such divisiveness made it difficult for new issues or implementation ideas to gain a position on the agenda since protecting policies and programs from changes proposed by the Bush Administration took priority. To their credit, *arts and aging* proponents had presented a new, positive framework for "creative aging" programs and for the image of older adults as creative community assets pursuing health and well-being (Binstock 2005b; Blanchard 2006). In addition, Cohen's study had demonstrated that the arts could muster the rigorous research and compelling evidence needed to make a persuasive case. Nevertheless, three cultural resolutions regarding the arts, lifelong learning, and library programs for the elderly had been grouped into competition with civic engagement issues that had stronger support. However, a number of top-fifty resolutions did make mention of the importance of design practices, particularly universal design, which facilitate aging in place.

WHCoA 2015: Healthy Aging and Age-Friendly Communities

The 2015 WHCoA marked not only a number of noteworthy anniversaries of aging policy but also significant changes in the organization and processes of the conference itself. That year was the fiftieth anniversary of the passage of the core federal policies concerning the aging: the Medicare, Medicaid, and Older Americans Acts. It was also the eightieth anniversary of the enactment of the Social Security Act. The four major themes of the 2015 WHCoA were retirement security, healthy aging, long-term services and supports, and elder justice.

The organization of the WHCoA was radically different from that of previous conferences. Neither President Obama nor Congress considered aging policy as a priority (Hooyman 2015, 701). Congress did not authorize funding for delegates to attend; nor did they provide any guidance on a framework. This suggested that the recommendations of the conference were likely to have less impact on the policy agenda than previous convenings. Without congressional funding, the conference had to be more modest. It became a smaller, invitation-only summit that invited the public to submit ideas to a White House website rather than attend as in-person delegates. Rather than hundreds of outreach and grassroots preconference activities, the White House took a very active role in structuring such activities.[11]

As usual, the NEA and the NCCA co-sponsored a preconference event that was titled *The Summit on Creativity and Aging in America*. In its final report, the WHCoA described the events as ". . . a summit on creativity and aging to explore the positive aspect of aging through arts participation and to promote the arts across policy and research disciplines" (WHCoA 2015, 30). Thus, while the arts summit was acknowledged by the WHCoA, it was not sponsored by the WHCoA. Via social media, the summit examined three topical areas: age-friendly community design; health and wellness and the arts; and lifelong learning and engagement in the arts (NEA 2016a). These did not align with the four major themes of the WHCoA: retirement security, healthy aging, long-term services and supports, and elder justice.

The arts summit advanced a set of thirty-eight findings pertinent to the arts and aging across its three topical foci. Many of these findings concerned a need to reframe, redefine, or broaden existing definitions and assumptions. These included a shift from *aging* to *longevity*, a shift to a *lifespan* or *intergenerational* perspective rather than a primary focus on older adults, and outcome measures that would be appropriate to both health and arts stakeholders. Calls were frequently voiced for better communication and understanding among the arts, health, and aging communities, as well as for rejecting *ageism* for a more positive perception of older people. Other persistent calls were for more and better research; more research collaborations across the arts, health, and aging sectors; sustainable business models and funding resources; and more cohesive and effective networks and partnerships across stakeholders. Finally, other findings pointed to gaps in leadership, particularly with regard to policy advocacy, mobilizing network development, and including the arts at various decision-making "tables" (NEA 2016a, 31–34). Altogether, the summit report seems to speak to the members of the *creative aging* community examining issues of concern to itself and trying to assess how it might improve its performance, strategy, and public perceptions while more effectively collaborating with the aging and health policy communities. The final report of the 2015 WHCoA reinforces this impression.

More so than previous WHCoAs, the 2015 WHCoA announced an extraordinary number of new public actions and initiatives undertaken by the Obama Administration across government and across the country designed to help older Americans live in retirement with dignity, maximize their independence and ability to age in place, and to be protected from elder abuse and financial exploitation (WHCoA 2015, 1–2). With regard to *creative aging*, the WHCoA 2015 final report simply acknowledged that "... the National Endowment for the Arts and the National Center for Creative Aging co-sponsored a summit on creativity and aging to explore the positive aspects of aging through arts participation and to promote the arts across policy and research disciplines" (30). Finally, in a discussion highlighting the positive potentials of age-friendly communities initiatives, the 2015 final report included the arts as one in a list of nine other types of aging programs, noting that "... participation in the arts [could] promote healthy aging and avoid isolation" (WHCoA 2015, 20).

An Objective Unattained

The decades-long efforts of the NEA (and the arts policy community) to find a way to frame arts programming as a legitimate, albeit partial, solution to problems identified on the aging policy agenda ultimately was an objective not attained. The NEA concentrated on the four WHCoAs held in 1981, 1995, 2005, and 2015 as focusing events where it sought to attach itself to the larger and more powerful aging policy community as a policy option and as a viable provider of aging services. The success of such a strategy needed a constellation of favorable circumstance in order to surmount numerous policy formulation challenges:

- It required the capacity to provide arts services for older adults that had a demonstrable record of effective programs provided by trained practitioners. Yet it took decades of innovation, pilot programs, and development among artists, arts organizations, and state and local arts councils to build the knowledge and training practices to provide this essential content.

- It needed the support of the arts community in securing a priority position on the arts policy agenda. But this policy consensus within the arts policy community remained elusive. More than any time previously, there is more support and interest within the arts policy today for linking the arts to healthy aging. However, as a matter of national policy as articulated by the NEA, programs specially designed for older Americans are not a distinctive grant category that merits its own review panels.
- It involved competing with other service options for older Americans that had vied and/or were vying for priority on the aging agenda and for access to limited authorized funding. In order to reach such a competitive position among many options in aging and/or health policy, the arts community worked for decades to develop a research record of evidence regarding the effectiveness of arts programming for conditions and purposes of concern to older adults.
- Finally, it needed political conditions that were conducive to treating the WHCoA as an agenda-setter that had the attention of Congress and the president, and thus the prospect of having its recommendations politically accepted and administratively implemented. Such supportive conditions were present during the earliest years of the WHCoA (in 1961 and 1971), years before the arts began to become active in aging issues. The conferences of 1981, 1995, 2005, and 2015 each experienced weak to hostile presidential attention, opposition and criticism in Congress, and/or conditions of budgetary constraints. Additionally, the NEA often faced significant political controversy and threats starting in the 1980s, which made it difficult for the agency to give the arts and aging a prioritized position on the arts policy agenda. Thus, building a window of opportunity where the definition of aging problems could be matched with feasible arts programming solutions amidst hospitable political conditions that could be catalyzed by a WHCoA "focusing event" proved unattainable.

A Change in Frame and Leadership: Creative Aging and the National Center for Creative Aging, 2001–2018

Starting in 2001, the NEA launched a third policy strategy—a "creative aging" initiative—in which the agency would continue to play an important, but different, role. The initiative introduced a new frame for the arts and aging issue: it announced the creation of the NCCA as the spokesman of the initiative, and it began a process of shifting leadership from the NEA to the NCCA. Although the NEA continued to partner with the NCCA on certain activities and was particularly engaged with interagency research projects, it was the NCCA that now became the voice and the leader of a national *creative aging* strategy. This discussion focuses on three key developments that propelled this third strategy. These developments interacted with each other extensively during the period between 2001 and 2018.

The recognition that the condition of the arts and aging movement had matured into a community of practice and a nascent arts advocacy community was the first key element of a *creative aging* strategy. The second element was the creation of the NCCA, which projected a shared identity for the movement, provided a key piece of administrative infrastructure, and could serve as a policy entrepreneur for shaping a reframed and positive arts policy for a potential aging constituency. The third significant change was the shift in the NEA's role from the leading advocate for *arts and aging* policy to acting as a think tank producing research and evidence to support the efficacy of *creative aging* programs. In the process, the NEA joined a group of public and private organizations committed to the training and professional development of teaching artists and specialized arts administrators that were essential to *creative aging* programming for older adults.

The Maturing of the Arts and Aging Movement

The many arts organizations and teaching artists that had been involved in the *arts and aging* movement since the mid-1970s had matured into a sizable field of practice that exhibited considerable self-awareness and had gained more acceptance within the general arts community. This evolution has been discussed in greater depth earlier in this chapter. Collectively, the *arts and aging* community of practice had learned to better understand the dynamics and expectations of the aging and health policy communities. It had also increased its capacity to provide quality arts programming for older adults oriented toward educational, community building, and healthcare goals across a variety of venues, institutional settings, and for older adults of differing physical and cognitive abilities.

Pioneers who had developed particular techniques and approaches to arts for older adults had sometimes won NEA grant support from various discipline programs. Examples included Susan Perlstein's "Living History" approach that served older New Yorkers located in all five boroughs and Ann Basting's "TimeSlips" storytelling program designed for individuals with dementia. Alternatively, members of the National Guild of Community Schools of the Arts have a long history of offering arts education programs for people of all ages. Initially, these focused on programs for children and youth. Arts education programs for older adults are a more recent concern and have often developed in partnership with local aging services organizations. Many of the experienced practitioners referenced above became leaders and exemplars of the *creative aging* initiative.

Despite the maturation of the field and the growing public awareness that the aging *baby boomer* population drew to the arts and aging movement, the field still lacked key dimensions of institutionalization. The NEA had never designated "arts and aging" as a grant category with its own peer panels. Established, arts-based professional associations had not recognized artists or arts organizations that specialized in arts and aging programming as constituting a subprofession or a subset of performing arts organizations, museums, or literary organizations. Finally, there were no national membership organizations that represented either the multidisciplinary arts and aging movement or the aging population that could benefit from and advocate for such targeted programming.

Without such characteristics as a recognized and institutionalizing field, the ability of the arts to function as an arts policy constituency was limited. The changing context of a growing population of aging *baby boomers* had attracted significant public attention and thus propelled the arts and aging movement toward becoming an emergent field with the possibility of being a nascent arts policy constituency. However, these possibilities needed a new frame for the arts and aging issue and entrepreneurial policy leadership dedicated to galvanizing the structuration and identity of the field. "Creative aging" became the spark to ignite both of these developments.

Creative Aging and the National Center for Creative Aging

In 2001, the NEA established the NCCA as a national service organization[12] to be a platform for policy entrepreneurship in the drive to activate the new policy frame of *creative aging*. The concept of "creative aging" grew out of the research and publication of Professor Gene Cohen's 2000 book, *Creative Age: Awakening Human Potential in the Second Half of Life*, which provided evidence and credibility to the connection of arts and aging and the mission of the NCCA. This was focused and elaborated in Cohen's subsequent report commissioned by the NEA and others entitled *The Creativity and Aging Study* (Cohen 2006). "Creative Aging" was hailed as "a new paradigm" (Hanna and Perlstein 2008, 3) that offered "an extraordinary opportunity . . . to transform the experience of old age in America" (Larson and Perlstein 2003, 145). It also opened additional possibilities for alliances and partnerships since it was very interdisciplinary: comprised not only of *arts and aging* interest and knowledge, but also education, health, and the humanities (Hanna and Perlstein 2008, 6).

The NCCA pursued its mission through public awareness campaigns, information and resources, education (onsite and distance learning), convenings, and partnerships. Multiple tools could be combined in a single project. For example, the NCCA announced a national public awareness campaign "The Art of Aging: Creativity Matters" in 2005. In the same year, "Creativity and Aging" was the theme of the arts mini preconference leading to the WHCoA. In 2006, the NCCA, the National Guild for Community Arts Education, and the New Jersey Performing Arts Center cosponsored the first national conference on "Creativity Matters." As a follow-up, the National Guild published a comprehensive, 262-page guide to arts and aging programming as the *Creativity Matters: The Arts and Aging Toolkit* (Boyer 2007). And in 2008, the NCCA collaborated with AFTA to publish a monograph—*Creativity*

Matters: Arts and Aging in America—which explained the background, goals, and key actors of the creative aging idea to the general arts policy community and beyond (Hanna and Perlstein 2008).

Between 2011 and 2017, the NEA conducted, sponsored, or collaborated in producing six research reports exploring the relationships between arts participation, older adults, and health patterns; arts and human development, lifelong learning, and individual well-being; the science and neurology of creativity; and community-engaged research on the arts and health[13] (NEA 2011; NEA 2013; NEA 2015a; NEA 2015b; NEA 2016b; Rajan and Rajan 2017). These research reports continued to add to the evidence base concerning creative aging and were used by the NCCA to inform advocacy, practice, and partnerships. The NEA and the NCCA also collaborated in developing two online tools for the creative aging field: a searchable directory of arts programs for older adults that articulated standards of effective practice and provided evaluation methodologies; and a free, self-guided training course for professional and teaching artists interested in working with older adults (Hanna, Noelker, and Bienvenu 2015, 272).

In 2013 and 2014, the NEA funded the NCCA to develop statewide communities of practice for thirty state arts agencies. Working in partnership, the NCCA and the National Assembly of State Arts Agencies (NASAA) drew together leaders in the arts, education, health, and human services, as well as traditional and folk artists. These states undertook activities, such as professional and resource development, asset mapping, expanded grant-making policies, and technical assistance (Hanna, Noelker, and Bienvenu 2015, 273). Most state arts agencies support training for teaching artists in *creative aging* techniques and skills. The training workshops or institutes commonly grant participants some sort of certificate or inclusion on the state's teaching artist roster. For example, the Maine Arts Council has a special roster of Creative Aging Teaching Artists, while New Hampshire incorporates *creative aging* teaching artists into its general roster of teaching artists.

The NCCA used convenings as a tool to cultivate the interest of private foundations in *creative aging* (Callahan and Mataraza 2011). The NCCA also held an annual national conference to foster cohesion of the *creative aging* field through the provision of professional development to professionals working in the fields of arts, aging, and healthcare. Starting in 2014, the NCCA convened an annual *National Leadership and Exchange Conference on Creative Aging*, including the 2016 conference that explored global perspectives on the practice of *creative aging*. The 2018 conference was canceled, and subsequent meetings have not occurred. Indeed, early 2018 proved to be the end of the era of national leadership of the *creative aging* movement. The NEA dissolved the NCCA in the spring of 2018 and a founding leader of the field, Susan Perlstein of Elders Share the Arts (ESTA), announced that her organization was closing after a forty-year history. The *creative aging* field would see other actors carry the cause of the *arts in healthy aging* forward in a more decentralized and diffused manner.

Decentralizing Creative Aging Policy and Diffusing the Arts into Healthy Aging, 2013 to Present

The fourth strategy designed to advance an arts and aging policy has only begun to shape a transition from an *arts and aging* formulation to an *arts in healthy aging* conceptualization. This transformation gestated for decades as a low-profile theme that ran beneath the more visible Special Constituency / NCOA advocacy building partnership and the WHCoA campaign for a place on the aging policy agenda. The arts community has a long, scattered, and often indirect record of interest in reaching older adults. Throughout the national arts policy trajectory traced here, and even earlier, individual artists and particular arts organizations have shown an interest in working with older adults. Some of these had even been able to secure small state or local grants from programs that set general eligibility parameters that applied to all potential grantees. This gave arts and aging activities "open access" to competitive public funding programs organized by artistic field or functional goal (Pankratz 1989, 25). Examples of such awardees have been included in many of the reports and directories noted in preceding sections of this chapter (e.g., Barret 1993; Lewis-Kane, McCutcheon, and MacDicken 1986; McCutcheon 1986b; Sunderland 1982).

However, such largely anecdotal listings of programming that spanned many disciplines and places of provision did little to reveal a collective identity and shared purpose. Systematic knowledge about early and scattered arts and aging programs was hindered by information collection problems and categorization confusion. Arts programs for older adults were variously regarded as crafts (rather than arts), were regarded as cultural enrichment programs, or were regarded as community arts. In the early 1980s, it was reported that ". . . the state and local arts community . . . provided most of the support for the growing arts and aging movement" and often worked in partnership with local aging agencies and groups (Sunderland 1982, 197). However, the NASAA grants information system did not require the collection of the age information regarding individuals benefiting from each grant, so these provided little information about arts-based programming for older adults (Pankratz 1989, 26).

Historically, national surveys of arts participation collected information on the age patterns of arts audiences, but only related individual participation with specific arts forms and genres, not specialized programming for specific age groups (e.g., older adults). These early arts for older adults programming activities included the visual arts, performing arts, literary arts, and folk/traditional arts. It was 2022 before a national survey could shed detailed light on and insight into the cultural participation and engagement preferences and priorities of adults aged over 55. This survey project brought LaPlaca Cohen—an arts management, marketing, and strategic planning consulting firm—and Slover Linett—a social research and evaluation firm for the cultural sector—together in partnership with E.A. Michelson Philanthropy (formerly Aroha Philanthropies) to result in *Untapped Opportunity: Older Americans and the Arts* (CultureTrack 2022).

A few years into the period focused on the "Creative Aging and National Center for Creative Aging," another strategic shift began to gather momentum as a more networked form of leadership emerged. This is resulting in a dense field network of *creative aging* practice and programming that can only be suggested here. The John F. Kennedy Center for the Performing Arts has expanded its role as an important field convener (Saunders et al. 2022). *Creative aging* program development organizations (such as Lifetime Arts and TimeSlips) have built curriculum and teaching models and expanded their work with foundation sponsors, arts service organizations, state and local arts councils, and libraries to design customized training and professional development capacity in *creative aging*. Some professional membership associations have taken on greater leadership roles in their fields for the advancement of *creative aging* (such as NASAA, the National Guild for Community Arts Education, and the American Alliance of Museums). A private foundation—E.A. Michelson Philanthropy—became a leading private foundation funder of *creative aging* program development. All three of the established national membership associations received grant funding from the Michelson foundation. A brief profile of two examples illustrates the network character that is emerging in the field of *creative aging*.

In recent years, the National Guild for Community Arts Education encouraged their members to learn about the *Catalyzing Creative Aging* initiative and apply for a place in a small cohort of ten museums or twenty teaching artists who received a seed grant of $7,000 starting with a first group in 2017–2018, a second group in 2018–2019, and a third cohort in 2019–2020. E.A. Michelson Philanthropy collaborated with the National Guild to select each grantee from a large pool of applicants, deliberately choosing grantees representing a broad geographic distribution and a "robust variety" of arts forms that belonged to a field constituency with which it could share their learning and experience and encourage others to become involved (Michelson and Bonner 2018). Lifetime Arts then provided a six-month program of sequential training and technical assistance through a series of workshops, webinars, and online and in-person consultants to increase the grantees' capacity to conduct high-quality, skill-based, participatory arts programs for older adults. All three initiative partners—the National Guild, E.A. Michelson Philanthropy, and Lifetime Arts—were fully engaged with one another in an ongoing learning experience and with attention to evaluation, model development, and sharing what was learned with the field.

E.A. Michelson Philanthropy and Lifetime Arts partnered in a similar multi-year initiative with NASAA, building on the original 2013–2014 *EngAGE* grants that the NEA awarded to fourteen state arts councils to redistribute as small grants within state arts communities to develop greater *creative aging* capacity among teaching artists and arts organizations (NASAA 2019a). In 2019, NASAA, in partnership with Aroha Philanthropies (as E.A. Michelson Philanthropy was named at the time), conducted a survey of its members concerning their *creative aging* work. Fifty-four of fifty-six state and jurisdictional members responded (98%), demonstrating the intense interest of state arts agencies in creative aging (NASAA 2019b). This survey provided valuable baseline information for the design of a new wave of funding from E.A. Michelson Philanthropy in 2021. This recent wave of funding provided a total of $1.457 million for awards to thirty-six state arts agencies to advance their creative aging development and services. Seventeen state arts agencies each received grants of $60,000, and another nineteen state arts agencies each received grants of $23,000. NASAA also convenes an annual *Creative Aging Institute* online, providing an opportunity for the network of state arts agencies to actively share experiences in *creative aging* development, training, and practice. Other interested state arts agencies as well as national arts and cultural organizations and individuals have been invited to attend for free. The four-part Institute of 2022 covered topics on embedding creative aging at the state level; being a community *elder artist*; dance reflections on intergenerational creativity; dismantling ageism; best practices for senior centers and libraries; reframing late-life potential through creative aging; online creative aging programs in reading, dance, and embroidery; Pennsylvania's *Academy for Creative Aging*; and case examples of several state arts agencies leveraging state investments in *creative aging*. Although targeted to state leaders and local practitioners, this annual Creative Aging Institute seems to help fill the void left by the discontinuation of National Leadership and Exchange Conference organized by the NCCA each year between 2014 and 2017.

Both new actors in the arts and healthy aging arose and an old arts policy advocacy goal saw progress. New interdisciplinary approaches reached beyond *creative aging* services for older adults. *Age-friendly community* initiatives (discussed in depth in Chapter 7 of this book) shifted their focus from the delivery of benefits to targeted individuals to engaging stakeholders from multiple sectors in a local geographic area to improve social and/or physical environments to be more supportive of the health, well-being, and ability of older adults to age in place (Greenfield et al. 2015). Another initiative expanded *creative aging* programming to the care partners of those with Alzheimer's disease or age-related dementia. Starting in 2015, the Pabst Steinmetz Foundation collaborated with a multi-sector group of Central Florida partners from education, arts, and healthcare to design and develop a creative caregiver guide that was launched at the NCCA 2015 Annual Leadership Conference in Washington, DC (Steinmetz 2015). Another initiative brought Health Resources Services Administration funding and Geriatric Education Centers together to integrate the arts into geriatric education and evaluation. These efforts not only reached medical students but also involved bringing older artists, teaching artists, creative arts therapists, state and local arts agencies, healthcare workers, and community-based training into the education of various healthcare providers working in clinical settings (Hanna, Noelker, and Bienvenu 2015, 273–275).

Finally, a long-sought policy advocacy goal achieved some purchase. AFTA is the leading national advocacy organization for the arts community. Every year, it organizes Arts Advocacy Day, which brings grassroots advocates and practitioners to Washington, DC to lobby their congressional representatives to support a number of issues of concern. A briefing book is prepared for all participants, and it includes a briefing paper on each issue on the arts policy agenda. Starting in 2010, AFTA began to include a briefing paper on *Arts in Health*, an indication that a cluster of arts and health issues had risen to a place on the arts policy agenda. As a talking point, the *arts in health* briefing paper declared: "creative arts in healthcare includes the professional disciplines of arts therapy, music therapy, dance therapy, drama therapy, and poetry therapy as well as artist-directed applications of visual, literary, educational and expressive purposes within a wide variety of healthcare and community settings for therapeutic, educational, and expressive purposes" (Americans for the Arts 2013). This definition opened up the possibility that arts services that were artist-directed and provided in community settings for educational and expressive purposes might become covered in the next reauthorization of the Older Americans Act. This was the goal that *arts and aging* advocates had pursued since the 1981 WHCoA. The fact that the premier arts advocacy organization in the United States was supporting that proposition suggested that a policy window might finally be opening, but this time in the domain of health policy. That "window" did open partially. When the Older Americans Act was amended through Public Law 116–121 in March 2020, the "definitions" Section 102, Subsection 14 regarding "disease prevention and health promotion" Clause E included "programs regarding physical fitness, group exercise, music therapy, arts therapy, and dance-movement therapy, including programs for multigenerational participation that are provided in (i) an institution of higher education; (ii) certain local educational agencies; and (iii) a community-based organization . . . ." The arts had finally taken a step forward in this long campaign. The Older Americans Act had finally named the arts (that is, the creative arts therapies) as recognized service programs for "health promotion."

Conclusion

Over the past five decades, the arts community has searched for a way to advance an *arts and aging* policy. Under the sometime reluctant leadership of the NEA, it first sought to find advocacy partners for the proposition that older adults comprised a special arts constituency. For an overlapping 14 years, the NEA worked with partners largely in the aging community to try to reframe arts and aging programming as a solution to certain health and social problems of older adults. From 2001 to 2018, the NEA slowly devolved its leadership role to the NCCA. Since 2018, national leadership has devolved to state and local arts agencies, to private foundations, and to national arts service organizations while the *creative aging* approach to lifelong education and healthy aging diffuses into other sectors of society.

These four overlapping strategies to formulate and enact a formal public policy designed to engage the arts in improving the quality of life of older Americans have achieved much progress, gained much knowledge and capacity, and generated growing public interest. However, these strategies were never fully mobilized, and an effective advocacy coalition capable of advancing public policy has not yet formed. The next step in this extended journey has just begun with a new national strategy for networked leadership to advance the *creative aging* field of policy and professional practice just beginning to take shape. Our recommendations for structuring and activating the nascent *arts in healthy aging* ecosystem are presented in Chapter 10 of this book.

4
How the Arts Support Health and Well-Being Outcomes in Older Adults

Introduction

This chapter builds on the foundations of the *creative aging* field provided in Chapters 1–3 by introducing the mechanisms through which the arts can support health and well-being outcomes in older adults. The chapter begins with discussing the sociocultural context within which older adults experience their own perception of health and well-being. This leads to an in-depth discussion of theories of human development in late life and the motivations that exist for older adults to participate in creative aging programs and activities. The chapter develops several systemic frameworks for analyzing the impact of arts participation on older adults' health outcomes and sense of subjective well-being and quality of life. Finally, the chapter addresses basic requisite design elements of *arts in healthy aging* programs.

The Sociocultural Context of Older Adults' Health and Well-Being

The term *social determinants of health* has come into common use to describe a wide array of inequities that can be analyzed as causal factors resulting in vastly different public health outcomes among population groups. Simply put, these causal factors are the economic and social conditions under which individuals live their lives. Five domains of social determinants of health are identified to be (1) economic stability; (2) education access and quality; (3) healthcare access and quality; (4) neighborhood and built environment; and (5) social and community context.[1]

The well-established social determinants of health are largely understood around the world to be economic and social constructs. The cultural contexts of health and well-being are relatively new to this framework, with a seminal publication from the authors of the *2014 Lancet Commission on Culture and Health* arguing that "the systematic neglect of culture in health and healthcare is the single biggest barrier to the advancement of the highest standard of health worldwide" (cited in Napier 2017, viii). In 2015, the World Health Organization (WHO) Regional Office for Europe initiated a new focus on culture in two strategic frameworks: the European policy framework Health 2020 and the 2030 Agenda for Sustainable Development. The

WHO expert group on the cultural contexts of health and well-being published its first policy brief, titled *Culture Matters: Using a Cultural Contexts of Health Approach to Enhance Policy-Making*, in 2017. As explained in the publication's executive summary, "with the adoption of Health 2020, WHO's strategic emphasis shifted towards a values base that emphasizes a life-course perspective, multisectoral and interdisciplinary engagement, and people-centred, whole-of-society approach to health and well-being. The 2030 Agenda and its Sustainable Development Goals reinforce this values base, and call for alternative ways of empowering and giving voice to marginalized groups" (viii). The authors of this white paper offer a compelling framework for understanding the cultural contexts of health and well-being as follows:

> In 2001, the United Nations Education, Scientific and Cultural Organization (UNESCO) defined culture as "the set of distinctive spiritual, material, intellectual and emotional features of society or a social group ... [which] encompasses, in addition to art and literature, lifestyles, ways of living together, value systems, traditions and beliefs." This definition stresses that culture is not limited to national, racial, ethnic or religious affiliation—it is comprised of overt beliefs and practices as well as the subtle and taken-for-granted conventions that frame our sense of reality, define what is normal and abnormal, and give our lives a sense of direction and purpose.
>
> Culture, in other words, is something all humans have and depend upon for making meaning. It sets the diverse and shifting parameters within which decisions and actions unfold in the context of families, communities, workplaces, peer groups and environments. The creative practice of culture in daily life influences how we perceive ourselves, one another and our place in the natural world. (Napier 2017, 1)

Arts in healthy aging embraces a broad conceptualization of the sociocultural context of older adults' health and well-being. A person's perception of their own health and well-being is embedded within a sociocultural context, including norms, beliefs, traditions, expectations, values, and ways of living. The social determinants of health are positioned within this much broader sociocultural context. This chapter identifies the mechanics of how arts programs can purposefully contribute toward a sociocultural context that supports public health and well-being for everyone over the age of 60.

Human Development in Late Life

As defined by the National Endowment for the Arts (NEA) in its publication on *The Arts and Human Development*, the term *human development* "describes a complex web of factors affecting the health and well-being of individuals across the lifespan. Together, these factors yield cognitive and behavioral outcomes that can shape the social and economic circumstances of individuals, their levels of creativity and productivity, and overall quality of life" (NEA 2011, 7). This definition is unsatisfying in that it lacks consideration of the cultural context of health, as well as both affective and sociocultural health outcomes. The causal factors that affect the health and well-being of an individual vary enormously by cultural background, geography and climate, political and economic system, the impact of media and communications, and more. Ultimately, however, one's individual assessment of quality of life may be best understood in the sense of *cultural well-being*, i.e., one's perception of his/her well-being as it aligns with one's sociocultural context and values. After all, "our experiences of health and well-being are fundamentally influenced by the cultural contexts from which we make meaning" (Napier 2017, xi).

Concepts, theories, and approaches in *adult development* are grounded in the field of *human development*, which is largely located within *developmental psychology*. Scholars in developmental psychology have traditionally focused their research on human development in earlier stages of life, and by the late twentieth century, publications still did not consider growth in the last third of a lifespan. Researchers lamented the dearth of empirical knowledge of late adulthood, with Levinson (1978, 38) writing that it "is obviously an oversimplification to regard the entire span of years after age 60 or 65 as a single era." As Cohen (2005, 29) explains, "the field of developmental psychology was largely based on theories that looked no further than the onset of adulthood, as though all of the important phases of growth were finished by that time."

The most frequently cited model of human development related to older adults comes from Erikson (1982), who built on the work of Peck (1956), Havighurst (1972), Puner (1974), and others. Erikson is seen to have "stood his well-known theory of human development on its end, reexamining it from the perspective of old age" (Martha Cliff, quoted in Carlsen 1991, 54). Erikson's model of the eight stages of life development, presented in Table 4.1, came to prominence in the field of gerontology in the late twentieth century. In the eighth stage, that of "old age," the key developmental task is seen to be examining one's past, coming to terms with one's

Table 4.1 Erikson's eight stages of life development

Stage of Life Development	Developmental Task	Virtue
I: Infancy	Basic trust vs. basic mistrust	Hope
II: Early childhood	Autonomy vs. shame, doubt	Will
III: Play age	Initiative vs. guilt	Purpose
IV: School age	Industry vs. inferiority	Competence
V: Adolescence	Identity vs. identity confusion	Fidelity
VI: Young adulthood	Intimacy vs. isolation	Love
VII: Adulthood	Generativity vs. stagnation	Care
VIII: Old age	Integrity vs. despair, disgust	Wisdom

Source: Adapted from Erikson (1982).

losses, and celebrating successes—thereby achieving a sense of *integrity*. However, Erikson adopts an ageist stance by viewing "old age" as a single stage for all older adults, with no variations in the developmental experience and little opportunity for growth. His research expanded throughout the 1980s, with research data demonstrating that people did not necessarily move through the eight development stages in a linear fashion. Instead, progression through the developmental tasks of each of the eight stages was better understood for individuals to be multi-directional and recurrent in nature, contingent on one's life circumstances (Erikson, Erikson, and Kivnick 1986).

With the juxtaposition of *integrity* with *despair*, Erikson positions a developmental task in "a dialectic that honors the losses of age at the same time it gives opportunities for the integrities of age" (Carlsen 1991, 59). For Erikson (1961, 161), *integrity* is seen as the ability of some older adults to "envisage human problems in their entirety" and "to represent to the coming generation a living example of the 'closure' of a style of life." Fowler (1984, 26) explains:

> Integrity seems to come with the considered feeling that one played the roles and met the challenges of each of the eras of the life cycle. It does not mean perfection; it does not mean the absence of regrets. It does mean having found a way to make one's life count in caring for—and hopefully enhancing—the ongoing flow of life. From the experiences one gathers, from the suffering and the gladness, one accrues the virtue Erikson calls wisdom.

A student of Erikson, Gene Cohen took the next crucial step in contributing to the human development literature "a new account of psychological development in the second half of life, a fundamentally forward-thinking and optimistic view about potential for lifelong growth, creativity, and emotional fulfillment" (Rollins 2013, 34). In his book *The Mature Mind*, Cohen (2005) uses the term *developmental intelligence* to refer to "the degree to which a person has manifested his or her unique neurological, emotional, intellectual, and psychological capabilities" (35). He explains:

> Developmental intelligence is defined as the maturing of cognition, emotional intelligence, judgment, social skills, life experience, and consciousness and their integration and synergy. With aging, each of these individual components of developmental intelligence continues to mature, as does the process of integrating each with the others. (35)

Cohen writes that he continued Erikson's work by dividing the expansive eighth stage into four phases of growth and development, as summarized in Table 4.2. As with Erikson's stages of human development, people pass through these phases at their own pace, and the phases can overlap significantly. According to Cohen (2005)'s model, older adults find in these phases a sense of liberation and freedom of expression, a desire for novelty, a motivation to share wisdom, and a desire to find meaning in their lives.

Table 4.2 Cohen's phases of late life

Phase	Age Range	Growth and Development Tasks
Midlife evaluation	40–65	Re-evaluation, exploration, and transition
Liberation	Late 50s–70s	Experimentation, innovation, and freeing oneself from earlier inhibitions or limitations
Summing up	Late 60s–80s	Recapitulation, resolution, and contribution Giving back to family, friends, and society
Encore	Late 70s to end of life	Living well to the very end, even in the face of adversity or loss

Sources: Adapted from Cohen (2005, 52–53) and Rollins (2013, 36).

In *The Mature Mind*, Cohen (2005, 32) argues that an "inner push" that we all have manifests as a range of developmental imperatives among older adults. He lists the following as most common:

- To finally get to know oneself and be comfortable with oneself
- To learn how to live well
- To have good judgment
- To feel whole—psychologically, interpersonally, spiritually—despite loss and pain
- To live life to the fullest right to the end
- To give to others, one's family, and community
- To tell one's story
- To continue the process of discovery and change
- To remain hopeful despite adversity

An individual's developmental drive in late adulthood will vary from person to person, and among the distinct phases of late life. In considering the list above, it is evident that these developmental imperatives are embedded within and reflect one's sociocultural context. Indeed, an older adult's sense of well-being goes far beyond basic health measures. *Cultural health and well-being* is perhaps best understood as one's perception of quality of life, which reflects a cultural context that shapes meaning and purpose.

Motivations of Older Adults to Participate in Creative Aging Programs and Activities

The "inner push"—or the developmental drive—that older adults seek to act upon varies significantly from one individual to the next. Maslow (1954)'s seminal work on *Motivation and Personality* may help to explain this variation. Maslow argues that humans have five levels of needs arranged in a hierarchy of importance. He contends that there are lower-order needs (physiology, safety, and society) and higher-order needs (esteem and self-actualization), and that only unmet needs act as motivators. Because these needs are arranged in a strict hierarchy—the well-known pyramid with basic needs at the bottom and self-actualization at the top—it is implied that an individual can only move to the higher-order needs if their lower-order needs are met.

A useful alternative to Maslow's hierarchy has been proposed by Alderfer (1969), who took the five needs articulated by Maslow and compressed them into three: *existence*, *relatedness*, and *growth*. Existence needs cover basic material and physiological desires, such as food, water, shelter, and safety. Relatedness needs encompass interpersonal relationships with friends and family, social groups, and being recognized as belonging to a group of people. Our desire to be accepted by others and to have some control over our lives also falls under relatedness. Growth needs are concerned with higher-order internal needs, such as one's creativity and the need to complete meaningful tasks. In contrast with Maslow, Alderfer argues that individuals can be concerned with more than one need, or group of needs, at a time. For older adults, an individual's perception of their own health and well-being will be largely determined by their ability to pursue human needs in the areas of relatedness and growth. Cohen (2005) frames an individual's motivation to meet higher-level needs as follows.

> People vary more in the "higher" drives of human development, such as spirituality and artistic expression, than in their more basic drives, such as those for comfort and security. Some people, for example, have a strong urge to be creative, whether in the classic arts or simply in whatever tasks or opportunities surround them. Others are not so consciously focused on creativity but feel a powerful drive to give of themselves to others. Some people are driven by a spiritual quest—a desire to find a spirituality that feels true to them and is compatible with their other beliefs about life. Of course, a person could feel each of these three drives equally powerfully. (Cohen 2005, 31)

In considering any of these theories of human development, it may be argued that *culture* speaks directly to many levels of needs and motivations. Clearly, basic biological requirements for human survival must be addressed before individuals have the capacity to pursue other needs. However, as soon as needs involve family, society, belongingness, and social stability, a broader set of influences on one's health and well-being is activated. Needs having to do with connectedness and interpersonal relationships can be well supported by participation in arts and culture activities, and access to one's own cultural heritage is viewed as crucial to an individual's well-being (United Nations Human Rights: Office of the High Commissioner n.d.). With widespread social isolation found among older adults in America, engaging the arts to promote community connections and social stability may serve as an intervention that will help individuals address human relatedness needs. Well-designed arts-based programs for older adults will also support physical and cognitive health throughout the aging process, as discussed later in this chapter. Moreover, with the inner drive that many people have throughout their lifetimes to pursue their personal growth, esteem, and self-actualization needs, positioning engagement in arts and culture as only a luxury for older adults is a mistake. Engagement in artistic expression, lifelong learning, and spiritual growth is a very real need experienced by many older adults in all sociocultural and economic groups.

Erikson (1982)'s and Cohen (2005)'s theories of adult development in late life provide a foundation for understanding the inner push—or the motivations—that older adults may have to pursue highly individual goals for health and well-being. If we understand motivations to participate in *creative aging* programs and activities to be largely driven by an individual's desires to pursue relatedness needs and growth needs, what would be the specific benefit or benefits that an older adult could hope to achieve through arts-based lifelong learning and arts participation?

To address this question, the concept of whole-person healthcare is very helpful. The basic premise of whole-person healthcare is that a person's health and well-being require attending to the body, mind, and spirit (Serlin 2007; Thornton 2013). The motivations to pursue beneficial individual outcomes in these three spheres (see Figure 4.1) will vary from person to person and over time, and there is also a considerable overlap among the well-being of the body, mind, and spirit.

As depicted in Figure 4.2, the motivations that older adult might have for participating in arts and culture programs for the health and well-being of their body, mind, and spirit are manifold. In the body (physical health) sphere, for example, some older adults might be seeking therapeutic benefits for specific diseases or conditions, such as found in arts programs designed to care for patients with Parkinson's disease or Alzheimer's disease. Crossing into the mind (cognitive health) sphere, older adults are found seeking to learn or develop specific artistic skills, such as learning painting techniques or technical skills on a musical instrument. In the mind sphere, many motivations are focused on lifelong learning, which also connects with the spirit sphere in overlapping benefits, such as stress relief or connecting meaningfully with others. The arts also provide many extraordinary benefits in the spirit (social and emotional health) sphere, when spiritually is viewed broadly as encompassing spiritual and religious beliefs, as well as the general pursuit of meaning and purpose in one's life. In short, there are many diverse motivations that older adults might have to participate in creative aging programs and initiatives. And, there is a full array of benefits that they can attain from creative aging activities that contribute toward their whole-person health and well-being.

Healthy Aging in All Phases of the Natural Aging Process

As a person moves through the various phases, or stages, of adult development in late life, they are doing so while experiencing the natural process of aging. The "inner push" that Cohen refers to and the cyclical process of moving through the stages of old age may be aligned with one's individual experience of physical, cognitive, and emotional changes that take place in this stage of life. Every individual experiences

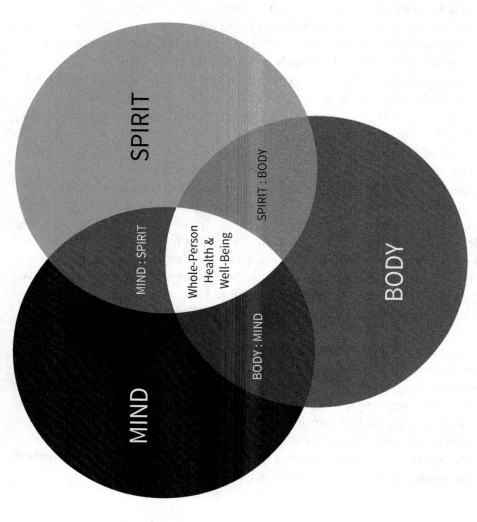

Figure 4.1 Whole-person health and well-being
Illustration by Stephanie McCarthy.

MIND : SPIRIT
- To deepen ties to one's community, family, and friends
- To provoke/influence social change and promote social justice
- To acquire a sense of self-satisfaction and well-being
- To engage in meaningful activities
- To recover from/to accept serious illness
- To relieve stress
- To better understand how spiritual or religious practices are enhanced by participation in the arts

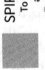

SPIRIT
- To achieve altruistic benefits of volunteering and community service
- To express spiritual beliefs
- To make or view art as a spiritual practice
- To pursue and find connections with loved ones
- To find hope and purpose
- To celebrate and commemorate
- To grieve
- To reflect on the meaning of one's life

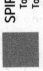

MIND
- To learn new things (joy of learning)
- To more fully engage in the world
- To enjoy social prestige/social connections
- To enjoy entertainment and distraction
- To learn strategies for appreciating and understanding the arts
- To learn new ways of communicating about the arts to others
- To learn the importance of the arts to society
- To learn how to be an arts advocate

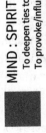

SPIRIT : BODY
- To deepen ties to one's heritage and legacy
- To express closure on one's corporeal existence
- To deepen ties to the natural world

BODY : MIND
- To learn or develop specific artistic skills
- To get training and experience in a new interest area
- To enjoy companionship and meeting new people
- To use arts participation as a way to understand and appreciate the relationship between the body and the mind

BODY
- To aquire physical and physiological health benefits of arts engagement
- To acheive therapeutic benefits for specific diseases and conditions
- To support healthcare for a partner or friend

Figure 4.2 Examples of older adults' motivations to participate in creative aging activities that support the health and well-being of the body, mind, and spirit

Illustration by Stephanie McCarthy.

living and aging as influenced by a unique set of factors, such as lifestyle, education, genetics, temperament, gender, social influences, and economic status.

This book explores opportunities for older adults to participate in *creative aging* programs and activities in three stages of late adulthood. Those in the age range of 60–75 are often referred to by terms such as *young retirees, early late adulthood*, the "*go-go years*," and even *late middle age*. One hopes at this age to be active, healthy, and able to participate in meaningful work, volunteer, and leisure activities with few health limitations. The second stage of late adulthood, the middle stage, extends roughly from age 75 to age 85. In this period, known as the "slow-go years," there are often some physical and/or cognitive limitations that may begin to affect the high levels of activity enjoyed previously. The third stage of late adulthood, beginning somewhere in the mid- to late 80s, tends to be the period of late adulthood in which healthcare needs become more important in daily life. Throughout these three stages of late adulthood, a majority of older adults maintain high levels of functioning in their everyday lives. One's individual experience of aging is related to declines in physical and mental health, and there is frequently a sharp increase in the number of health-related challenges after the mid-80s (Barnett et al. 2012; Rollins 2013).

Numerous physical and biological changes take place during the natural aging process, although older adults who practice healthy behaviors and take advantage of clinical preventive services are more likely to remain healthy and live independently. Physical changes that take place during aging often result in balance problems, slower reflexes, shortness of breath, fatigue, and an increase in blood pressure. In older age, there is also a decrease in muscle strength, speed, and endurance. Most older adults experience some sensory loss, especially in vision and hearing. By age 65 or 70, 90% of adults have some vision loss, and nearly two-thirds of Americans aged 70 and older are deaf or hard of hearing. Diminished taste and smell may make eating less enjoyable for older people (Boyer 2007, 4–5; NCCA n.d., 10–11).

> Older adults are also disproportionately affected by chronic diseases, which are associated with disability, diminished quality of life, and increased costs for health care and long-term care. Today about 80 percent of older adults have at least one chronic health condition and 50 percent have two or more. Major chronic health conditions of older people include heart disease, arthritis, diabetes, cancer, hypertension, and high blood pressure. (NCCA n.d., 11)

The cognitive, social, and emotional changes that take place during the natural aging process may be even more significant to older adults who wish to participate in the arts. As life expectancy increases, people do not necessarily know what they wish to do—or have the financial means to pursue the activities they desire—in their retirement years. Many older adults worry about medical expenses and long-term care. In addition, social connections change with relocations in older age and the mortality of friends and family. The death of loved ones frequently leads to sadness, anger, and loneliness. At some point in their aging process, the older adult may have to give up driving, which further limits their activities and engagement in their communities. Despite these challenges,

> ... older adults as a whole experience greater emotional balance than younger people. Developments in the brain's limbic system, which produces and regulates emotional responses, lead to calmer emotions, better judgment, and a positive outlook. However, emotional losses, chronic illness, pain, medications, and changes in income and surroundings may make an older adult at risk for depression. Depression is characterized by persistent sadness, discouragement, loss of self-worth, insomnia, and an increased concern with aches and pains. It is often under-diagnosed and untreated in the older population. (NCCA n.d., 11)

Many adults experience short-term memory loss, although intellectual ability remains strong among healthy older adults. Older adults frequently need more time to learn new things due to the natural cognitive changes that affect memory, reasoning, and abstract thinking. Most older adults and their families worry about dementia and Alzheimer's disease. Cognitive impairment can be very mild, where one experiences significant and persistent memory deficits but is otherwise functional and independent. *Dementia* "refers to a global loss of cognitive and intellectual functioning, caused by damage to the brain that is severe enough to interfere with social and occupational performance. It is not a disease itself, but a group of symptoms that characterize several diseases and conditions" (Rollins 2013, 35). Dementia is characterized by severe memory loss, problems with speech and hearing, difficulty with concepts of time and space, and severe shifts in mood. *Alzheimer's disease* is a progressive disorder that is the most common form of dementia, accounting for more than 60% of the cognitive function disorders in the aging population (Boyer 2007, 5–6; NCCA n.d., 11).

The authors of this book acknowledge both the challenges and opportunities that are present in the natural aging process. However, it is imperative to understand that the aging process is not only about the gradual decline of health, but this is also a phase of life that is a time for growth, creativity, and well-being. Throughout the decades of late adulthood, carefully designed arts programs can both diminish the negative impact of health conditions and provide meaningful opportunities for adult development. The pages that follow explain how participating in arts and culture programs after the age of 60 can contribute to healthy aging.

At its core, healthy aging is best understood as one's ability to achieve whole-person health, which encompasses the body, mind, and spirit. The WHO defines *healthy aging* as "the process of developing and maintaining the functional ability that enables well-being in older age" (WHO 2015, 28) and *functional ability* as the "attributes that enable people to be and to do what they have reason to value" (28). These WHO definitions suggest that an understanding of healthy aging thus requires an understanding of what it is that people "have reason to value" into very old age, and how they can attain and maintain these valued aspects of their lives. Functional ability can be viewed as a crucial asset—or a multifaceted output—that can lead to desired impacts or outcomes.

Cultivating older adults' functional ability through arts-based programs intentionally designed to promote health and well-being is the central focus of this book. Indeed, in the field of *creative aging*, arts-based interventions that contribute to healthy aging either explicitly or implicitly seek to support the functional ability of older adults. The National Center for Creative Aging states in their manual on *Designing and Delivering Arts Programs for Older Adult Learners*:

> Throughout the aging process, the arts can play a vital role. Participation in the arts stimulates the senses, enlivens individuals mentally and emotionally, and promotes physical and cognitive health. The arts provide opportunities for healing, self-expression, and learning amid physiological, cognitive, and social losses, such as illness or the death of close friends and family members. [The arts] allow older adults to maintain and form social bonds that can bolster health and well-being. And they offer an avenue of exploration and expression for the perspectives, stories, and creative impulses of older adults. (NCCA n.d., 11–12)

Understanding an older adult's functional ability as the capacity and motivation to do what they have reason to value requires an understanding of how individuals can experience healthy aging within a complex set of social, economic, and institutional forces. Each individual possesses a unique sociocultural context of health and well-being, within which the social determinants of health—introduced earlier in this chapter—play a crucial role in setting the conditions for an individual's basic health status. Importantly, it is also within the cultural context of health and well-being that each person will locate the norms and values for what is viewed as a desirable quality of life.

Figure 4.3 depicts a model of the dynamic relationship within which an older adult assesses their state of general health throughout the aging process. The model also illustrates how a person's functional ability leads to the individual developmental drive to pursue quality of life, particularly with regard to one's interpersonal relationships and desire to find meaning and purpose in life.

Health outcomes can be identified in any combination of physical, cognitive, social, or emotional measures. However, a person's sense of health and well-being goes far beyond basic health status and the attainment of existence needs, such as food, housing, economic security, and safety. The field of adult development shows us that healthy aging has to do with optimizing an individual's functional ability to pursue what he or she values in the higher-order relatedness needs and growth needs. Assuming that basic health and basic existence needs are met, the engagement of older adults in diverse activities that offer meaning, purpose, social connections, and life satisfaction can become a mutually reinforcing system of supporting one's functional ability. Carefully designed programs and activities can help develop older

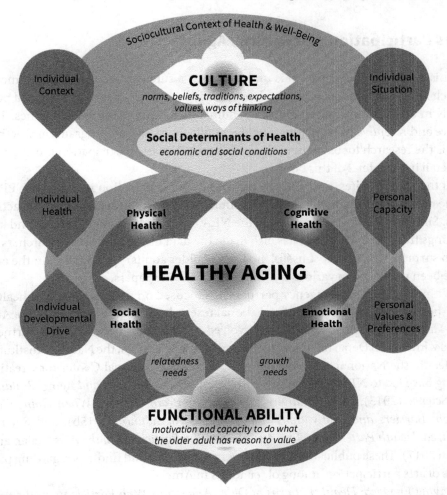

Figure 4.3 The sociocultural context of healthy aging
Illustration by Stephanie McCarthy.

adults' abilities to learn and explore/discover, to build and maintain relationships, and to contribute to culture and society. These kinds of abilities are the key to one's subjective sense of quality of life.

The model shown in Figure 4.3 assumes choice and is developed from numerous assumptions about the older adult's capacity to engage in diverse developmental tasks. Tremendous variety in the sociocultural context of health and well-being exists, and these social conditions will contribute to very different levels of individual capacity and desire to pursue relatedness needs and growth needs. Many other factors, such as genetics, also play an important role in influencing functional ability. However, this model is useful in that it clarifies the context within which an individual experiences healthy aging, and it illustrates the dynamic relationship between a person's functional ability and individual developmental drive.

Arts Participation and Healthy Aging

In this book, arts participation is understood as a subfield of cultural engagement, which refers to all the ways in which people of all ages can engage actively and passively in arts, culture, heritage, and the humanities throughout their lifetimes. The *active* and *receptive* participation of older adults in arts-based programs and activities is the research focus of the authors; this model of arts participation is explained in detail in Chapter 2 of this book.

In the United States, the NEA's Survey of Public Participation in the Arts (SPPA) is the nation's largest periodic survey of adult involvement in arts and cultural activities. Since the survey began in 1982, the NEA has issued summary reports and key findings from each SPPA and has also made the data files available to researchers. It is no surprise that the most useful analyses of older adults' participation in the arts have been published in various NEA reports and white papers.

Within the NEA's interagency partnerships focused on various aspects of health, well-being, and lifelong learning, a national research agenda articulated as *The Arts and Human Development* (2011) has evolved over the past decade. NEA's partnerships with the US Department of Health and Human Services, the National Institutes of Health, the National Academy of Sciences, and the National Center for Creative Aging have led to NEA publications with titles, such as *The Arts and Aging: Building the Science* (2013); *How Creativity Works in the Brain* (2015a); *When Going Gets Tough: Barriers and Motivations Affecting Arts Attendance* (2015b); and *Staying Engaged: Health Patterns of Older Americans Who Participate in the Arts* (Rajan and Rajan 2017). These publications provide very useful data and findings regarding patterns of arts participation among older adults in America.

Staying Engaged: Health Patterns of Older Americans Who Participate in the Arts examines data from an existing longitudinal study (the Health and Retirement Study) on the health benefits that derive from older adults' participation in the arts. Key findings are that older adults who both create and attend arts report better health outcomes, and that greater frequency of arts attendance and arts creation is also positively linked to health outcomes (Rajan and Rajan 2017). Importantly, this publication also distinguishes between active and passive participation in the arts, which the authors refer to as *creating art* and *attending art*. As they explain:

> Creating Art includes the process of generating, conceptualizing, and making works of art such as (but not limited to) dancing, painting, singing, woodworking, and knitting. Attending Art includes activities that invite older adults to observe, analyze, and interpret works of art, such as (but not limited to) attending a play or going to an art museum or festival. (Rajan and Rajan 2017, 5)

A broad understanding of both active (creating) and receptive (attending) arts participation is similarly proposed by Fancourt and Finn (2019) in their WHO scoping review titled *What is the evidence on the role of the arts in improving health and well-being?* In their review of more than 3,000 studies that identified a major role for the arts in the promotion of health and well-being across the lifespan, they delimited their study to arts participation in five broad categories:

- Performing arts (e.g., activities in the genre of music, dance, theater, singing and film);
- Visual arts, design and craft (e.g., crafts, design, painting, photography, sculpture and textiles);
- Literature (e.g., writing, reading and attending literary festivals);
- Culture (e.g., going to museums, galleries, art exhibitions, concerts, the theatre, community events, cultural festivals and fairs); and
- Online, digital and electronic arts (e.g., animations, filmmaking and computer graphics). (Fancourt and Finn 2019, 1)

Rajan and Rajan (2017) note that most existing research on the relationship between arts participation and older adults' health has focused on the active creation of art in participatory visual arts and performing arts programs. Cohen and colleagues (2006)'s seminal work *Creativity and Aging Study*, for example, used a small-scale experimental design involving choral group singing to demonstrate greater improvement in health and well-being among older adults in the arts intervention group when compared to the control group. The researchers also concluded that social engagement was enhanced because arts programs include interpersonal interaction.

> Results of [Cohen's 2006] study of older people participating in a weekly music, visual arts, or multidisciplinary group arts activities showed improvement to physical, social, and emotional well-being, including fewer falls, decreases in medication and doctor visits, reported decreases in loneliness and depression, and increased involvement in community activities; the control group of nonparticipants showed a decline. (Rollins 2013, iv)

Noice, Noice, and Kramer (2013) and Fraser, Bungay, and Munn-Giddings (2014) built upon Cohen's studies to provide further documentation of the positive impact of the participatory arts on improving and maintaining good health in the last third of one's life. However, scant research is available that specifically focuses on receptive arts participation, such as visiting art museums or attending live performances. Even less is known about how and whether creating art and attending art may work together to benefit the health of older adults (Rajan and Rajan 2017, 7).

An NEA study on the barriers and motivations that affect arts attendance provides helpful insight into the ways older adults choose to attend arts events, arts exhibits, music performances, dance performances, and theater performances. The report notes that retirees (as older adults are categorized in this publication) are "significantly more likely than other adult attendees to mention experiencing high-quality art among major motivations for arts attendance" (NEA 2015, 35).

Other strong motivations for older adults' attendance include celebrating cultural heritage and supporting community. For retirees, the greatest barrier to attendance is the difficulty accessing the location. In addition, "the difficulty of finding someone to go with becomes an increasingly common concern as interested non-attendees age, particularly among retirees who want to attend a performance" (35). Social isolation is a very real barrier to older Americans' arts participation, as is poor physical health.

An exploration of existing research on the arts and health begs the conceptualization of some kind of model that unpacks the various dimensions of this relationship. In the most comprehensive meta-review of literature on this topic completed to date, Fancourt and Finn (2019) synthesize across thousands of research publications from around the world to develop a logic model that links arts engagement with health outcomes. In their model, they identify nine components that serve as inputs into a logic model design. They then identify an array of responses, or measures of various kinds, in four groups: psychological responses, physiological responses, social responses, and behavioral responses. The outcomes of this logic model are then analyzed in the domains of prevention, promotion, management, and treatment. This model is a little confusing in that it does not adequately address the inputs and outputs of an art in health program, and it conflates outputs with outcomes. In addition, the potential short-, middle-, and long-term outcomes of an art in health program are not identified.

A modified illustration of this model as relevant to older adults is provided in Figure 4.4. Expanding on the Fancourt and Finn model (2019, 3), Figure 4.4 presents a logic model that is more thorough in its relevance to the design and evaluation of creative aging programs (Slater 2016). The basic elements of this model—i.e., the *inputs* of creative aging program design, the *outputs* of cultivating older adults' functional ability, and the *outcomes* of healthy aging—will be expanded upon and developed throughout the chapters of this book. Whereas Figure 4.4 focuses specifically on health outcomes, outcomes in other domains of healthy aging are addressed in other chapters of this book.

Any arts-based program that is intentionally designed and implemented to contribute to the health of older adults will need to track its efficiency and efficacy in achieving desired outcomes. The *outcomes* of any program have to do with changes that can be reasonably attributed to participation in the program. Short-term effects from arts in health programs are measured as psychological, physiological, social, and behavioral changes among the program participants. Psychological outcomes are generally understood as enhanced self-efficacy, coping, and emotional regulation. Physiological changes commonly measured are a lower stress hormone response, enhanced immune function, and higher reactivity. Improved social health pertains to a person's reduced loneliness and isolation, enhanced social support, and improved social behaviors. And behavioral changes measured as health outcomes include metrics, such as an increase in exercise, adoption of healthier behaviors, or skills development (Fancourt and Finn 2019, 3). All of these measures map onto the

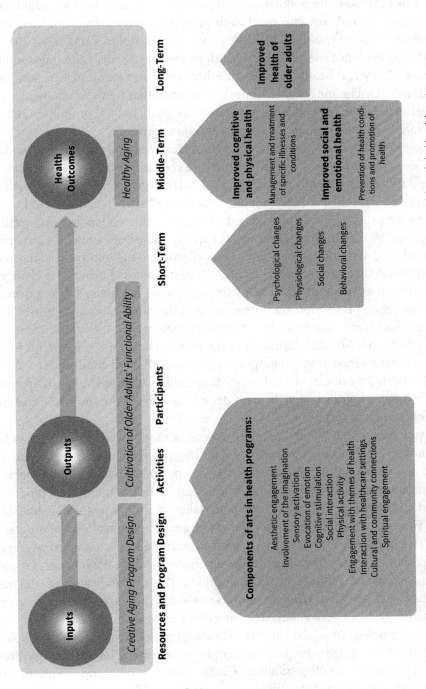

Figure 4.4 Example of a logic model framework for how creative aging programs contribute to older adults' health outcomes Illustration by Stephanie McCarthy.

four dimensions of health that were introduced previously, namely, the desire to improve the cognitive, physical, social, and emotional health of older adults.

As seen in other specific population groups, arts programs for older adults are yielding important and cost-effective health outcomes. Several excellent literature review publications are readily available (e.g., see Hanna, Rollins, and Lewis 2017). Overwhelming evidence attests to these health and wellness benefits for older adults in the areas of physical health, cognitive health, social and emotional health, and end-of-life care. Discussions of specific health outcomes that are well documented in existing scholarship are embedded throughout this book, but a thorough synthesis of this scholarship[2] goes beyond the scope of this book project.

In the logic model, short-term outcomes from creative aging program participation may lead to medium-term results, which are seen as people develop repeated actions and routines in their lives. In Figure 4.4, this category of outcomes for older adults has to do with the management and treatment of specific illnesses and conditions and the provision of improved end-of-life care. Prevention and promotion outcomes may be even more significant as there is robust evidence of participation in arts-based activities and programs contributing to the improved social and emotional health that leads to healthier lifestyles. Outcomes of behavioral changes can be evaluated as older adults' healthy living choices. Examples of the positive outcomes in health prevention are numerous, and the prevention of cognitive decline, frailty, and premature mortality are well documented in the extant literature (Fancourt and Finn 2019, 24–26). Ultimately, policymakers and the general population are most interested in the long-term changes in health conditions of older adults. This ultimate impact, or the long-lasting change attributed to participation in creative aging programs, may be best defined simply as the improved overall health of older adults.

The eleven "components" of arts in health programs, modified from the nine identified by Fancourt and Finn, provide a useful list for *creative aging* program designers. As illustrated in Figure 4.4, these components may best be understood as either program inputs (i.e., activities to be integrated into the design of the program) or as program outputs when these specific activities are undertaken during program implementation. The Fancourt and Finn logic model is silent on other inputs into the program design. It also does not suitably discuss outputs as both the activities undertaken and as participation measures. For program design and evaluation, the outputs are best understood as what the program has actually done and as clear indicators of who has been reached by the program. This is a significantly different measure from outcomes, which has to do with what has changed because of the program (Slater 2016).

The basic, linear logic model depicted in Figure 4.4 presents a useful starting point for discussing *creative aging* program design. However, many issues are raised regarding its applicability to older adults as a distinct population group. Given the diverse needs and interests of older adults, the components of arts in health programs will need to be customized, be combined, employ different art forms, and provide a range of functional engagement. The individual choices and preferences of distinct groups of older adults will drive decision-making regarding these program design elements and will largely determine the nature of the program activities. In other words, authority for program design needs to be shared between the organization providing the program and the actual participants in the program. This suggests that the standard logic model needs to be adapted to somehow integrate *outputs* within *inputs*. Moreover, the focus on improving and supporting *functional ability* might be best understood as both the main *output* of creative aging programs (that is, what the program is actually doing for participants) and the main indicator of short-term *outcomes* for program participants.

We conclude that using a traditional unidirectional logic model (*inputs* lead to *outputs*, which lead to *outcomes*) is wholly inadequate for creative aging program design. The chapters of this book systematically address these challenges, and a more well-developed logic model to inform creative aging program design, implementation, and evaluation is offered in the final chapter of the book.

Subjective Well-Being in Older Adults

Both the WHO's biopsychosocial approach to *health* and the growing focus on the *social determinants of health* position health firmly within society and culture. Health involves general health promotion, illness prevention, and the treatment or management of illnesses that occur. The capacity to self-manage one's health lies at the core of this understanding of health. A person's health has to do with being well, both in terms of individual experience and lifestyle and as a member of social and cultural groups (Fancourt and Finn 2019, 2). The terms *well-being* and *wellness* are often used in tandem with *health* to represent this holistic approach.

The aim to improve older adults' health and well-being is what healthy aging is all about. However, whereas a robust literature exists on the efficacy of arts programs in improving physical, cognitive, social, and emotional health, there is a scarcity of literature and models that address more comprehensive well-being in older adults. This gap in the literature is notable, given that older adults' functional ability to pursue the things that they value most (i.e., the functional ability to pursue their relatedness needs and growth needs) is largely concerned with one's subjective sense of well-being.

The things that an individual values the most are embedded within one's culture—i.e., within one's beliefs, traditions, norms, expectations, and ways of living. In using this sociocultural lens, it can be argued that deeply held American sociocultural values are enshrined in our nation's founding documents. For example, the *Declaration of Independence* names inalienable human rights of life, liberty, and the pursuit of happiness. Translated into a healthy aging framework, these universal values may be understood as the basic human desire to preserve health and to have the freedom to pursue quality of life. In a very general sense, then, older Americans' individual sense of functional ability may be understood as this set of sociocultural values. It follows that older adults are seeking both health and quality of life that are congruent with their cultural expectations for well-being.

A person's well-being, then, can be understood as a person's assessment of their quality of life. In a WHO project that sought to conceptualize quality of life in cross-cultural terms, *quality of life* was defined as:

> An individual's perception of their position in life, in the context of the culture and value systems in which they live, and in relation to their goals, expectations, standards and concerns. It is a broad ranging concept, affected in a complex way by the person's physical health, psychological state, level of independence, social relationships, and their relationship to salient features of their environment. (Camfield and Skevington 2008, 765)

Camfield and Skevington note that a sixth domain of spirituality, religiousness, and personal beliefs was later added to these five domains by this WHO working group. These six domains within which people assess their individual quality of life contain subjective, existential, and objective elements. As explained by Ventegodt, Merrick, and Andersen (2003, 1031), these three separate groups are each concerned with an aspect of a "good life" for that individual. The *subjective* quality of life has to do with how good a life each individual feels he or she has. The *existential* quality of life pertains to how good one's life is at a deeper level, especially with regard to meaning, purpose, and spirituality. The *objective* quality of life means how a person's life is perceived by the outside world, within a distinct sociocultural group.

For individuals, overall well-being is generally understood as overall *life satisfaction*. Ventegodt, Merrick, and Anderson (2003, 1033) suggest that "satisfaction is a mental state; a cognitive entity" and that "being satisfied means feeling that life is the way it should be." They differentiate life satisfaction from *happiness*, which "comprises an individual's whole existence and is signified by a certain intensity of an experience, which is also the case with unhappiness" (1034). Being happy, they argue, is not just being cheerful and content. Happiness is something deep within the individual and is usually associated with dimensions, such as love.

Because a person's overall assessment of well-being is perceived at the individual level, the field of healthy aging is generally concerned with subjective well-being. *Subjective well-being* is "an umbrella term for different valuations that people make regarding their lives, the events happening to them, their bodies and minds, and the circumstances in which they live" (Diener 2006, 400). Life satisfaction, positive affect, and negative affect are three major indicators of subjective well-being (Diener 1984). Life satisfaction, then, is best understood as a subordinate component of subjective well-being and as the individual assessment of one's quality of life (Camfield and Skevington 2008). Life satisfaction is evaluative in nature. Individuals across cultures assess various aspects of life in this factor, such as health, finances/income, job satisfaction, leisure satisfaction, access to education, taking pleasure in life, finding life meaningful, consistency at the matter of reaching goal satisfaction, positive individual identity, physical fitness, economic security, and social relationships (Prasoon and Chaturvedi 2016, 28). Life satisfaction reflects an individual's evaluation of the extent to which basic needs are met and the extent to which a variety of other goals are viewed as attainable (Bradley and Corwyn 2004). Positive life satisfaction is related to better physical and mental health, longevity, and other positive outcomes (Beutell 2006).

In this book, the term *subjective well-being* is used to represent the individual assessment of quality of life, life satisfaction, and happiness that comprise a person's sense of overall well-being. This framing of subjective well-being connects directly to the WHO concept of functional ability, which has to do with the intrinsic capacity of the individual, relevant environmental characteristics, and the interaction between them. When an older adult's functional ability is nurtured, they will have the capacity to more fully engage in the relationships and activities that are valued, leading to a feedback loop that supports subjective well-being.

Figure 4.5 provides a representation of the constituent elements of subjective well-being for older adults. One's functional ability derives from the variables included in Figure 4.3. Figure 4.5 assumes that an older adult has met their existence needs and is focused on pursuing the social relationships and developmental tasks that they have reason to value.

Five domains of subjective well-being are included in this model, comprising *evaluative well-being, eudemonic well-being, affective well-being, hedonic well-being,* and *cultural well-being*. In this constellation of five domains, complex sets of evaluative criteria contribute to an individual's assessment of the quality of relationships, their state of self-actualization and esteem, and their emotional state and sense of individual identity. If a person has a positive perception of their well-being, they will be better prepared to pursue Erikson (1982)'s developmental tasks of old age: *wisdom* and *integrity*.

The two most complex constituent spheres of subjective well-being are *evaluative* and *eudemonic* in nature. Evaluative well-being connects most directly with older adults' motivation to pursue relatedness needs. Through interpersonal relationships, older adults continually assess their sense of life satisfaction, leisure satisfaction, and social and cultural participation. Evaluative well-being also contains an older adult's assessment of their legacy and contribution to family, friends, and society. Evaluating one's life and contributions to others in a summative manner involves important cognitive processes of recapitulation and reminiscence.

In contrast, eudemonic well-being is focused more on the older adult's higher-order growth needs and self-actualization. In this domain of well-being, an individual will continually assess whether he or she is realizing their life potential. This domain has to do with meaning, purpose, and spirituality. Well-being in a eudemonic sense is activated through learning, growth, development, creativity, innovation, exploration, and innovation. Evaluating one's meaning and purpose in life often involves an assessment of liberation, novelty, experimentation, and development. At the end of life, one's individual sense of spirituality and transcendence may become the primary focus of eudemonic well-being.

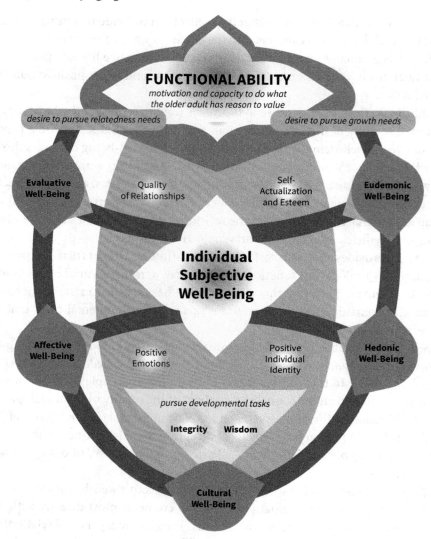

Figure 4.5 Domains of subjective well-being in older adults
Illustration by Stephanie McCarthy.

Two additional domains of well-being that have a single subjective measure are important to consider. *Affective well-being* has to do with whether an individual's mood is positive or negative. *Hedonic well-being* is assessed as pleasure (either positive or negative). *Cultural well-being* is included in Figure 4.5 as an important reflection point in evaluating subjective well-being. Cultural well-being brings together evaluative, eudemonic, affective, and hedonic assessments. Ultimately, it is through the evaluation of one's own well-being within a sociocultural context that an individual determines whether or not they are living a good life.

To summarize, healthy aging is determined by outcomes in four areas of health (physical, cognitive, social, and emotional) and in five domains of well-being (evaluative, eudemonic, affective, hedonic, and cultural). An older adult's functional ability can be cultivated in many different ways so that the individual has an improved capacity to pursue the relatedness and growth needs that he or she has reason to value. Arts-based programs designed to improve functional ability can, therefore, lead to significant outcomes in older adults' health and well-being. The implications of the logic model introduced in this chapter are crucial for *creative aging* program design.

Basic Design Elements of *Arts in Healthy Aging* Programs

Leaders in America's *creative aging* movement are most interested in understanding and promoting the ways in which older adults can take advantage of arts-based programs and activities to attain the healthy aging outcomes that this field has to offer. The explicit argument here is that meaningfully engaging the creative mind through well-designed active and receptive arts-based programs will lead to significant positive outcomes in an older adult's health and well-being. Many researchers around the world are investigating the relationships between arts engagement and whole-person health. Although some of this scholarship is referenced in this book, this has not been the main focus of our study. Instead, we are interested in studying how *creative aging* programs can be designed and implemented so that their participants receive the maximum health benefit. In other words, the emphasis of this book is on *arts in healthy aging* policy and program design.

Currently, there are very few resources that contribute to the intentional design of programs that contribute to a holistic understanding of healthy aging. The most advanced program that aims to build individual capacity to achieve an array of healthy aging goals is the National Council on Aging (NCOA)'s *Aging Mastery Program*, first introduced in Chapter 1 of this book. The *Aging Mastery Program* currently offers the most developed framework available for translating one's desire to pursue evaluative, eudemonic, affective, hedonic, and cultural well-being into concrete action steps. Figure 4.6 depicts the six focus areas of this program in the center sphere. As profiled throughout this book, *creative aging* programs can contribute significantly to these six focus areas, with the possible exception of "Finances + Future Planning." Each of these six program areas represents an important value for relatedness and growth expressed by many older adults. It follows that building functional ability in these six areas will contribute significantly to the quality of life experienced by individual older adults. The distinct goals of the *Aging Mastery Program*—again, perhaps with the exception of the financial security goal—are also similar to goals articulated for many successful *creative aging* programs. The well-structured and mainstream focus of the *Aging Mastery Program* would be wise for the creative aging field to consider as arts-based programs intended to promote healthy aging continue to grow.

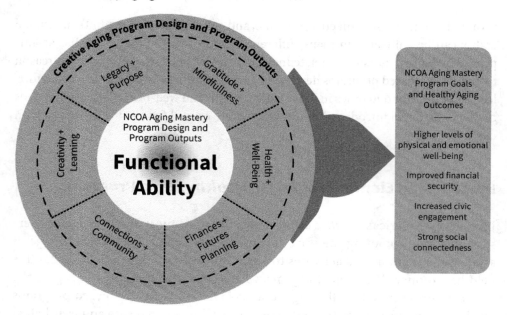

Figure 4.6 Creative aging programs in support of program outputs and outcomes of the National Council on Aging's *Aging Mastery Program*
Illustration by Stephanie McCarthy.

When mapping *creative aging* programs onto the NCOA's *Aging Mastery Program*, as depicted in Figure 4.6, these programs appear to build functional ability in two specific ways. *Creative aging* programs tend to be oriented toward being education focused or toward being therapy focused. One may conceive of *creative aging* programs along a continuum, as illustrated in Figure 4.7, although a wide array of mixed program goals, design elements, and outcomes may exist. At their core, all *creative aging* programs engage various elements of arts learning, arts practice, arts participation, and creative expression. It follows that the primary—or intrinsic—benefits of participating in a *creative aging* program are to advance one's own artistic practice, knowledge, and creative capacity.

However, specific *creative aging* programs also tend to lean toward achieving lifelong learning outcomes (an education-focused approach) or toward achieving health outcomes (a therapy-focused approach). Numerous prospective secondary instrumental benefits exist, and these program benefits are what professionals in the *creative aging* field tend to emphasize. These instrumental benefits may be best understood as improved functional capacity to achieve improved health and subjective well-being. Instrumental benefits refer to the specific health-related changes or supports that derive from participation in the program. These secondary outcomes posit that engaging with the arts in various ways can lead to specific benefits for the program participant. Education-focused benefits may include specific outcomes, such as advancing one's technical skills in playing the piano, working with clay, or writing specific forms of poetry, among other arts skills, as they support the older

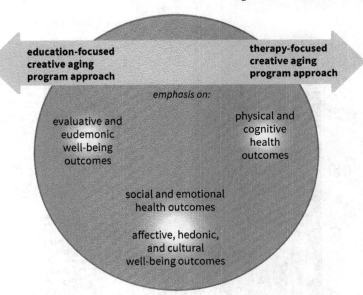

Figure 4.7 A continuum of creative aging program approaches and outcomes
Illustration by Stephanie McCarthy.

adult's overall educative purposes. Concrete therapeutic outcomes include the kind of physical benefits that patients with Parkinson's disease can gain from participating in a specially designed dance class.

It is possible to connect basic program design with intended outcomes across health and well-being. Education-focused programs emphasize lifelong learning that characterizes the growth and life satisfaction goals associated with evaluative and eudemonic well-being. At the opposite end of the continuum, carefully designed arts in health programs and creative arts therapy programs can support specific physical and cognitive health outcomes. A wide array of additional health and well-being outcomes connect these two poles.

Individuals will have many different kinds of motivations to participate in this full array of *creative aging* programs (see Figure 4.2). Older adults interested in lifelong learning outcomes may be propelled to participate by growth needs, such as self-actualization and skill development. Representative motivations that apply across diverse creative aging programs are the inner drive for exploration, expression, enrichment, and social connections. Health-related motivations to participate may focus on specific physical or cognitive outcomes, the desire to address social or emotional health, and developmental tasks, such as the evaluation of one's life and reflection on one's legacy.

Program designs that adopt an education-focused approach and a therapy-focused approach can also be used to imagine the representative types of engagement that could be found across the creative aging continuum, as depicted in Figure 4.8. In beginning our research, we identified from anecdotal evidence that there seemed to be a targeted age range for different types of creative aging programs, ranging

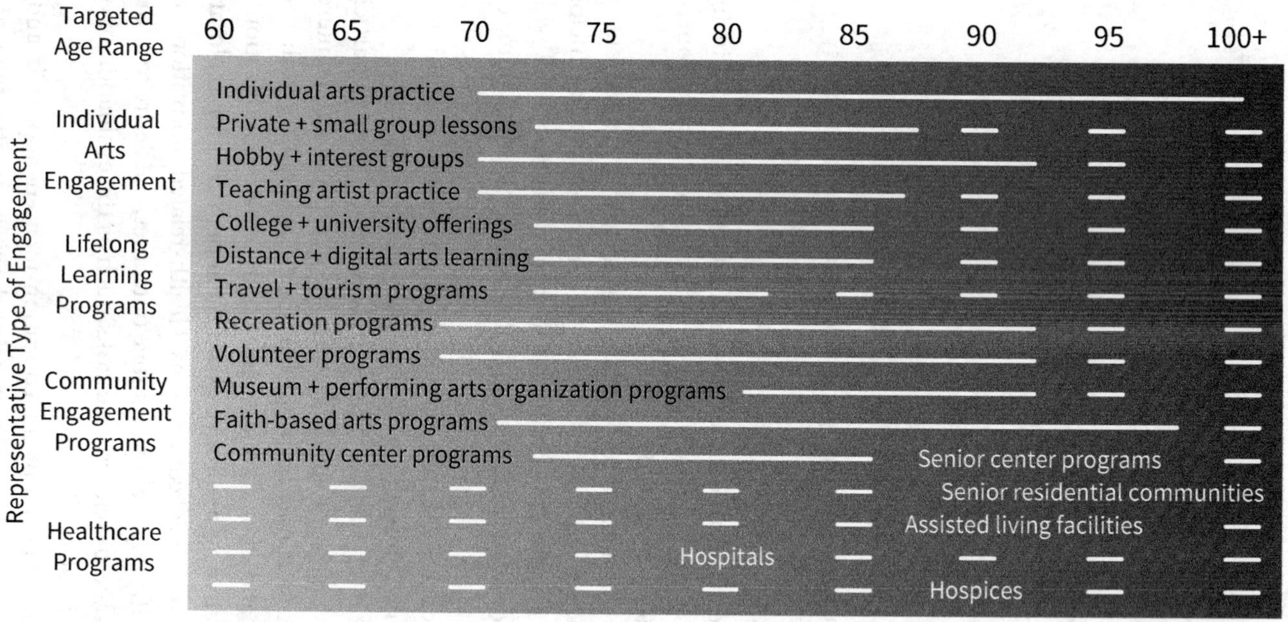

Figure 4.8 Representative types of creative aging programs
Illustration by Stephanie McCarthy

from age 60 to 100+. In Figure 4.8, different types of engagement are characterized as individual arts engagement, lifelong learning programs, community engagement programs (which refers to arts participation taking place in community organizations of all kinds), and healthcare programs (which refers to arts-based programs for health and well-being that are offered in formal healthcare facilities as well as skilled nursing facilities). The solid lines in Figure 4.8 represent what is envisioned as the targeted main age range focus for each type of program. The dashed lines illustrate that it is expected that the programs would also be offered to the age range, but perhaps not as the program's primary focus.

Naturally, participation within *creative aging* programs will vary tremendously from person to person and from organization to organization; however, Figure 4.8 illustrates a spectrum of lifelong learning and cultural engagement programs intended for adults over the age of 60. This range extends from active participation in community-based arts classes and arts groups to the other end of the spectrum where one finds receptive participation in arts initiatives that are designed for well-being in hospitals and hospices.

Creative aging practitioners working for a community organization, a residential facility, or a healthcare institution who are interested in developing arts-based programming to benefit the health and well-being of their older participants, residents, or patients have many choices to make in designing a specific program or activity. One way to think about this, as depicted in Figure 4.9, is to position the program design by the program's goal(s)— intended outcomes in education, well-being, and/or health—as well as by the targeted type or location of engagement. It is often helpful to think about the representative type of engagement along a natural aging timeline. This can help program entrepreneurs and administrators to position their *creative aging* initiative in a way that works best for the intended clients and to also complement other existing programs in a community.

It is important to acknowledge that many barriers exist that might prevent older adults from participating in *creative aging* programs. Despite the many possibilities for older adults to engage in lifelong learning and the arts in their communities, there is not equity in access. Many barriers to participation stem from socioeconomic status, a person's educational background and experience with the arts, perceived racial and ethnic barriers, disabilities and health conditions of all kinds, a person's geographic location, and a lack of social support for cultural engagement. There are also many barriers due to general ageism throughout the nation. *Arts in healthy aging* policy and practice must be responsive to all these barriers.

Another way to think about program design is from the lens of the program participant. For a variety of reasons, older adults and their care partners may be searching out arts programs that call for receptive participation or active participation—or a combination of these. Also, depending on the state of health of the program participant, older adults may benefit from programs where they have more or less autonomy in selecting whether or not to engage in the activity, and in the way they

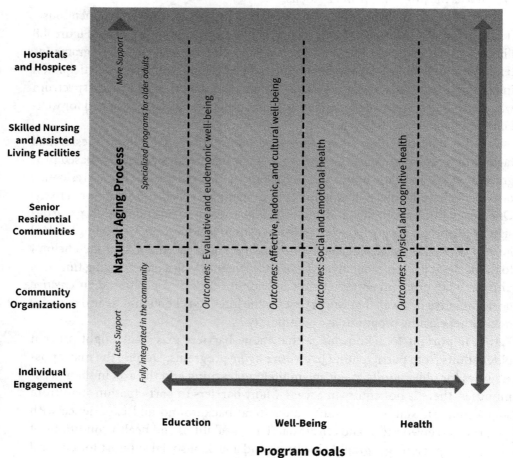

Figure 4.9 Creative aging program design by program goals along the natural aging process. Illustration by Stephanie McCarthy.

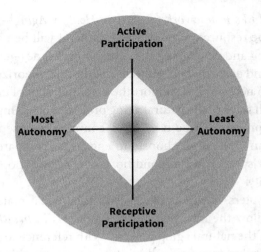

Figure 4.10 Program design by nature of participation and level of autonomy
Illustration by Stephanie McCarthy.

actually participate in the program or activity. The way in which such a program might be positioned by receptive versus active participation and by more or less autonomy is provided in Figure 4.10. Without a doubt, we all want as much choice, as much agency, and as much autonomy as possible when we choose the ways we spend our time and engage in the world around us. Older Americans' choice to participate in *creative aging* programs and activities is no exception.

Conclusion

This chapter has provided information, resources, and tools for policymakers and practitioners to better understand the many ways in which the arts can support health and well-being outcomes in older adults. The chapter began by explaining the sociocultural context of older adults' health and well-being, including the influence of the social determinants of health. Concepts and theories pertaining to human development in all the stages of late adulthood were then presented. The basic human need and desire to grow and to be creative may be best understood as the many motivations that older adults act upon when they choose to participate in the arts. The chapter concisely discussed how arts participation can support healthy aging in all phases of the natural aging process. Several conceptual tools were offered to help readers understand the linkages between the sociocultural context of health, domains of health, functional ability, and domains of subjective well-being. The chapter introduced four sets of health outcomes (physical, cognitive, social, and emotional) and five domains of well-being outcomes (evaluative, eudemonic, affective, hedonic, and cultural). Several typologies and instruments for designing arts programs to support specific health and well-being outcomes were also provided.

Reflecting on the *8Ps Framework for Arts in Healthy Aging*—first introduced in Chapter 2—all of the resources provided in Chapter 4 will be useful for those systematically designing and developing the actual *program* design, consisting of *purpose, place, people,* and *participation*. However, additional theorizing and conceptual foundations are also necessary to support the careful design of *arts in healthy aging* programs along each stage of the natural aging process. For example, a very different program design approach will be used for a community-based intergenerational program in which an older adult chooses to engage, as compared with a program designed to support specific health conditions of a distinct population group in a long-term care facility.

The next five chapters of this book develop theoretical material and program design tools that follow the intended outcomes of *arts in healthy aging* programs along the decades of the natural aging process. With reference to Figures 4.7–4.10, a focus on lifelong learning may gradually shift to a focus on older adults' health and well-being goals. Over time, as chronic health conditions emerge, the arts can be used to support specific therapeutic goals. And at the end of life, the arts can provide pathways to address the final tasks of life and support the family's well-being. Chapters 5–7 address concepts, theories, and approaches for successful arts-based lifelong learning in community settings. Chapter 8 presents opportunities for arts programs to support the needs of older adults in residential and clinical care settings. Chapter 9 focuses specifically on arts programs in hospice and end-of-life care.

5
Centering the Learner in Arts Education for Older Adults

Introduction

Perry Johnson is a resident of Eugene, Oregon. Born in 1949 and raised in Eugene, he is now retired from his job as a detailer with a local auto dealership. Primarily a painter, Johnson also draws and takes photographs. He has recently begun to make portrait sculptures from clay. Johnson regularly attends the Oregon Supported Living Arts and Culture Program. This program provides classes and a place for artists to work, along with others, with an emphasis on access and inclusion. This emphasis on access and inclusion is crucial to Johnson's participation. The program offers classes and workshops, as well as guidance on seeking out opportunities to exhibit in professionally oriented venues.

Johnson's vividly colored paintings include portraits of family members, particularly his mother and eight brothers. Johnson is one of three triplets, and his brother, Terry, is an artist who concentrates on paintings of automobiles. Perry Johnson[1] also paints images of the "Three Stooges," his work at the auto dealership, Eugene's landmarks, Pacific Northwest cityscapes, and notable personages, including John Lewis, Martin Luther King, Jr., and George Floyd. Johnson recently painted a self-portrait where he situates himself within the Black Lives Matter (BLM) movement and the closing of the Oregon Supported Living Arts and Culture Program in response to the COVID-19 pandemic. Johnson portrays himself, smiling, from mid-chest up, within a vivid multicolored environment consisting of a fruit tree, a fir tree, and a blazing sun shining down on him. References to the BLM and the COVID-19 pandemic are in brightly colored text.

In a review of Johnson's work, Carnes (2015) describes Johnson as having "a gift. His work is inquisitive and multidimensional, at once rooted in a folk art tradition while branching out towards something more visceral and visionary. Employing color, shape and text, Johnson's pieces are composed, developed and hauntingly autobiographical."

In 2019, Johnson's work was juried into the *Eugene Mayor's Art Show*—a highly competitive exhibit of Eugene artists. Johnson's *Artist Statement* provides insight into his approach to the arts. In his statement, he is described as "an orderly and dedicated artist....a quiet man... who loves having his artwork on display and the attention he has received for his notable style and point of view" (Mayor's Art Show

2019). In terms of visibility, a high point in Johnson's life as an artist was his inclusion in *We.Construct.Marvels.Between.Monuments.*—an exhibit at the Portland Art Museum in 2018. This exhibit was one in a series of exhibits focusing on regional artists with a particular emphasis on people who have faced barriers to exhibiting their work in galleries and museums.

Johnson is not unique in beginning his engagement with arts and education in later life following his retirement. Johnson's story introduces in this chapter—the first of three—a focus on learner-centered arts education for older adults. Issues and perspectives drawn from the fields of folklore, adult education, gerontology, and arts education (among other related fields) will be considered. Folklore in particular is useful in assisting the field of creative aging in embracing a nuanced conceptual understanding of the importance of culture in people's lives. In doing so, this chapter responds to Boyer's (2007, 34) recognition that people of all ages can and should be able to participate in arts education programs throughout their lives. This chapter also builds on Boyer's recognition of the field of folklore, and the subfield of folk arts, with their "emphasis on passing traditions and skills from one generation to another, honoring elders, and preserving history," and in doing so provides "a model for other arts disciplines that are just starting to think more broadly about arts education" (Boyer 2007, 34).

Readers are encouraged to consider the issues and perspectives discussed in this chapter to specific programmatic offerings they may be associated with. Recognizing that arts education occurs formally and informally, this chapter emphasizes a learner-centered approach to arts education that centers the learning experience within a larger context of institutional and organizational educational programming (museums, community arts centers, eldercare settings, religious institutions, etc.). It is posited that creative aging programs committed to the motivations, factors, perspectives, and orientations outlined below and in the preceding chapters can look to the field of folklore, in part, to theoretically ground learner-centered creative aging programs and practices. In this regard, the chapter considers what constitutes *arts* within a diverse multicultural, multiethnic, and multiracial society dedicated to a democratization of arts participation. The intersection of folkloristic and folklore in education approaches with the *life course* perspective from gerontology will be shown as being mutually reinforcing. The chapter concludes by contextualizing the foci of this chapter within the larger field of adult education, particularly adult education that is informed by learner-centered andragogy and transformational learning perspectives. Recommendations are offered for designing arts education programs that include older adults.

Chapter 6 provides a more expansive discussion of andragogy and transformational learning. This next chapter presents adult learning within a lifelong learning context coupled with a discussion of factors contributing to age-friendly educational environments. Subsequently, Chapter 7 investigates the systemic network associated with the locations available to older adults, such as Perry Johnson, who wish to participate in the arts within an arts education context.

Examples of Motivating Factors for Older Adults' Arts Participation

Earlier chapters delineate the motivations and benefits of older adults engaging with the arts. These motivations and benefits are identified using a holistic approach to whole-person health associated with the body, mind, and spirit. Motivations integral to this tripartite orientation to motivation include cultivating physical and psychological health benefits of arts engagement (body); skill development in continuing or new interest areas in the company of others (mind); deepening ties to one's community, participation in social change, finding meaning in activity, acquiring a sense of self-satisfaction and well-being (mind–spirit); and expressing spiritual beliefs, to pursue and find connections to loved ones, deepen ties to heritage and legacy, find hope and purpose, celebrate, grieve, reflect on meaning of one's life, and express closure on one's corporeal existence (spirit).

To increase understanding and appreciation of these motivational factors, consider the following two additional examples and how these factors are evidenced in older adults' lives and arts making.

Marion Sykes

A second example comes from folklorist John Kay and his fieldwork supporting his scholarship associated with "folk art" and aging (Kay 2016). Although born and raised in Chicago, Marion Sykes[2] lives in Chesterton, Indiana. According to an interview, Kay first encountered Sykes' hook rugs when invited to a hooked rug fair. For Kay, Sykes' rugs stood out from the rest. They stood out, in part, because of their story telling. Kay (2016, 46) describes Sykes' work as "her memories and her art to produce rugs that are beautiful to see and pleasant to recall; they are visual distillations of storied events and/or often-remembered locations. Sykes' life has not been without challenges. These challenges include being placed in an orphanage at three after the death of her mother and an abusive and dysfunctional marriage. However, her creative process carries her memories back to 'happier times.'" Sykes, when asked by Kay about the focus of her rugs, stated that,

> That's why I put nice [scenes] . . . it's hard for people to realize, they figure you should get over it. But when you're young and you've been hammered all those years, you don't. It doesn't erase your mind. You get over it in a way—but you don't treat kids like that! You don't make people feel bad. (Kay 2016, 53)

The stories that Sykes' rugs tell are associated with her life in Chicago and the lives of her children. For example, Sykes' rugs depict scenes of festivals, urban street life, neighborhoods, family trips to parks and zoos, Halloween, swimming, and snowball fights. About Sykes' rugs, Kay (2016, 50) observes that, "current memory research reveals that the practice of retrieving autobiographical memories is a type of problem-solving process through which seniors select, change, and reorganize information to meet specific needs of their current situation."

While Sykes is described as having always been "crafty," she did not create hooked rugs until her eighties (Burke 2017). She describes herself as self-taught having learned rug hooking from a magazine. She uses recycled materials provided by her daughter to make her rugs, at times dying her materials with Kool-Aid and other readily available dyes to create desired colors (Kay 2016). About her approach to rug hooking, Sykes told Kay that, "I make sketches until I feel that it'll work. Make many sketches and make a part of it and add a little more. And then finally, it'll seem to fit and come in place, you know. And I think about what happened at that time" (Kay 2016, 51).

Collete Maze

In May 2021, French pianist Collette Maze, at the age of one hundred and seven years, released her sixth album, a compilation of her Claude Debussy recordings. Maze, born in 1914, has been playing the piano since the age of five. In an interview with National Public Radio correspondent Eleanor Beardsley (2021), Maze describes a difficult life and the importance of the piano and her chosen repertoire to living through the difficulties. Over the course of her life, Maze witnessed two world wars, including the occupation of her country by the Nazis during the Second World War. Maze's professional aspirations were not supported by her family, and she was also a single mother. About the importance of music in her life, Maze says in her interview, "I always preferred composers who gave me tenderness . . . . Like [Robert] Schumann and [Claude] Debussy. Music is an affective language, a poetic language. In music there is everything—nature, emotion, love, revolt, dreams; it's like a spiritual food."

Maze describes being brought up in a musical family. Her grandmother was a pianist and her mother was a violinist, both amateurs. In her interview with Beardsly (2021), she describes being drawn to music to compensate for a lack of love from her mother. She recognized music as a "guiding force" in her life. Despite women being discouraged from becoming professional musicians, Maze did qualify to provide piano lessons and did so for twenty years. Fabrice Maze, Collette's son, describes Maze's difficult relationship with her family. In his view,

> The problem is Colette was an artist in an excessively classic family that did not understand her, so she was completely isolated . . . . And despite that, she persevered and did take her destiny in hand. She did not want to be in conformity with the family tradition. She

decided she was an artist, a musician, not a housewife, so she married the piano... to the detriment of all the social conventions of the day. (Beardsly 2021)

When she reached her nineties, Maze was encouraged by her son to be recorded. In part, according to Fabrice Maze, this was because Maze uses a "specific technique and method" taught by French pianist Alfred Cortot (1877–1962). Based on her work with Cortot, according to her son, "the way she's touching the piano is very special.... It's very rare. The way she is playing Debussy is very unique." In the interview with Beardsly (2021), Fabrice Maze observes that his mother

> decided she was an artist, a musician, not a housewife, so she married the piano.... I always knew the piano—from morning to night—she was always at the piano. She sort of breathed through the piano.... And for me, it was important that she could record, to leave a trace—to leave a message. Now she's existing through her piano, and her piano was her life.

Maze herself observes: "You have to look at life from all sides... and there's always an angle of joy.... Youth is inside us.... If you appreciate what's beautiful around you, you will find a sense of wonder in it" (Beardsly 2021).

The connections between the work of these older artists with the body, mind, and spirit are evident across these three examples. All three artists have pursued skill development through classes (Johnson and Maze) or through other instructional resources (Sykes). All are members of larger communities appreciative of their work. In Johnson's and Sykes' work, there are obvious connections to family and heritage. Maze's recordings connect her to the legacy of her teachers, as well as the composers whose work she is interpreting. All these artists have faced significant psychological challenges in their lives that their artistry responds to.

At the outset, it is important to recognize that it would be incorrect to believe this is the first time Johnson or Sykes and certainly not Maze (who has played the piano for over one hundred years) has been creative, or that creativity in the last decades of life is somehow more accessible or attainable. It is also important to note that while Johnson, Sykes, and Maze are receiving attention beyond their own communities, the implication here is not that participation in creative aging should be aspirational in this way. The point here is to show that these artists are responsive to the motivations identified in earlier chapters for why people are drawn to creativity in aging.

Creativity, Culture, and Folk Groups

There are myriad definitions and explanations for *creativity*, and many of these have been discussed in earlier chapters. For the purposes of this chapter, it is important to emphasize the seminal work of Gene Cohen in articulating the importance of creativity for all people, including older adults. Cohen (2000, 12)'s definition of "creativity as an equal opportunity attribute" resonates with the purpose of this book and chapter. Keeping in mind the above examples, Cohen recognizes creativity as "built into our species, innate to everyone of us . . ." (12). Creativity is multi-varied in how it manifests and "is the flame that heats the human spirit and kindles our desire for inner growth and self-expression" (12). Cohen sees creativity as a universal human attribute that manifests in myriad ways dependent on the context in which it occurs. If there is a uniqueness to creativity in later life, it is how it occurs in combination with life experience encouraging "a dynamic dimension for inner growth with aging" (17).

Johnson, Sykes, and Maze demonstrate that engaging with the arts by older adults is motivated by a combination of factors that can be broadly identified based on the motivations delineated in earlier chapters, such as a desire to create, cultivate community, embrace one's heritage, and find meaning in one's life. It is important to recognize that these motivations encourage engagement with the arts in informal settings, such as at home, at work, and in one's neighborhood, or in formal settings, such as museums, performing arts centers, festivals, and community arts centers. In the latter settings, engagement often occurs within the context of educational programming.

As Johnson's, Sykes', and Maze's lived experience and creative work affirms, creativity does not occur in a vacuum. Creativity is inextricably linked to *culture*: "a people's way of being, knowing, and doing" (The Smithsonian Center for Folklife and Cultural Heritage 2021). Earlier chapters address definitions of culture and the importance of recognizing the cultural context with which any given older adult is associated. Of particular importance are those definitions of culture associated with UNESCO referenced in Chapter 2. *Learning for Justice*, an education program associated with the Southern Poverty Law Center, amplifies this earlier material by affirming that culture is a "shared system of meanings, beliefs, values and behaviors through which we interpret our experiences. Culture is learned, collective, and changes over time. Culture is generally understood to be 'what we know that everyone like us knows'" (Learning for Justice: Our Multicultural Self 2021). It is within culture that "individuals and groups come together to generate creative and symbolic forms commonly referred to as art" (Blandy 2008, 174). As Pocius (2003, 56) observes, "all creation is culturally based."

In Chapters 1 and 2, attention was given to defining a number of concepts, theories, and fields of study associated with this book and that contribute to the theories and practices informing creative aging. Significant to the discussion here is that in addition to one's cultural identification, it is also important to consider those affinity groups to which people belong. Useful to extending the understanding of the communities that older adults may belong to is the *folk group*. As mentioned earlier, *folklore*, as a term, has been in usage for almost three hundred years. As the use of the term became more commonplace and complicated, the academic field of folklore emerged. Along with the emergence of folklore as a field of study so too did a debate about what folklore is and how it manifests. The American Folklore Society's project *What is Folklore?* succinctly defines *folklore* as "our cultural DNA. It includes the art, stories, knowledge, and practices of people. While folklore can be bound up in memory and histories, folklore is also tied to vibrant living traditions and creative expression today" (American Folklore Society 2022).

Folklore is based in culture in that it refers to the "informal or unofficial level of cultural understanding" garnered through customs, experience, and observation (McNeill 2013, 2). The *folk* in folklore is *all* people. Lore can be considered the knowledge that people hold to be important. This knowledge manifests in those expressive forms through which people "communicate and interact" (McNeill 2013, 5). Examples include: the arts broadly defined, jokes, how people celebrate holidays and other special events, participation in sports, rituals, slang, political messaging, and hobbies.

People find commonality in and outside of their cultural milieu and form groups around common interests and pursuits. Within the field of folklore, such groups are commonly referred to as *folk groups* (Toelken 1996, 31). Folk groups form around an infinite number of possibilities. Readers of this chapter and book are all members of one or more folk groups. One obvious example are those people who identify with the creative aging movement. Other identifiable folk groups may form around shared interests, such as cooking, reading, birding, knitting, teaching, religious beliefs, and gardening. Folk groups are associated with those experiencing or treating a particular health challenge. Folk groups are also commonly associated with occupations. Participants in particular art forms are also folk groups. The size of a folk group can range from two people to an indeterminate number.

The Arts, Making Special, and Expressive Culture

Anthropologist Ellen Dissanayake's (2013, 127) view of art as "making special" is at the intersection of culture, folk groups, and art. Dissanayake proposes a *psychobiological* view of art (122) in which art is behavioral, psychological, necessary for human survival, and cultural. It is through art that the ordinary becomes extraordinary (127). Like Cohen (2000), Dissanayake believes art to be integral to who we are as humans. This can easily be seen in the lives and works of Johnson, Sykes, and Maze and the ways in which their artistry reflects their humanity, assists them in coming to terms with life challenges, and the way that they have been able to take these challenges and make them "special" through their artistry. Dissanayake concludes that "art is a human universal" and is "integral to our lives" (135). For Dissanayake, art "emerges for our fundamental nature as humans and for untold millennia has been essential to our life in the world" (135).

The relationship between art and culture as theorized by Dissanayake (2013) is further nuanced through the discussion of folk groups above and the *expressive culture* emerging from both. Expressive culture, identified and documented in folklore and anthropology, is particularly useful in considering the ways in which people express themselves visually, auditorily, kinesthetically, and through the olfactory and gustatory systems. As such, expressive culture includes sensory experiences associated with the visual, performing, literary, time-based, environmental, culinary, and heritage arts. Expressive culture also includes what is referred to as the *fine arts*, *traditional arts*, and *folk arts*. Burstein (2014, 132) describes expressive culture as associated with the everyday and a "way to embody culture and express culture through sensory experiences as dance, music, literature, visual medium, and theater." Likewise, Feintuch (2003) considers what is often referred to as *art*, a concept that he recognizes as a "notoriously slippery" (2), as necessary to understand and appreciate

> culture's expressive realm—the forms, processes, emotions, and ideas bound up in the social production of what Robert Plant Armstrong has called "affecting presences," aesthetic forms and performances in everyday life—music, verbal art, play, material culture, celebration, ritual, and display. (1–2)

Like Dissanayake, Feintuch recognizes art, despite its slipperiness, or the "capacity for aesthetic experience," as universal (2) and "at the center of many conversations about socially based creativity, about the ways in which individual and symbolic action is grounded in . . . culture" (3). Consequently, for the purposes of this chapter and book, it is important to recognize that references to art should be understood to mean the plethora of ways that expressive culture will manifest. Definitions of "art" will differ in multicultural, multiethnic, and multiracial societies.

The Arts and the Life Course

The preceding discussion associated with art and expressive culture brings our attention to the field of gerontology and the importance of what is referred to in theory and practice as the *life course*. Examining the work of a fourth artist assists in comprehending this theoretical perspective and its application through the creative process.

Aminah Brenda Lynn Robinson

Aminah Brenda Lynn Robinson (1940–2015) was raised in a housing development project in Columbus, Ohio. Built on an area referred to locally as the "Blackberry

Patch," that neighborhood, as well as life in the housing project, was centered on family and community. This included fostering Black cultural traditions often communicated in the form of stories particularly from "Big Annie," Robinson's formerly enslaved great-aunt Cordelia.

From her mother, Helen Zimmerman-Robinson, Robinson "learned how to sew, weave and master seamstress skills, working with buttons, fabric, needlepoint, ribbons and yarn." From her "father, she learned to work with raw materials and scraps of items, ranging from charcoal, glass, leather and seashells to animal hides, clay, rope and wood . . . She also worked with a concoction of brick dust, glue, lime, mud, pig grease, red clay and sticks that her father taught her how to make; they called this creation 'hogmawg' and it was used to develop two-dimensional and three-dimensional pieces" (Black Listed Culture 2022). Robinson[3] described art "as a way of life," and her art as a way to tell "Black people's stories" (Opam 2021). Robinson kept journals and in one she wrote that "By the time I reached 9 years old, I was deep into transforming and recording the culture of my people into works of art . . . . My works are the missing pages of American history" (Opam 2021).

In 1957, Robinson was a student at the Columbus Art School. In 1974, she was able to purchase a home on Sunbury Road not far from the place that she grew up. Upon her death at age 75, Robinson gifted her home and estate to the Columbus Museum of Art. Robinson's home incapsulates the course of her life. Every room is a testament to her story telling through paintings, journals, drawings, puppets, and handmade furniture, as well as numerous other examples of expressive culture. The site contains a plethora of materials that she collected over the years through which she would tell her stories.

Robinson coined the term *rag on* to express her desire that her work would continue on in the minds and work of others (Columbus Museum of Art 2021). To "rag on" means attending to detail, making *Gupa* (imaginary figures), knowing Black history and culture, imagining what it would be like to be inside a picture, finding sources of creative inspiration, knowing our neighborhoods, participating in social action, and remembering and passing on memories (Columbus Museum of Art 2021). About memories, Robinson wrote, "Memories, woven together like threads of treasured family cloths, are protected and loved through generations; the sharing of memories becomes the story of all our lives" (Columbus Museum of Art 2021, 13).

Within the field of gerontology, Robinson's recognition of her lived experience, as represented in her art, is referred to as the *life course*. An extensive body of literature associated with the life course perspective exists within gerontology and the subfield social gerontology, as discussed in Chapter 2 and below. Quadagno (2005) provides a primer on social gerontology and the life course perspective. First, she asks us to remember that it was not until the last century that old age was even thought to be normal or possible for most people. Quadagno describes social gerontologists as those who examine questions associated with how biology shapes the social experience of aging and vice versa. Important to social gerontology are familial relationships, other personal relationships, the economics of aging, orientations to retirement, perspectives on mortality, and short- and long-term care for older adults. Also considered within social gerontology are how conceptions of aging will differ across and within cultures, how such conceptions will influence social expectations associated with older adults, and similarities and differences between *functional age* (what an older adult can do) and *subjective age* (how an older adult compensates for what they cannot do). Within the life course, emphasis is placed on history, as well as individual choices and decisions. Early life will influence later life. Social roles are not static, but will evolve and transition over the course of one's life (Elder 1994).

The subfield critical gerontology also contributes to the life course perspective. Katz (2005, 85) identifies *critical gerontology* as providing "an important critique of prevailing social policies and practices around aging, while promoting the rise of new retirement cultures and positive identities in later life." Katz also credits the voices of critical gerontologists with bringing to the fore "age-based inequality, poverty, and injustice as widespread structural problems" (89). Katz views critical gerontology as a "humanistic orientation" (89) where "ideas become critical when they overflow their contextual boundaries, resist theoretical stasis, and accommodate emancipatory projects aside from professional pronouncements about their value and utility" (91). Within this process, Katz views critical gerontology as being derived "from the gerontological tradition of fracturing, transfiguring, borrowing, and recombining theoretical ideas from outside aging studies" (15).

The importance of cohorts and generational differences are important to social gerontologists and critical gerontologists in defining the life course. Ryder (1965, 845) defines a *cohort* as the "aggregate of individuals who experienced the same events within the same time interval." Uhlenberg and Miner (1996, 208) view "cohort aging" as "the continuous advancement of a cohort from one age category to another over its life span." This advancement will be unique to any given cohort. Five cohorts associated with the last century have relevance to our current century. These include the *swing generation* (1900–1926), the *silent generation* (1927–1945), the *baby boomers* (1946–1964), *Generation X* (1965–1979), and the *millennials* (1980–1995). Currently, the *swing*, *silent*, and the *baby boom* generations are experiencing older age with the *Generation X* cohort fast approaching elderhood.

Cohorts are not discreet. Cohorts are linked through family and kinship. Important to understanding cohorts is that they are defined by the peculiarities of how one's own life is lived in relationship to larger social events, such as war; local, regional, national, and international political economies; pandemics such as the current COVID-19 pandemic; social movements such as the Civil Rights or Feminist Movements in the United States; the interpretation and application of state and federal law; public policy initiatives; and the availability of education (Uhlenberg and Miner 1996).

Also influencing the life course perspective are socially based theories of aging (Elder 1994). Riley and Foner (1988) posit that aging is a social process and that this process coupled with "age as a structural feature of changing societies and groups" creates an "age stratification system" (243). According to Riley and Foner, age stratification theory emphasizes how age is "defined as an element of social organization" instead of a "search for optimal aging" (24). In this view of aging, there is no norm. Instead, the emphasis is placed on the structures created for older adults within society and culture. Ethnicity, race, gender, political economies, and social class influence the social structures, as well as the inequities that may exist within these social structures. Policy is recognized as significant to shaping social structures for aging (24). As such, policy, along with any resulting initiatives or programs, should assume that within a multicultural, multiracial, multiethnic, socioeconomically diverse society, such as found in the United States, it is impossible to impose a "single developmental logic" to the life course. The diversity across life courses is well documented through cross-cultural studies, and

> the life course regimes of typical modern Western societies have been shaped according to white, masculine, heterosexual, middle-class values, and cultural patterns. Hence, the critics point out as well that life course politics constitute a critical arena of struggle whereby race, gender, sexual, and class divisions intersect with those based on age. (Riley and Foner 1988, 189)

Katz (2005, 195) suggests that "growing older differs substantially depending on the social, cultural, and historical contexts within which it is experienced." In this regard, Riley and Riley (1994, 154) argue that "what is now viewed as 'natural' or 'normal' life course—in which early adulthood is devoted to the acquisition of human capital, middle age is dominated by labor force participation, and old age is a time for leisure—rest on social convention rather than on biological necessity." They contend that "education, paid work and leisure should be pursued in tandem across adulthood" generating "higher quality lives for society members and better use of the talents of society members for societal goals." Such an approach "would largely eliminate age stratification, bringing an end to one form of institutionalized inequality" (Riley and Riley 1994, 155).

While members of each of the cohorts described above experience a common number of significant historical events within their lifetimes, cohorts should not be thought of as homogeneous, but as having significant differences in relationship to cohort size, race, ethnicity, gender, cultural differences, education, and demographical differences around important life events, such as marriage, children, social mobility, and so on. In addition, not every member of a cohort experiences life in the same way. As Katz (2005, 32) argues, a "life course is characterized by a number of overlapping, often disparate conditions associated with the blurring of traditional chronological boundaries and the integration of formerly segregated periods of life.

Fixed definitions of childhood, middle age, and old age are eroding" (32). Moreover, "many older people are not the exemplars of senior citizenry idealized by current imagery and do face tremendous emotional and health problems that require sustainable support, effective care solutions, and informed public sympathy" (194).

It is helpful to consider O'Rand (1996)'s discussion of the theory of cumulative disadvantage and the inequality that exists within cohorts. In O'Rand's view, the inequities people experience over the course of their lives will accumulate and build on each other over time, contributing to individuals being disadvantaged in their ability to participate fully in culture and society. Important to this book and chapter is that inequality and cumulative disadvantage within the cohorts served by creative aging programs means that such programs are not currently accessible to all based on those factors contributing to any given person's cumulative disadvantages.

Novelist, short story writer, and folklorist Zora Neale Hurston poetically recognizes the course of her life, and by extension the life course perspective, in the following quotation from her 1942 autobiography *Dust Tracks on the Road*.

> Like the dead-seeming, cold rocks, I have memories within that came out of the material that went to make me. Time and place have had their say.
>
> So you will have to know something about the time and place where I came from, in order that you may interpret the incidents and directions of my life. (Hurston n.d., 1)

Within the field of gerontology, Katz and Campbell (2005) describe the relationship of the life course perspective to art and creativity. They view both art and creativity as influenced by age and the way that one's life is lived within culture and society. Examining the lives of well-recognized artists, such as Michelangelo and Titian, they observe that "creativity continues, grows, and renews itself across the life span and throughout an artist's life in immeasurable ways" (101). Important to this book is their observation that as late as 1993, only a generation ago, Betty Friedan was concerned with what she was seeing as a dismissal "of the possibilities of late-life creativity and personal change" (105). The field of creative aging generally and this book specifically provide ample evidence of the wrong-headedness of such viewpoints.

Consistent with the life course perspective is the scholarship of folklorist Jon Kay. Kay has studied and written extensively on the expressive culture of older adults. In his fieldwork, Kay (2016, 3) witnessed the myriad ways that "elders . . . use, and/or display objects to recall, reflect upon, and share their lives." For older adults, "material forms of life stories, as a strategy for coping with some of the difficulties they face as they age. Often deployed to express their personal or cultural identities, these distinctive objects also help maintain and forge connections with family and friends, and assist in distilling and telling their own meaningful life stories" (3).

Kay (2016), based on his extensive cross-cultural fieldwork, concludes that the art objects emerging from the expressive culture of older adults can be considered *life-story objects*. Kay defines *life-story objects* as "those material items that elders keep, display, and arrange that relate to and help communicate one's personal memories and stories" (6). He does caution that reducing life-story objects "to mere works of art or storytelling props fails to appreciate the complex and diverse narrative nature of these creations and the process that brought them into existence" (6). Life-story objects are multifunctional, "they are objects to reflect upon; props for explaining events and their meanings; the product of a pastime . . .; mnemonic devices . . .; and a material legacy to leave to family and friends" (6). Based on his research, Kay also posits that life-story objects are not isolated or static forms of expressive culture but are objects through which older adults "recall and remake their world" (105). This perspective is affirmed in the research associated with the importance of *reminiscence* for older adults and the role of life experience to education (Merriam 1990).

Folklore and Creative Aging

Kay (2016)'s fieldwork and identification of life-story objects created by older adults only begins to suggest what the field of folklore can bring to creative aging programs. *What Folklorists Do: Professional Possibilities in Folklore Studies*, edited by Timothy Lloyd, suggests myriad possibilities in this regard. Lloyd (2021), in his introduction to the book, identifies several characteristics of folklore relevant to the development and implementation of creative aging programs with an educational emphasis congruent with a learner-centered approach that recognizes the importance of a broad-based definition of art, culture, folk groups, and expressive culture. Folklore "constitutes a significant proportion of all cultural expression" and in doing so contributes to "understanding the identities and values people and communities create, and the extent and operations of human imagination; and that folklore shapes and is shaped by everyday life in our own (or any) time and place . . ." (xiii). The field of folklore engages multiple definitions of culture and creativity. Folklore is a "listening discipline" exercised through fieldwork for the purpose of understanding "the intersections of artfulness and the social world, community-based creativity in a global economy, and both communication and conflict within and across religious, geographic, and ethnic divides" (xiii). Within the field, "lay and expert knowledge" are complementary, leading to a fuller understanding of diverse forms of expressive culture. In combination, such knowledge also provides "insights to the creation, analysis and evaluation of cultural policy" (xiii).

Folklorists recognize that older adults are participating in a "culture of aging in addition to other cultural groups that they may be a part of" (Kirshenblatt-Gimblett et al. 2006, 32). Historically, this culture of aging, according to Kirshenblatt-Gimblett et al., is the source of a variety of cultural forms, such as folktales, games, and customs foundational to folklore (32). They describe older adults as "active and present and experts on what the later period in the life cycle is all about. To focus on elders in the present is to discover their creative cultural responses to advancing years, with all the challenges age brings, and to rethink our assumptions about the nature of memory, tradition, and old age" (32). They identify "age [as] one of the variables that helps define culture for an individual in any given time and place. We progress through the life cycle individually, but we are bound into communities by sharing in the life cycles of others" (33). As noted above, Kirshenblatt-Gimblett et al. also see the cohort as important to the culture of aging and emphasize that, "there are things one generation of elders can understand and communicate with each other that are inaccessible to other cohorts. Only people who entered the stream of history together can share their view of the same moment in time" (34).

The Arts, Education, and Folklore

Relevant to the preceding discussion of older adults' expressive culture, the arts, and life-story objects are Greene (2001, 5–6)'s observations on the relationship between arts, aesthetics, and expressive culture. While acknowledging that *aesthetics* is often used to describe a field of philosophical discourse about "perception, sensation, imagination, and how they relate to knowing, understanding, and feeling about the world" (5), *aesthetics* is also understood to consider "the kinds of experiences associated with reflective and conscious encounters with the arts" (5). For Greene, this second meaning of aesthetics offers a "focus on the way in which a work of art can become an object of experience and the effect it then has in altering perspectives on nature, human beings, and moment-to-moment existence" (5). For Greene, *education* "is a process of enabling persons to become different, to enter the multiple provinces of meaning" leading to "knowing, seeing, and feeling in a conscious endeavor to impose different orders upon experience" (5). It is through this process that we learn to "make the culture's symbol systems our own" (6). Education is thus "an intentional undertaking designed to nurture appreciative, reflective, cultural, participatory engagements . . . enabling learners to notice what is there to be noticed . . . . When this happens, new connections are made in experience: new patterns are formed, new vistas are opened. Persons *see* differently, resonate differently . . ." (6).

Furthermore, according to Greene, education is "integral to the development of persons—to their cognitive, perceptual, emotional, and imaginative development" (7). Educational experiences should provide an opportunity "to seek greater coherence in the world . . . an effort to move individuals (working together, searching together) to seek a grounding for themselves, so that they may break through the 'cotton wool' of dailyness and passivity and boredom and come awake to the colored, sounding, problematic world" (7). Greene (1995, 1) emphasizes the importance of understanding "lives in narrative form, as a 'quest'" facilitating people to "create a self." Within this context, teachers and students are "conducting a kind of collaborative search, each from her or his lived situation" (23). In this search for one's lived situation, educators must recognize that some students "face fearful obstacles due to inequities. . . . The facts of race, class, and ethnic membership need to be taken into account along with the necessity of extensive social and economic restructuring" (18).

Analysis of the ways in which lay and expert knowledge contributes to the conceptualization of education programs across the lifespan is found in the work of folklorists Lynne Hamer and Paddy Bowman (2011). They situate a folkloristic orientation to education within the progressive education movement of the early twentieth century and this movement's members' commitment to the democratization of culture as advanced by John Dewey. Dewey promoted "democracy as beginning at home and in neighborly communities, and a democratic culture as characterized by trust, tolerance, and humor, as well a recognition of the inherent value of each individual" (John Dewey, cited in Hamer and Bowman 2011, 6).

Hamer and Bowman (2011, 12–13) identify five goals for educational programs informed by folklore:

1. Value of "their own familiar individuals' folk groups and their vernacular, everyday artistic expressions."
2. Assist students to see the significance of their expressive culture in relationship to "history, politics, and economics."
3. "Critically observing differences, as well as intersections, between elite and popular culture and the folk culture of their communities."
4. "Recenters authority outside institutions" "challenging the exclusive legitimacy of official knowledge and these challenging institutions to include the heterogeneous authorities and bring into the classroom community knowledge as authorative and community people as teachers."
5. "Based on students' participation in real learning situations . . . the work is inherently collaborative as well as interdisciplinary . . . creating knowledge."

The perspectives introduced thus far from the fields of folklore, gerontology, and aesthetic education are consistent with two different, but complementary, approaches to adult education: *andragogy* and *transformative learning*. McGarth (2009), in her review of research on adults and learning, defines *andragogy* as "based on the experience of the learner and the role that it plays in the classroom" (103). In her view, the educator who aligns with this perspective "assumes that the student has a bank of experience accumulated over their lifetime" (103) that must be recognized in the learning environment if adult learners are expected to participate. Also important to andragogy is that the facilitator must recognize that they, and their adult students, bring knowledge and experience to the learning environment. In the andragogic model, the "teacher" is more of a facilitator or guide, and not a manager of content (102). Equity between facilitator and student is assumed. Knowles (1998, 65), an early theorist and advocate associated with andragogy, goes so far as to say that "adults resent and resist situations in which they feel others are imposing their will on them."

Transformative learning, according to Taylor and Laros (2014, 136), emerges from a critique of andragogy for the purpose of strengthening "theory, research and practice" within the transformative approach. Transformative learning, such as andragogy, emphasizes the agency and independence of the adult learner, recognizes the importance of authentic dialogue between the adult learner and the facilitator, recognizes that there are multiple ways of knowing, and respects that the adult learner brings to the learning environment a conception of self that is informed by their life course. Where transformative learning differs from andragogy is the importance placed on critical reflection (137). Mezirow (1991) identifies three foci for reflection: content, process, and premise for reflection. Taylor and Laros (2014) amplify Mezirow by concentrating on critical reflection of adults as associated with the purpose of the educational experience, the focus or object of the reflection, and the process of reflection.

Miller (2020)'s comprehensive literature review of transformative learning in the arts argues for the importance of artistic and creative ways of knowing. She concludes that transformative learning in the arts, broadly defined, is both possible and desirable. Rather than the more typical focus on specific arts forms, Miller addresses arts forms within the following categories: imagination, improvisation, and creativity (341–342); arts-based learning (342–343); expressive, embodied, and performing arts (344–345); visual arts and symbols (345–346); storytelling and film (346–347); and community arts and social change (347–348). In this way, the author is able to address the interrelationships between arts forms with regard to what they can bring to the learning experience.

Conclusion

This chapter focused on issues and perspectives drawn from the fields of folklore, adult education, gerontology, aesthetic education, and arts education, among other related fields, which should inform learner-centered arts education programs in which adults, particularly older adults, participate. As introduced in Chapter 2, this chapter focused on several of the individual choice categories for arts participation by older adults, including mode of participation, purpose of participation, place of participation, skill, and content as associated with a person's life course. Particular attention was given to the field of folklore because of its unique perspectives on expressive culture, broadly defined definitions of arts rooted in lived experience, and natural inclinations to pass on traditions, heritage, and skills to others. The field of folklore is also uniquely able to guide learner-centered arts education for older adults across formal institutions and organizations. This approach is informed by participants' everyday life, culture, and folk group membership. As Cohen (2009) observed, the folk arts make "a strong case for the increased appeal of art in the second half of life" (51). Important to his identification of the importance of folk art (or the related concept of expressive culture) is his conclusion that "folk art is ultimately egalitarian in how it cuts across social strata with a heavy representation of artists from lower socio-economic backgrounds" (51). This perspective is mutually reinforcing the life course perspective associated with critical and social gerontology. Lastly, this chapter contextualized adult learning, including learning by older adults, within the larger field of adult education as informed by andragogy and transformational learning perspectives.

Based on the discussion above, the following items should be considered in the design and implementation of arts education programs that are learner centered and within which older adults will participate:

1. People of all ages should have the opportunity to participate in arts education.
2. Creativity is innate and can be cultivated.
3. What constitutes the meaning of *art* will differ in multiracial, multicultural, and multiethnic societies.
4. The literature associated with the fields of folklore, aesthetic education, arts education, adult education, and gerontology stresses the importance of learner-centered education programs for older adults.
5. Learner-centered arts education for older adults should consider the learner's culture and membership in folk groups and how these perspectives inform the learner's engagement with the arts, as well as the learning environment.
6. Each older adult will experience common and idiosyncratic life experiences based upon their life course and cohort. This life experience, and the way that it is expressed, will shape the older adult's experience with the arts. This life experience is expressed implicitly or explicitly by the older adult in their art and responses to the arts.
7. Aging is a social process influenced and shaped by race, ethnicity, culture, folk group, history, and politics, among other sociocultural factors. These factors are contributing to social inequalities and accumulative disadvantage that should be addressed in social and educational policy associated with older adults. Given predicators that show that early experiences with the arts will influence engagement with the arts across the lifespan, such policy should be conceptualized within a lifelong learning perspective.
8. Lay (older adult participant) and expert (professional) knowledge should contribute to the design and implementation of arts education experiences for older adults.

9. Older adults bring to the education environment criticality, intentionality, and purpose that should be respected and acknowledged if the older adult is to benefit from participation.

These conclusions associated with the older adult learner and learner-centered arts education programs should be kept in mind as readers engage with Chapter 6 and its focus on the conceptualization and implementation of age-friendly, learner-centered educational environments.

6
Creating a Learner-Centered Transformative Arts Education Environment for Older Adults

Introduction

Concerned with the invisibility of lesbian, gay, bisexual, or transgender (LGBT) older adults, an interactive theater program for this constituency was initiated through the Transforming Theatre Ensemble at Michigan State University (Hughes et al. 2016). Older adults identifying themselves as LGBT and healthcare providers were brought together to talk about improving health services for the LGBT community. Participants in this conversation also engaged in a transformative theater process, based in practices associated with the *theater of the oppressed*, to address the bias and discrimination experienced by the members of the LGBT community when seeking healthcare. Foundational to this educative process was the belief that "theatrical frameworks offer the opportunity to observe human behavior, peel back the layers of defensiveness, rationalization, fear, and guardedness" personified by characters in a play for the purpose of portraying "their humanity" (294). Participants collaboratively developed a script for public performance. The resulting play, *Aggie's Story*, focused on Aggie, her breast cancer diagnosis, and her partner Cheryl, as they navigate a healthcare system that is microaggressive and marginalizing in response to their personal relationship and sexual orientation. Following each performance of *Aggie's Story*, a dialogue between the characters and the audience occurred revealing multiple perspectives on what Aggie and Cheryl experienced. Through an evaluative process involving producers, actors, and audience, those involved in the production concluded that participating in transformative theater "is a promising method of engaging audiences to examine their biases, and move them toward provision of more inclusive, culturally competent care of older adults who are LGBT" (303).

Aggie's Story exemplifies the learner-centered approach to arts education for older adults proposed in Chapter 5. This argument for a learner-centered approach was supported by theory, issues, perspectives, and practices drawn from the fields of folklore, adult education, gerontology, aesthetic education, and arts education, among other fields associated with older adults, education, and the arts. Particular attention was given to the field of folklore because of its unique perspectives on expressive culture, broadly defined definitions of the arts rooted in lived experience, and natural inclinations to pass on traditions, heritage, and skills to others. Arts educators informed by the field of folklore are uniquely able to guide learner-centered arts education for older adults across formal institutions and organizations that are informed by participants' everyday life, culture, and folk group membership. In turn, a folkloric perspective is mutually reinforcing of the life course perspective associated with critical and social gerontology.

Chapter 5 also introduced the importance of pairing learning by older adults with transformative education theory. Transformative learning was discussed as supporting learner-centered approaches and a holistic approach to whole-person health associated with the body, mind, and spirit. Chapter 5 concluded with recommendations for the design and implementation of learner-centered arts education programs for older adults. These conclusions are associated with the nature of creativity; the myriad ways in which the arts manifest in multicultural, multiracial, and multiethnic societies; aging as a social process; the importance of the individual and collective life experience of older adults in relationship to arts making; and the importance of the voice of the older adult in shaping the learning experience.

The purpose of Chapter 6 is to identify what is specifically required of learning environments, such as what was designed for the creation of *Aggie's Story*, for a learner-centered orientation to arts education for older adults to succeed. Referencing the *8Ps Framework for Arts in Healthy Aging* introduced in Chapter 2, this chapter addresses most directly those portions of the model that are associated with person-centeredness, participation/purpose/place, and people/programs. Chapter 6 emphasizes the importance of lifelong learning and provides a continued investigation of what transformative learning can bring to aging creatively through arts education. This chapter recognizes the multiplicity of formal educational settings and organized learning opportunities with which the readers of this volume are associated. Learning opportunities may be in the form of structured classes and workshops or self-directed experiences as facilitated by an arts educator.[1] The educational experience may include arts making or responding to the arts, or both. This chapter also recognizes that the settings within which arts education occurs will have their own education missions and curricular approaches. For these reasons, this chapter should be read as less of a how-to manual and more of a literature synthesis that can be used by arts educators to work within the educational missions and curricula of their institutions and organizations for the purpose of designing learning environments responsive to the desire of older adults to shape their learning in the arts toward personal transformation. In addition, this chapter should not be read as a critique of prevailing approaches currently in use within creative aging programs.[2] A comprehensive study of approaches used for arts education within creative aging programs has yet to be published. However, readers will find below references to the use of the transformative approach to arts education documented in the literature. This chapter also recognizes the heterogeneity of adult learners and the myriad life courses that will be evident in any group of adult learners.

Lifelong Learning

Human beings have the capacity to learn throughout their lifespans. Jarvis (2008, 20) describes this predilection for lifelong learning in humans as a

> combination of processes though out a lifetime whereby the whole person—body (genetic, physical and biological) and mind (knowledge, skills, attitudes, values, emotions, beliefs and senses)—experiences social situations, the perceived content of which is then transformed cognitively, emotively or practically (or through any combination) and integrated into the individual person's biography resulting in a continually changing (or more experienced) person.

The stimulus igniting the learning and transformation described by Jarvis begins with a "disjuncture" or that the "harmony between us and the world has been broken" (25). This is recognizable in the motivations for creating and performing *Aggie's Story* referenced above. Keeping *Aggie's Story* in mind, the disjuncture evident in the healthcare available to older adults who identify themselves as LGBTQ+ motivated a creative response based on self-reflection, conversation, investigation, exploration, and performance. These processes contribute to what Jarvis identifies as the preconscious and conscious formation of attitudes, beliefs, and values; meaning creation; tacit knowing; and identity (28–29). Significant to this description of learning is an emphasis on the sociocultural contexts in which learning takes place, as well as how this learning informs a "person's biography" or life course.

Recognizing the potential for adult learning, the emphasis within the United States "from the beginning of the twentieth century was on a lifetime of learning for individual development with 'good' citizenship as consequence" (Wilson 2008, 515). Adult learning emphasizes self-development, community participation, and "emancipating and transforming individuals and/or society, and sometimes all these together" (512).

As learners, those older adults participating in the creation and performance of *Aggie's Story* were perceived as capable, engaged, independent, and creative. As Wolf (2008, 57) concludes, older adults "are no different from learners of any age. They are curious, able, and constantly in need of adaptation and assimilation." Findsen and Formosa (2011, 75), following an analysis of a significant body of literature that considers intelligence; cognitive processes and functions, such as attention, memory, language, and problem-solving; and wisdom, conclude that

> a definite answer of the effect of age on people's cognitive development is near to impossible to attain. Whilst intellectual ability varies extensively from one person to another, the variations from study to study in content and methodology make absolute comparisons unworkable. Yet, it is clear that barring physiological and psychological impediments people can and do have the ability to continue learning well into extreme old age. Indeed,

older persons actually possess a number of compensatory factors—such as the integrity of crystallized intelligence, the accumulation of knowledge and experience, the persistence of curiosity, and the ability to put new information in a highly meaningful context.

However, maintaining older adult learning as described above may at some point require support for the individual's *functional ability*. This is an issue that will be discussed in more detail below.

In relevant published scholarship, questions do arise about older adult learners and whether the approach to facilitating learning among older adults requires a distinct theory. Tam (2014, 817), through a systematic analysis of the literature, reaches the conclusion that "the view that older learners are simply different from learners of other age groups does not provide a strong premise for a separate theory." Tam does not imply, however, that there are no differences between the preferences of older adults and younger learners based on the social, psychological, physical, and motivational transitions associated with aging. These preferences, according to Tam's research, are influenced by coping with and transcending the physical and psychological changes associated with aging, a heightened desire to bring meaning to one's life, and a desire to serve others. These are important preferences that do support the transformative learning approach introduced in Chapter 5 and discussed in greater detail below.

As discussed in Chapter 4, with reference to Erikson (1982) and Cohen (2005), these transitions can be grouped into developmental phases across the lifespan. Of particular importance to learning by older adults are Cohen (2005)'s four phases of later life where emphasis is placed on midlife evaluation/re-evaluation (40–65 years of age); a desire to experiment, innovate, and free oneself for reified notions of the self (late 50s–70s); reexamination of one's life toward sharing the wisdom resulting from this process with others (late 60s–80s); and discovering what it means to live and die well at the end of life (late 70s to end of life). Across these phases, the older learner is assessing their quality of life, life satisfaction, and happiness overall. This sense of well-being, as discussed in Chapter 4, comprises evaluative, eudemonic, affective, hedonic, and cultural well-being. Intrinsic to each of these are motivational factors stimulating an older adult's desire to learn. It is for this reason that any arts education program designed for older adults requires ongoing dialogue between learners and educators resulting in the basic elements of program design as evident in the creation and performance of *Aggie's Story* and as discussed in Chapter 4 and below. Learning within such programs will be the "process in which older adults 'individually and in association with others, engage in direct encounter and then purposefully reflect upon, validate, transform, give personal meaning to and seek to integrate their ways of knowing'" (Mercken cited in Tam 2014, 815).

This motivation to learn on the part of older adults is resulting in what has been described as a "remarkable surge of interest in learning activities, educational centers, programs, and curricula designed to enhance the lives of older adults" (Wolf

2008, 57). Encouraging this flourishing of opportunities for learning by older adults is, according to Wolf (2008),

> the lengthening of the life course, improved health and economic status among retirement-aged adults, higher rates of prior education among those reaching later life, the rising popularity of the notion of lifelong learning (whether formal or non-formal) as both a person and public good, developmental and neurological theories advancing the appropriateness and the benefits of continued learning, and greater opportunities for learning and teaching in mid and later life through such diverse organizations as colleges and universities, churches, synagogues and mosques, senior centers, public libraries, day health centers, hospitals, unions and residential housing groups. (Manheimer cited in Wolf 2008, 59)

Centers for lifelong learning are encouraging "self-efficacy," "intellectual stability and maintenance," "socialization," "integration and meaning making" (Wolf 2008, 60). Supporting Wolf's perspective is Lawton and LaPorte (2013)'s investigation of arts education and older adults. They conclude that "quality community-based arts education programs for older adults should exploit the broad range of interests and cognitive abilities of participants by utilizing adult education theory, brain research, and the best practices of adult arts education programs" (311). Based on their analysis of the literature coupled with case study research, Lawton and LaPorte equate effective older adult education practices with transformative learning theory.

Transformative Learning Theory

Transformative learning theory emerged in 1975 with the publication of *Education for Perspective Transformation: Women's Re-Entry Programs in Community Colleges* by Mezirow.[3] Mezirow identifies four types of learning: "the acquisition of new knowledge and skills, the elaboration on existing knowledge and skills, the revision of meaning schemes (beliefs and values), and the revision of meaning perspectives (a larger view of the world)" (Mezirow cited in Kroth and Cranton 2014, 1). This "revision of meaning perspectives" is essential to transformative learning.

As referenced in Chapter 5, transformative learning for adults emerged from "andragogy." Wilson (2008, 516–517) describes *andragogy* as

> a fundamentally humanist-progressive orientation centered on individual experience and development, to transformational theory, a fundamentally critical humanist development theory centered on critical rationalist thought (not that much of an ideological shift), a growing number of adult educators in the US academy began to recreate (some argued, returned to) a space in the study of adult education for a more radical transformationist stance that made space for the class, gender, race, sexual orientation, and diaspora interests.

Transformative learning, as described above and by Lawton and LaPorte (2013), occurs "with the help and support of educators, counselors, coaches, and other helping professionals, or it can occur informally in individual's lives, often without being recognized or named as transformative learning" (Kroth and Cranton 2014, 10). While not mentioned specifically by Kroth and Cranton, arts educators are among those who should be identified as "helping professionals." The role of the helping professional, including arts educators, within the formal transformative learning process is to facilitate the learner's interaction with views that may differ from their own leading to "critical self-reflection, exploration, questioning, and possibly a shift in perspective" using arts materials or in their response to artworks (10).

Transformative learning theory as it first emerged in the work of Mezirow resulted in additional theorizing and applications of the theory to various adult learning contexts. Washburn (2021, 308) goes so far as to use the metaphor of the "crazy quilt," with its random patterns and embellishments, to describe present-day transformative learning theory. Mezirow and Taylor (2011) took stock of the state of this evolution of transformative learning theory in their edited volume *Transformative Learning in Practice: Insights from Community, Workplace, and Higher Education*. In this volume, Mezirow (2011) returned to his conception of *transformative learning* as "a critical dimension of learning in adulthood that enables us to recognize, reassess, and modify the structures of assumptions and expectations that frame our tacit points of view and influence our thinking" (18).

Mezirow (2011) reemphasizes that the roots of his transformative learning theory are associated with

> Paulo Freire's concept of "conscientization," consciousness raising in the women's movement, the theory of transformation of psychiatrist Roger Gould, the writings of Jürgen Habermas and Harvey Siegal, and the transformative experience of . . ., Edee Mezirow, as an adult returning to complete her undergraduate degree at Sarah Lawrence College in New York. (19)

Mezirow

> embraces Habermas' critical distinction between instrumental learning and communicative learning. Instrumental learning involves controlling or managing the environment of other persons, including improving performance . . . . Communicative learning involves understanding what others mean when they communicate with us. (20)

With regard to "meaning," Mezirow identifies

> three types of meaning perspectives—epistemic (about knowledge and how we obtain knowledge), sociolinguistic (understanding ourselves and social world through language), and psychological (concerned with our perception of ourselves largely based on childhood experiences). (Mezirow cited in Kroth and Cranton 2014, 4)

> **Box 6.1 Ten phases of transformative learning**
>
> 1. A disorienting dilemma
> 2. Self-examination
> 3. A critical assessment of assumptions
> 4. Recognition of a connection between one's discontent and the process of transformation
> 5. Exploration of options for new roles, relationships, and action
> 6. Planning a course of action
> 7. Acquiring knowledge and skills for implementing one's plan
> 8. Provisional trying of new roles
> 9. Building competence and self-confidence in new roles and relationships
> 10. A reintegration into one's life based on conditions dictated by one's new perspective
>
> Source: Mezirow (2011, 19).

Mezirow (2011)'s emphasis on the importance of discourse involving "dialectical and critically reflective thinking leading to a best tentative judgement" (20) leads to his definition of *transformative learning* as "learning that transforms problematic frames of reference to make them more inclusive, discriminating, reflective, open, and emotionally able to change" (22). As delineated in Box 6.1, Mezirow posits ten phases to transformative learning leading to a sudden or incremental personal change. Keeping in mind the older adult learners as they progress through these ten phases, Findsen and Formosa (2011, 74) argue that "older adult learning must be less concerned with mastery and competence, and more with aiding learners to develop a reflective mode to thinking, contemplate the meaning of life, come to terms with their past, and hone their quest for self-fulfillment and spiritual advancement."

Significant to this chapter is Mezirow (2011)'s reassessment of transformative learning as posited through the phases of learning represented in Box 6.1. He acknowledged that this original conceptualization does not adequately consider "imagination, intuition, and emotion" (27) and that "intuition may substitute for critical self-reflection" (28). Imagination, intuition, and emotion are integral to the arts and must be considered if transformative learning theory is to be applicable to adult arts education, including creative aging programming. As will be shown below, scholars have taken the arts into consideration and have modified transformative learning theory accordingly. Taylor (2011) asserts that transformative learning must recognize the importance of an individual's life experience (life course) within the context of affective and relational ways of knowing. Taylor emphasizes that "learners rarely change through a rational process (analyze-think-change). Instead, they 'are more likely to change in a see-feel-change sequence'" (Brown quoted in Taylor 2011, 10) and that

> expressive ways of knowing provide the means to evoke experiences for greater exploration, help learners become more aware of their feelings and their relationship to

sense making, and help concretize an experience allowing the learner to reexperience the learning experience through creative expressive representation. (Brown quoted in Taylor 2011, 11)

Amplifying Brown and Taylor's perspective on the importance of "expressive ways of knowing" is Dirkx's use of the Jungian concept of "individuation" to describe transformative learning as an imaginative, intuitive, emotional, and soulful experience (the way of *mythos* rather than *logos*) (Dirkx cited in Kroth and Cranton 2014, 5). *Mythos* is associated with "symbols, images, stories, and myths, paying attention to the small everyday occurrences of life and listening to individual and collective psyches" (Kroth and Cranton 2014, 5). The importance of this perspective to transformative learning is further articulated by Boyd who argues that "discernment rather than reflection, is the central process of transformation . . . symbols, images, and archetypes lead to personal enlightenment as people bring the unconscious to consciousness" (Boyd cited in Kroth and Cranton 2014, 5).

Kroth and Cranton (2014, 9), motivated by their desire to provide practitioners with a broader and more applicable definition of *transformative learning* and recognizing transformative learning theory as consisting of multiple perspectives, propose a "unified or integrated" theory of transformative learning as

a process by which individuals engage in the cognitive processes of critical reflection and self-reflection, intuitive and imaginal explorations of their psyche and spirituality, and developmental changes leading to a deep shift in perspective and habits of mind that are more open, permeable, discriminating, and better justified. Individual change may lead to social change, and social change may promote individual change.

Mezirow (2011), like Kroth, Cranton, and others, also recognized the need for a more expansive definition of his original theory. Mezirow identifies O'Sullivan (2002)'s as the most comprehensive approach building on his (Mezirow's) original theory. O'Sullivan (2002), like Kroth and Cranton (2014)'s later conceptualization of transformative learning theory, recognizes an integrative approach emphasizing a "deep cultural shift in the basic premises of thought, feeling, and action" (28). Acknowledging the myriad definitions of transformative learning existing at the time, O'Sullivan (2002, 11) defines *transformative learning* as

experiencing a deep, structural shift in the basic premises of thought, feeling, and actions. It is a shift of consciousness that dramatically and permanently alters our way of being in the world. Such a shift involves our understanding of ourselves and our self-locations, our relationships with other humans and with the natural world; our understanding of relations of power in interlocking structures of class, race, and gender; our body-awareness; our visions of alternative approaches to living; and our sense of the possibilities for social justice and peace and personal joy.

O'Sullivan (2002)'s attempt at proposing a unified theory is important to combine with Kroth and Cranton (2014)'s formulation because of its expansiveness in affirming people's relationships with the natural world, power relationships, class, race, and gender, as well as the "joy" that can be experienced within the transformational process.

The unified or integrated theories of transformative learning, as proposed by O'Sullivan (2002) and Kroth and Cranton (2014), recognize the importance of the individual's relationships with culture and society. Bailey-Johnson (2012) writes on the intersectional quality of these relationships. She states that, "as social beings, we all reason and negotiate from our cultural base, our history, and our experiences" (261). Such positionality, informed by factors such as gender, race, and so on, "intersect[s] with other positions—such as class, age, and sexual orientation—to affect and order our everyday lives, invariably permeating our educational institutions. Classes, practices, programs, and research reflect what students and teachers have experienced and believe about ourselves and others" (263).

Bailey-Johnson (2012, 268) concludes that positionality or intersectionality precedes and fosters transformative learning. This learning, according to Bailey-Johnson, is adaptive. Positionality should not be perceived as confining, but contributing to "discourse or dialogue that easily moves between the rational and the intuitive to perhaps create a synergy of knowing that is based on and values both logic and instinctive ability as ways of understanding and affecting change" (269). Bailey-Johnson argues that transformative learning can be "sculpted" by learners and educators through "testing and adjusting" (269). For this sculpting to occur, the learning environment should be one of positional consensus, bounded by "common experiences and common goals" and "trust and open dialogue" toward the development of a culturally sensitive "discourse that transcends regular discussions and is informed by research while valuing positional experiences and intuition-based knowledges" (270). In doing so, transformative learning must "stretch past its comfortable location in a traditional Western teaching and learning environment" (270). One example of this stretching is Johnson (2021)'s use of transformative learning theory combined with indigenous ways of knowing in environmental education.

Given the emphasis on the culture of the learner in this volume and within transformative learning theory, creating a culturally responsive learning environment must be a part of the design of any transformative learning environment. Fareed (2009)'s model is applicable here. Although Fareed's model was developed specifically for communities of color, the processes associated with the model can be more broadly applied. Fareed's model includes strategies consistent with transformative learning, such as reflecting on lived experience, peer learning, and the documentation of learning (119). Four main goals and outcomes are associated with the model:

1. Creating "Culturally Sensitive Learning Environments" (121–122) leading to the formation of cohesive and collaborative learning groups.

2. Encouraging "Culturally Inclusive Learning Experiences" (123–124) leading to the creation and appreciation of cultural objects.
3. Creating "Opportunities for Critical Reflection and Learning Through Critical Questioning on Culturally Shared Meaning" (124–125) leading to a participant's recognition of their "own purposes, values, feelings, and meanings rather than act on those of others" (Mezirow cited in Fareed 2009, 130).
4. Assessing "Personal and Group Learning and Change Using Evaluation Methods That Allow Freedom of Expression" (125–127) and which are approved by the learning group. Arts-based methods of evaluation should be considered.

Transformative Learning, the Extrarational, and the Arts

Transformative learning as theorized by Mezirow (2011) was centered on a rational frame of mind. Rightly, this narrowness in approach was the subject of critique resulting in an expansion of the theory to include imaginative, intuitive, and emotional ways of knowing and learning. Lawrence (2005) envisions the pairing of the arts with transformative learning as extending "the boundaries of how we come to know, by honoring multiple intelligences and Indigenous knowledge" (3). In turn, this makes possible for learners to "uncover hidden knowledge that cannot be easily expressed in words" leading to a "deepening understanding of self and the world" (3). Lawrence (2012), in addressing the relationship of transformative learning to the arts, posits an *extrarational process* "which does not reject rationality but is a more inclusive concept" that "goes beyond rationality" (472). For Lawrence, the "extrarational describes a process of meaning-making expressed through symbol, image, and emotional expression" (472). This is the realm of the arts. As mentioned above, it is by engaging with the arts that individuals can discern the relationships between and among things leading to "contemplative insight," "personal illumination," "and seeing them in their relational wholeness" (Boyd and Myers cited in Lawrence 2012, 472). Lawrence does not reject Mezirow's ten phases of transformative learning as cited in Box 6.1. Rather, she views the arts as "ways to carry out these phases, such as using popular theatre techniques to act out alternative scenarios, or writing poems that explore and express new ways of being" (482).

Aggie's Story, as referenced at the start of this chapter, is only one example of transformative learning through the arts. An early effort is Hogan, Simpson, and Stuckey (2009)'s collection of essays, *Creative Expression in Transformative Learning: Tools and Techniques for Educators of Adults*. The contributors to this volume explicate how transformative learning, including creative expression, cultivates multiple ways of knowing—affective, spiritual, imaginal, symbolic, somatic, and artistic/creative—that lead to greater possibilities for personal transformation. More recently, Miller (2020)'s systematic and methodologically rigorous literature review of transformative learning theory and the arts within adult education is both foundational to practice and supportive of the need for additional research. Miller's literature review revealed foci associated with transformative learning as it supports imagination, improvisation, and creativity; arts-based learning / activities; expressive, embodied, and performing arts; visual arts and symbols; storytelling and film; and community arts and social change. Miller concludes that transformative learning assists "with self-expression, perspective transformation, better understanding of the 'other,' and dealing with difficult or complicated emotions" (349). She also concludes that "one of the most important aspects of this type of learning is meaning making, which the arts help to process in a unique way. When adults experience a transformation and suddenly their life world has new meaning and purpose, it can be a powerful experience that has many ripple effects in their lives" (349).

Then, how can Mezirow (2011)'s ten phases of transformative learning be considered and applied to an extrarational perspective focused on meaning making through the arts? Assistive in thinking through this are the five approaches to creative learning identified by Hogan, Simpson, and Stuckey (cited in Miller 2020, 341): "(1) imagining new possibilities, (2) deep learning of course content, (3) self-awareness, (4) purposeful change, and (5) social change/increasing awareness of others." It is important to acknowledge, however, that for arts activities to be transformative, "educators need to create spaces and activities to make use of these experiences, reflect on them, and help to bring about change as a result" (Miller 2020, 349). When the arts are involved, the learning process includes imagination, intuition, emotion with discernment, and reflection—all elements that are integral to personal transformation. It is "discernment rather than reflection" that leads "to personal enlightenment as people bring the unconscious to consciousness" (Kroth and Cranton 2014, 5).

Figure 6.1 represents Mezirow (2011)'s ten phases as modified to encourage an extrarational process and perspective. It is important to keep in mind that there is no one way to move through these phases when applied to arts activities. People will move through these phases sequentially and/or in a nonsequential manner, and repetition of phases may also occur as the creative process unfolds. As Fleige (2017, 324) observes, "transformation and learning though the arts is possible but takes its time, taking steps, going through phases, or even going in circles, taking over new views and making new experiences."

For older adults, Mezirow (2011)'s phase 1. *disorienting dilemmas* can be associated with the recognition of personal limitations, deaths of loved ones, moves to new living arrangements, discrimination as in the example of *Aggie's Story*, and other significant experiences for which there is no "rational response to one's feelings and actions" (Lawrence 2012, 472). Mezirow's phases 2.–4. *self-examination, a critical assessment of assumptions, and recognition of a connection between one's discontent and the process of transformation* include the extrarational (symbolic, imaginative, and emotional) with rational critical self-reflection (Lawrence 2012, 472). It is within these phases that Lawrence (2012, 472) proposes cultivating discernment or a "sifting through these various forms of meaning-making" leading to

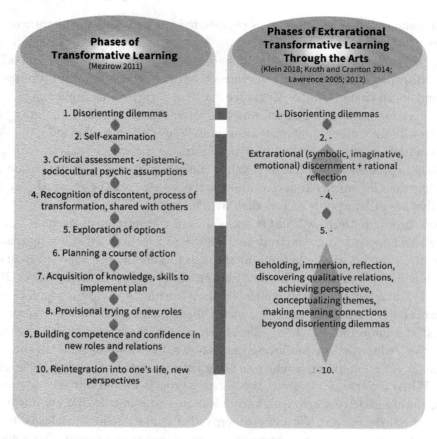

Figure 6.1 Phases of transformative learning and extrarational transformative learning through the arts
Illustration by Stephanie McCarthy.

"contemplative insight, a personal illumination gained by putting things together and seeing them in their relational wholeness" (Boyd and Myers cited in Lawrence 2012, 472). Amplifying possible ways to move through these phases through arts and arts making is a framework proposed by Klein (2018) that includes processes associated with *beholding, immersion, and reflection. Beholding* (mindfulness, curiosity, observation) (Greene 2001, 53 cited in Klein 2018, 6) allows for sensing "what we sometimes describe as the qualities of things, to make out contours, shapes, angles, even to hear sound as sound" toward having "an aesthetic experience with the world around you" (Klein 2018, 6). *Immersion* is described as "noticing detail," "seeing relations between parts," "seizing the whole as the whole," and "prolonged engagement with an image, space, or artwork" (Armstrong cited in Klein 2018, 6). Mezirow's phases 5 through 10, *acquiring knowledge and skills for implementing one's plan, trying new roles, building competence and self-confidence in new roles and relationships, and reintegrating into one's life new perspectives* are captured in Klein's concept of *reflection* focused on achieving perspective, conceptualizing themes, and making connections beyond the initial experience (Klein 2018, 6). During these phases, the older learner's experience is associated with "qualitative thought" or the "process in which significant relationships are intuitively grasped" (Constantino cited in Klein 2018, 11).

Amplifying Klein (2018)'s reference to qualitative thought, as applied to Mezirow (2011)'s and Lawrence (2012)'s extrarational phases within the context of the arts and arts education, is Ecker (1963)'s identification of the artistic process as qualitative problem-solving. Ecker builds on John Dewey's observation that "all thinking depends upon the awareness of qualities" (284). About artistic problem-solving, Dewey wrote: "the artist has his problems and thinks as he works.... The artist does his thinking in the very qualitative media he works in, and the terms lie so close to the object that he is producing that they merge directly into it" (Dewey cited in Ecker 1963, 286). Like Mezirow's and Lawrence's phases, "qualitative problem solving is ... not a neat progression of steps but a single continuous means-end progression, sometimes hesitating, groping; it may be rethought, move forward again, start over, in short, it is *experimental* behavior" (288). Ecker (1963) observes that people will bring to qualitative problem-solving in the arts a recognition of qualities as associated with "technique, style, or theme" (284), "the construction of future qualities," the identification of intended outcomes publicly available to others," "problem solving taking place in the artist's medium," and that describing the qualitative relationships in the work does not require anything "beyond what is evident in the art." Creative judgement occurs "within, before, during, and after" the qualitative problem-solving process (285–286). Ecker (1963, 289) summarizes his methodological conception of the artistic process as "a mediation in which qualitative relations as means are ordered to desired qualitative ends. Thus, to choose qualitative ends is to achieve an artistic problem. Whenever qualitative problems are sought, pointed out to others, or solved, therein do we have artistic endeavor—art and art education."

Transformative Learning and the Role of the Arts Educator

It is evident that the arts educator possesses a significant role in the transformative learning process as described above. Gleaned from the analysis of literature referenced in Chapter 5 and within this chapter, arts educators committed to facilitating transformative arts experiences for adults generally, and older adults specifically, will be advancing the aims within the transformative learning environment leading toward transformative experiences as shown in Box 6.2.

These aims can serve as the basis for transformative arts education curricular design with corresponding arts activities for older adults. The discussion that follows is most applicable to those older adults who can independently, or with minimal support, participate in arts education experiences in community-based settings. While transformative learning is possible by all older adults, specialized programs

> **Box 6.2 Aims within the transformative learning environment leading toward transformative experiences**
>
> **The transformative learning environment and experience should:**
> 1. Recognize that the learning process focuses on the whole person, their intersectionality, and their cognitive and affective capabilities leading to the potential integration into a person's understanding and appreciation for their life course;
> 2. Seriously consider the sociocultural context that the learner brings to their educational experience;
> 3. Affirm that older adults have the capacity to learn;
> 4. Involve the older learner as a co-creator of the learning environment;
> 5. Provide opportunities for older learners to evaluate / reevaluate their life course;
> 6. Provide opportunities for the older learner to discover meaning in their life;
> 7. Cultivate the older adult's desire for well-being;
> 8. Encourage self-efficacy and socialization;
> 9. Recognize and respond to any physiological or psychological barriers to learning;
> 10. Encourage expressive ways of knowing—emotional, spiritual, imaginal, symbolic, somatic, artistic, and creative.

for older adults experiencing significant memory loss or other significant health issues that compromise functional ability and require clinical care are addressed in Chapter 8. Within community-based settings, such as senior citizens centers, universities, performing arts centers, museums, religious institutions, and community arts centers, transformative learning may occur in singular workshops associated with an older adult's arts interests or educational experiences associated with a series of related classes or workshops with each building on the preceding experience. Because transformative learning is recommended for adult education generally, older adults may be participating in programs designed to be intergenerational and/or in programs specifically designed for older adults. What follows also recognizes that transformative learning can occur across art forms, but that there are also distinctive characteristics associated with each art form and that these distinctions must be taken into consideration within curricular development and the learning environment.

Also of importance in achieving the aims identified in Box 6.2 is that while aging, in and of itself, is not a disability or functionally limiting, prerequisite to achieving the curricular aims identified is that arts educators will need to work with older learners around any short- or long-term disabilities or functional limitations they may be experiencing. *Universal design* (UD) and *universal design for learning* (UDL) are promising in this regard. UD and UDL, widely recognized as strategies for meeting the learning needs of all students, emphasize that the needs of learners are diverse and therefore the learning environment should be designed in such a way that there is flexibility in the ways that older adults can make choices about how they engage, what constitutes success, and that access to the materials associated with learning is accessible. The seven principles of UD are shown to support successful aging, namely, equitable use, flexibility of use, simple and intuitive use, perceptible information, tolerance for error, low physical effort, and size/space for approach/use. "Of all the design theories that attempt to accommodate the aging process, the philosophy of universal design may be the most desirable option" because of its emphasis on accessible built environments and flexible instructional strategies (Carr et al. 2013, 6). Supporting the creation of UD and UDL environments is Pierce (2019)'s creation of a sensory design assessment tool for enhancing vision, auditory, tactile/touch, movement/space, and oral/olfactory experiences. Also helpful in this regard is *Design for Accessibility: A Cultural Administrator' Handbook* (National Assembly of State Arts Agencies and National Endowment for the Arts 1994) that promotes inclusion through understanding the law regarding access for people experiencing disabilities, architectural access, and effective communication strategies for a variety of arts and humanities activities. Also relevant is Storey (2022)'s articulation of instructional strategies for supporting people's self-determination and self-advocacy and for promoting functional skills in community settings.

Associated with the curricular aims identified in Box 6.2 are assessment strategies congruent with transformative learning through the arts. Cranton and Hoggan (2012) acknowledge that the literature associated with transformative learning has not fully explored assessment strategies for transformative learning. In response, they describe strategies, such as student self-evaluation, interviews with students, the creation of narratives by students about their learning, observations by instructors, surveys of student perspectives, checklists, student journals, metaphor analysis, conceptual mapping by learners, and arts-based techniques, such as the creation of "photography and collage, creative writing, music, improvisation, body movement, and visual imagery" (Hoggan, Simpson, and Stuckey cited in Cranton and Hoggan 2012, 527). Searle et al. (2021, 339) amplify the arts-based approach with an emphasis on the "disorienting dilemma, the qualities of self-reflection, and liberatory actions." Particularly important to their arts-based approach are the "holistic assessment processes the authors enacted with learners" (339).

A prerequisite to working with older adults in relationship to the aims represented in Box 6.2 is that arts educators should hold the competencies represented in Box 6.3. In short, Love (2011, 431) identifies the arts educator's role when working within a transformative learning framework as that of a "mediator" assisting students to "engage with the arts as 'portals' for deep analysis and empowered creation" for the purpose of supporting older learners to "foster the control that they may be consciously or unconsciously lacking through continuous encouragement to take responsibility for their learning by choosing those methods and resources by which they want to learn" (Findsen and Formosa 2011, 107).

> **Box 6.3 Prerequisite competencies for working with older adults within the transformative arts education learning environment**
>
> **Arts educators should be familiar with:**
> 1. Transformative learning theory as applied to the arts;
> 2. Characteristics of the aging population generally and the older adults they are working with specifically;
> 3. The significance of the "life course" and how learning activities can utilize life courses individually and collectively;
> 4. The sociocultural context in which they are working and their students are learning;
> 5. Listening to and talking with older adults about their needs and personal / educational desires;
> 6. Open classroom/studio/performance spaces within which an extrarational approach can be cultivated through the integration of multiple ways of knowing and learning;
> 7. The similarities and differences between critical reflection and discernment and how to facilitate each;
> 8. Any biases they may hold about older adult learners;
> 9. Skill development with art processes as secondary or supportive of personal transformation through the arts;
> 10. Facilitating self-directed learning in the arts;
> 11. Building a community among learners;
> 12. Providing appropriate supports to the older adult to maintain functional ability to the greatest extent possible.

Conclusion

This chapter argues that transformative learning theory is congruent with a learner-centered orientation to arts education for older adults. Initiating this discussion was the case example of the theater production *Aggie's Story*—a response by an LGBT community of older adults and healthcare professionals to discrimination that people who identify themselves as LGBT may experience in seeking healthcare. This case example emphasizes the importance of supporting the self-efficacy of older adults and their desires in this stage of life as significant to transformative learning.

Recognizing that older adults will participate in a multiplicity of community-based arts education settings, what was proposed within this chapter is applicable to a variety of arts educational contexts. To assist readers in planning transformative arts education, transformative curricular aims and competencies were articulated. In Box 6.3, these competencies appear as a list of recommendations for arts educators to guide their co-creation and/or adaptation of curricula and arts-based learning activities for older adults. Two leading national examples of rigorously developed lifelong learning programs for older adults are provided in Box 6.4.

> **Box 6.4 Examples of lifelong learning programs for older adults**
>
> **Program Example—*Lifetime Arts***
> Lifetime Arts supports the field of creative aging nationwide through professional development, technical assistance, information, and support. Since 2008, Lifetime Arts programs have fostered lifelong learning through the arts for independent older adults in community-based settings.
> Source: lifetimearts.org
>
> **Program Example—*Osher Lifelong Learning Institutes***
> Since 2001, the Osher Foundation has invested in expanding its network of (currently) 125 lifelong learning programs that serve the continuing education interests of older adults on university and college campuses across the country.
> Source: osherfoundation.org/olli.html

To further assist readers in the development of transformative arts education experiences, two additional case examples are offered. The first case, "I Know a Thing or Two," a storytelling program offered by Lauren Jost to fifteen older adults over a nine-week period at the Brooklyn Public Library Central Branch, is documented on the Lifetime Arts website as a "Creative Aging 101 Case Study" (Jost 2022). Jost facilitated this program in such a way that participants could reflect upon their life course as a source for their creative storytelling. The oral and written literacy levels of the participants varied. Jost began each session by asking participants to share a memorable life story verbally. This was followed by the participants choosing an experience or memory as the inspiration for poetry or creative writing. Informing the participants' writing was Jost's introduction of writing skills, such as "point of view," "first person narrative," and "dialogue." Participants chose a "favorite" piece of writing for a public presentation to family members and as a part of a published book. Within this case, co-creation of the learning environment is evident as is Jost's awareness of the various life courses and literacy levels of the participants. Also evident, and in keeping with the transformative learning environment, was that skill development was secondary to the overall goal of personal reflection through storytelling.

A second case is documented in an "informal" case study of the "Arts and Minds" programs at The Studio of Museum of Harlem (Halpin-Healy 2015). Designed for participants experiencing memory loss and their care partners, this program embraces "interpretation as a creative act" (175). The program is explicit in linking the museum's self-definition as "the nexus for artists of African descent locally, nationally, and internationally, and for work inspired and influenced by black culture" with transformative learning (175). Participants talked about the art in the museum's galleries followed by "expressive art making" (172). The twenty participants in this program were diverse in terms of "race, religion, age, level of education, sexual orientation, and health status" (175). Care partner participants were described as holding "professional" credentials in healthcare. In keeping with the transformative learning experience, participants were invited to interpret their responses to works in the galleries as related to their own life courses and cultural backgrounds. Important to the interpretive process was a facilitative approach that moved beyond liking or disliking a work to this deeper engagement. After their experience in the museum galleries, participants were prompted to respond to the work in the studio in ways like the conversation in the gallery. Integral to this dialogue was a "horizontal relationship between teacher and student" creating "a dynamic exchange of experience and knowledge" (184).

These case examples, and the transformative learning theory and practice evidenced in each, are a desired and appropriate response to Cohen (2000, 10)'s assertion that the "creative spirit has the power to change our lives at every age, and to do so in quite different ways as we get older." Amplifying Cohen's observation about creativity is Erikson (1988, 135)'s belief that the arts "sustain and nourish us all, restoring trust, hope, and compassion" and through which "we honor simultaneously the struggle of the process undertaken, the stamina and authority of the artist, and the integrity of the vision manifested."

To fully realize the promise and possibilities of creativity and the arts as recognized by Cohen (2000), Erikson (1988), and the additional scholars referenced above, extant arts curricula for older adults should be examined through the lens of transformative learning theory to assess its ability to encourage individual and collective transformation. New co-created curricula should be developed and published along with research studies examining effective practices for program delivery and evaluation. Continuing case study research will be vital in this regard. Also important going forward is the necessity of affirming and elevating the expertise of arts educators working with older adults. Funders of arts programs for older adults should be cognizant of the power of the arts to be transformative within the educational context, the importance of the older adult shaping their learning, and the diverse life courses that inform personal and collective transformation. It is also imperative to examine arts policies at local, regional, and national levels that support arts participation generally for older adults, transformative arts education specifically for older adults, and the professionalization of those providing transformative educational experiences.

7
Older Adults, Community Arts Participation, and Age-Friendliness

Introduction

Perry Johnson was introduced in Chapter 5 as an artist who initiated his work in the visual arts as an older adult. As noted in Chapter 5, Johnson regularly attends the Oregon Supported Living Program (OSLP)'s Arts and Culture Program in Eugene, Oregon. This program provides classes, a place for artists to work, and guidance on exhibiting professionally. Johnson's artistry is characterized by vividly colored paintings of family members, figures from popular culture, and notable personages, including John Lewis, Martin Luther King, Jr., and George Floyd. Johnson frequently exhibits his work in Eugene. His paintings were also featured in a 2018 exhibit at the Portland Art Museum in Portland, Oregon.

Johnson was among several artists featured in Chapter 5 to emphasize the capacity and motivation by older adults to participate with art and the importance of the "life course perspective" and the creation of "life-story objects." However, to fully understand Johnson, and the work of other artists, one must also recognize those other people, organizations, and businesses that support their work in the arts within their communities.[1] For Johnson, this includes the OSLP Arts and Culture Program, the educators and support staff associated with this program, the locations from which Johnson procures his materials, those family members and friends who affirm the importance of his arts engagement, the collectors who buy his work, and those largely nonprofit organizations within which his work is shown. Also important to Johnson's artistic endeavors are his housing; the transportation options available to him; healthcare; and safe spaces in which to live, pursue his art, and use his leisure time. Also integral to Johnson's work, and the work of other artists, is how it is understood and appreciated by aestheticians, critics, sociologists, gerontologists, arts educators, and the like.

The OSLP Arts and Culture Program is part of a larger network of community-based organizations existing in Eugene. By keeping in mind this community that Johnson inhabits, thinking of older adults as networked within their communities, and exploring the larger networks that Johnson's art and artistry are a part of, it is possible to investigate, understand, and appreciate the larger arts and culture sector within which older adults can, and do, participate in the arts. Within Johnson's community, participation is associated with myriad organizations and institutions. In some, arts participation is a primary emphasis (e.g., the Lane Arts Council, the Maude Kerns Art Center, the Very Little Theater, and the John G. Shedd Institute

Arts in Healthy Aging. Patricia Dewey Lambert, Doug Blandy, and Margaret J. Wyszomirski, Oxford University Press.
© Oxford University Press 2024. DOI: 10.1093/oso/9780192847607.003.0007

for the Arts), whereas in others, it is a secondary emphasis (e.g., the Eugene Parks and Recreation, the Eugene Public Library, and residential settings for older adults, such as Cascade Manor). In some settings, older adults participate alongside multiple generations of participants, whereas in others, the programs are designed specifically for older adults. It is also important to recognize that *how* an older adult participates may change over time due to a variety of circumstances, including health, transportation options, personal interests, and program availability. As has been discussed elsewhere in this book, the motivating factors contributing to arts participation may vary over time. What all of these settings and programs have in common is a commitment to those living in the Eugene area. Many of these Eugene-based organizations, and the professionals associated with them, are part of larger regional, national, and international networks advancing the availability of arts and cultural activities. Locally and regionally, organizations, such as the Oregon Arts Commission, the Oregon Cultural Trust, the National Endowment for the Arts (NEA), and the Alzheimer's Association, among others, constitute the network. The systemic community-based network described above in relationship to Eugene is not unique. It is representative of what is referred to nationally and internationally as "community arts."

Building on the initial discussion of the arts and cultural sector in Chapters 1 and 2, this chapter considers this sector in greater detail with an emphasis on enhancing arts participation by older adults to the greatest extent possible. This is accomplished by first contextualizing the arts and cultural sector within the larger array of community-based services available to older adults. Following this contextualization, this chapter orients readers to the choices that older adults can make within the arts and culture sector and where their arts participation will occur. Emphasis will be placed primarily on nonprofit organizations that offer arts and cultural programming to local people within the context of what is understood to be community arts. Recognizing barriers to full participation discussed throughout this book, this chapter discusses how such organizations can emphasize "age-friendliness." This chapter will also assist the older adult and those professionals or family members supporting the arts participation by older adults by providing a series of evaluative questions associated with program offerings within the community. Relevant research and practice-based literature are referenced throughout. Other sectors within which older adults will participate in the arts and culture, such as residential and/or healthcare settings, are discussed in greater detail in Chapters 8 and 9.

Community Resources Available to Older Adults

Overview of Community Resources for Older Adults

The arts and culture sector is just one of the many sectors providing educational and other leisure time opportunities, services, and resources to older adults. Other sectors serving older adults include those associated with healthcare, housing, transportation, and financial planning, among others. Across these sectors, the current generations of older adults, particularly the *baby boomers*, are reexamining their options and preferences, which in turn is motivating those serving older adults to initiate changes within these sectors (Wacker and Roberto 2014). The ability for older adults to participate in these sectors is significantly influenced by an older person's economic stability, education, overall health, and the availability of support systems allowing participation by family and friends (93). Also, influencing participation will be the life courses that each older adult will bring to their participation, as discussed in Chapters 5 and 6.

Wacker and Roberto (2014, 10) observe older adults participating in a continuum of services within a "dynamic and interactive system" that includes community resources, support services, and long-term care services. Wacker and Roberto's definition of this continuum of services includes intergenerational programs and education programs with a variety of foci, including the arts and culture, located in recreation and senior centers. However, as these authors note, participation will be dependent upon the older adult being able to access other supports associated with housing (independent or residential), mental health, physical health, and care partners as appropriate. While each older adult has a life course unique to them, Wacker and Roberto acknowledge that the educational attainment among older adults does differ particularly as associated with race and ethnicity. In looking to the future, Wacker and Roberto observe increasing levels of educational attainment to at least the high school level along with a concurrent increase in those with at least some higher education. Wacker and Roberto perceive of older adults participating in lifelong learning as having entered an emancipatory period in their lives where personal growth intersects with learning within community and through technology. The focus is on older adults actively participating "in all realms of life" (100). With their access to leisure time, older adults will pursue opportunities associated with relaxation, entertainment, and personal development. Involvement will be both serious and casual (118). Wacker and Roberto have identified several models of senior centers responding to this increase in leisure time as being multigenerational, wellness-oriented, civic-centered, and the arts within lifelong learning (126–128). Participation may occur in inclusive programs that are open to all older adults or targeted to particular subgroups of older adults living in a community.

Participation in services available to older adults will also be impacted by location. For example, the number of older adults living in rural areas of the United States is increasing due to "declining birth rates and migration patterns among younger adults" (Tuttle et al. 2020, 2). Older adults in rural areas have fewer financial resources than their urban counterparts with "low to moderate incomes" as compared to higher incomes among urban dwellers (2). Also significant is that older adults living in rural areas are "more likely" to experience disabilities, cardiac issues, and lung disease (3).

The Community-Based Arts and Culture Sector

Recognizing that engaging in arts and cultural opportunities requires participation and support from multiple sectors, it is important to discuss the community infrastructure supporting the arts and culture sector in more detail and as particular to community-based arts or what will be referred to here as "community arts." Congdon and Blandy (2003), based on a review of the literature and their own experience as arts educators working in community, define *community arts* as "first and foremost community-based, community focused, and integral to the everyday life of the community" (242). They emphasize that community arts are not unique to the United States but are also evident in the United Kingdom, Australia, France, and Canada, among other international locales. Significant to their definition is the strong relationship between community arts and the cultures that exist within community. Also significant to their definition is that although "communities are often identifiable through shared purposes and history, . . . community and art are not static" (242). Related to the elasticity of community arts is that they are shaped and informed by "politics, economics, and the desire for social justice" (243). This is evident in the histories of community arts where reference is made to this history has continued to the present day with the influence of the Disability Rights Movement, Black Lives Matter, LGBTQ + activism, and advocacy efforts associated with older adults.

> social reformism (for instance, abolitionism, utopianism, and feminism) in the nineteenth century, immigration policy in the early twentieth century, the New Deal in the 1930s, the civil rights movement and the War on Poverty in the 1960s, and the environmental movement for the 1970s onward. These forces in turn encouraged such specific arts oriented initiatives as the public works projects in the 1930s, the first community arts councils in the late 1940s, the National Endowment for the Arts in the mid-1960s, and the so-called culture wars of the 1990s. (243)

In the present day, community arts[2] consist of a vibrant and engaged collective of advocates, practitioners, and participants associated with organizations, such as Imagining America, the National Art Education Association's Community Arts Caucus, and the National Guild for Community Arts Education. Education for community arts workers is available at institutions of higher education, such as the Maryland Institute College of Art, Rutgers, and Lesley University. Community arts are also linked to community and cultural development. As such, existent and possible community arts initiatives will be linked with public and private agendas fostering organizational partnerships linking the arts, culture, economics, and social justice (Congdon and Blandy 2003, 244). Scholars associated with community arts publish in academic journals and books associated with fields, such as community and regional planning, education, folklore, the health professions, and aging, and use arts-based, qualitative, and quantitative research methodologies. Discussed later in this chapter will be a review of some of this research supporting positive health outcomes and well-being associated with participation in arts programs generally and community arts programs specifically.

Community arts can be both an organizational description and a description of programming. Organizationally, this includes organizations, such as the OSLP Arts and Culture Program referenced above, which have missions to serve the community from a broad-based perspective and respond to all or some of the multiple orientations to the arts and culture that exist within the community. Community arts programming also exists within organizations that have a comprehensive mission extending beyond community-based needs, but do include within their mission programs that are representative of a community-based orientation. One example in Eugene, Oregon is the "Reflections and Connections" program at the University of Oregon's Jordan Schnitzer Museum of Art for people experiencing memory loss and their care partners (Oakman and Blandy 2021). Box 7.1 is illustrative of the types of community-based arts and cultural programs either specifically designed for older adults or multigenerational programs in which older adults can participate.

Community arts organizations and programs exist within the larger arts and cultural sector, introduced in Chapters 1 and 2 of this book. In the United States, a first comprehensive effort to define this sector, which included a broad-based definition of the arts consistent with community arts, was initiated by the American Assembly and published as *The Arts and the Public Purpose* in 1997. Significant to this definitional work by the assembly was the breadth of interests and expertise represented in the assembly. Those people contributing to the definition of sector were artists, arts administrators, businesspeople, foundation representatives, politicians from across the political spectrum, policymakers, and academics, among others. Margaret Wyszomirski, one of the co-authors of this book, was among this group. Foundational to the work of this assembly, and consistent with community arts, was the belief that the arts in the United States reflect the cultural pluralism within American society and that participation in arts experiences is something that most children, youth, and adults engage with in one form or another. This pluralistic perspective of the arts and arts participation was foundational to the assembly's poetic description of the sector as

> diverse as rhythm & blues and symphony orchestras, movies and mambo, abstract expressionism and the dozens, singing commercials and stand-up comedy, Charlie Parker and Georgia O'Keeffe, advertising logos and Bruce Springsteen, Balanchine and Bill "Bojangles" Robinson, Superman and Carlos Santana, Buster Keaton and the Vietnam War Memorial. As happily profane as Harpo and as sacred as a kachina doll, as eclectic as jazz itself, as unpredictable as the rhythms of William Carlos Williams, as sweeping as Oklahoma, our national art, as an immeasurable whole, remains a form or motion, rather than any kind of stasis or purity. (9–10)

Box 7.1 Examples of community-based arts programs for older adults

Program Example—*Encore Creativity*
The nation's largest choral arts organization for adults aged 55+, Encore Creativity's mission is to "provide an excellent and accessible artistic environment for older adults." The organization offers multiple professionally led choral programs, music education programs, and therapeutic programs that address cognitive change.

Source: encorecreativity.org

Program Example—*Stagebridge*
Located in Oakland, California, this performing arts organization—the oldest arts organization of its kind—has been devoted to older adults and lifelong learning in the performing arts since 1978.

Source: stagebridge.org

Program Example—*Dance for PD*
An award-winning program founded by the Mark Morris Dance Group in 2001 and now serving more than 300 communities in twenty countries, Dance for PD (Parkinson's disease) offers therapeutic dance classes for people with Parkinson's disease.

Source: danceforparkinsons.org

Program Example—*Meet Me at MoMA*
The Museum of Modern Art (MoMA)'s well-known program titled "Meet Me" provides a forum for dialogue through looking at arts for individuals with Alzheimer's disease or other forms of dementia and their family members or care partners.

Source: moma.org/visit/accessibility/meetme/resources/#history

Program Example—*StoryCorps*
StoryCorps, which is well known for its national recording initiatives since 2003, seeks "to preserve and share humanity's stories in order to build connections between people and create a more just and compassionate world." One intergenerational program, named "The Great Thanksgiving Listen," specifically encourages young people to record an interview with an older adult.

Source: storycorps.org

Program Example—*The Naropa Community Arts Studio*
Founded by professor and art therapist Michael A. Franklin, this community-based studio, which focuses on service as a spiritual practice, is open to local participants "who are marginalized and unlikely to have access the humanizing practice of engaging in artistic behavior in community." Art experiences are facilitated by graduate students in Naropa University's Transpersonal Art Therapy Program, working toward their preparation to become socially engaged art therapists.

Source: naropa.edu/programs/graduate-academics/clinical-mental-health-counseling/transpersonal-art-therapy/about-the-program/

The assembly also described the locations where people experienced the arts as broadly as the arts experienced. Arts experiences occur "in museums, concert halls, parks, and alternative spaces; they also inhere in the objects and buildings we use every day, and in the music we listen to in our cars, workplaces, homes, and streets" (10). These descriptions are all consistent with community arts. Tantamount to what and where of the arts experience was the assembly's identification of what US citizens were gaining from their arts experiences. Again, as poetically described by the assembly, arts experiences

> calm us and excite us, they lift us up and sober us, and they free our spirit from the relentless mill of daily obligations; they entertain as well as instruct us; they help us understand who we are as individuals, as communities, and as a people. Their beauty or rage can fill us with emotion. In grief or celebration, and also in the subtler modes of irritation, amusement, sexiness, or depression, in great works or in the humblest objects or diversions, they tell our personal and national stories. (10)

The assembly identified three arts and culture subsectors: the informal/unincorporated sector, the nonprofit sector, governmental entities, and the commercial or for-profit sector. Community arts organizations and programs are most readily available within nonprofits and government entities; however, other organizational forms can also accommodate such programs.

Across the subsectors identified by the assembly, four public mandates for advancing public participation in the sector were posited, all of which are consistent with community arts: recognizing the arts and culture as significant to democracy and a collective identity; contributing to individual and collective quality of life, economic well-being, and community livability; contributing to an educated citizenry; and providing opportunities for creativity, relaxation, and entertainment (see Chapter 2 for a more detailed discussion). Among those recommendations made by the American Assembly, one is of particular significance to this book. This recommendation is that "America's education and arts communities should make the fullest possible range of resources available to provide serious and rigorous arts education to young people (K-12), adults and to older citizens" (8).

Amplifying what occurs in the arts and culture sector, including within community arts organizations, is the NEA Office of Research and Analysis study *How Art Works* (2012), which was also first introduced in Chapter 2 of this book. Foundational to the NEA study was the recognition that engaging with the arts is "an essential contributing factor to health, happiness, and prosperity" with benefits that accrue separately to individuals and communities" (9). The study's conclusion cautions that "these benefits are not all equally distributed. Nor are they always reliably present" (9). Within the arts and culture sector, and consistent with community arts, art works as "an artifact, an action, or an ongoing process" (9–10). Like the

American Assembly's conceptualization of the arts in the United States, the NEA study emphasizes that

> There are a multitude of individual-level and community-level outcomes associated with arts engagement. None is privileged (in the sense that one more important or more valuable than others), not all need be present in every circumstance, and the outcomes may register subjectively or objectively. Our system anticipates many subtle influences of arts engagement, over time and differentially over people. (10)

The NEA study of how art works includes several component parts that are associated with the arts and culture sector as conceptualized by the American Assembly and within the community arts field as described above. These include the inherent desire on the part of children, youth, and adults to be creative and expressive. The field also comprises institutions and organizations—such as museums, performing arts centers, educational institutions, and community arts centers, among others—within which arts participation occurs. In alignment with the purposes of this book is the affirmation by the NEA of the importance of education in arts across the lifespan (12). Arts education should "invite us to critique what we know, to challenge the conventional, and to consider change. In this way, the arts help the citizenry analyze, interpret, and debate the conditions of national life" (13).

The two initiatives cited above by the American Assembly and the NEA, which describe the arts and culture sector, are primarily focused on the organizational and institutional structures within which children, youth, and adults participate in the arts. In keeping with the person-centeredness emphasized throughout this book, it is important to also consider how older adult participants define an arts and culture sector through their own participation. In this book, Chapter 2 presents and introduction to choice-based arts participation, and data from past NEA studies on older Americans' participation in the arts and culture sector are included in Chapters 2–4.

The most recent national study on choices made by older adults regarding their participation in America's arts and culture sector was published in late 2022 when Culture Track, in partnership with E.A. Michelson Philanthropy, released the report *Untapped Opportunity: Older Americans and the Arts* (Culture Track 2022). For this report, 28,300 people over the age of 55 were surveyed in 2021 for the purpose of discovering their preferences and behaviors as associated with the arts and culture. Fifty-six percent of respondents were aged 65 and above. The methodology associated with the data presented in the study was combined and weighted, providing a representative demographic sample of the US population. Those surveyed were representative of all regions of the United States, as well as urban, suburban, and rural residents, and comprised diverse self-reported educational attainment, race and ethnicity, and gender identification. The goal of this research was "to inform and inspire transformational approaches to cultural engagement across the spectrum of that age that promote lifelong connection, learning, and creativity" (8). Also important to this research was to investigate "how engagement with arts and culture activities evolves over our lifetimes" and to "challenge limiting misperceptions of the priorities and desires of older adults, and in so doing, deepen sector-wide conversations and commitments to intersectional inclusion, diversity, equity, and access in the arts" (8).

Unlike the reports from the American Assembly and the NEA cited above, this research occurred during the "global pandemic," and the findings from this report reflect the experience of older adults during the pandemic. In this regard, one finding from this research is that "age and experience provide vital perspectives for navigating unprecedented times. While the pandemic has left everyone feeling less connected, older adults are more likely to have a positive attitude than younger generations, with some feeling more hopeful" (11). Other important findings affirm the desire on the part of older adults to have "fun" and "connect with others" (12). Given these findings, it is not surprising that this research revealed that, "for older adults, creative and cultural activities provide meaningful ways to connect with others, find personal fulfillment, and expand their understanding of our shared world" (15).

A very significant finding associated with this research is that "older and younger adults choose to participate in the same kinds of arts and cultural activities" (18). Whereas the American Assembly and NEA reports define the arts and culture sector based in institutional and organizational structures, this study's person-centered approach focuses on types of arts and cultural activities, many of which can be associated with community arts, as attending "fairs and festivals"; "parks, zoo, aquarium, or botanical garden"; "musical performance"; "historic site or tour"; "theater"; and "museums" (18). While in-person participation is preferred over online, "more than half of older adults had participated in digital cultural activities one year into the pandemic, a higher proportion than may been presumed" (21). Those older adults participating in arts and cultural activities identified learning "something new" as a "leading benefit" (23).

Other significant findings in this Culture Track research, relevant to arts and cultural participation by older adults within community arts contexts, are associated with expectations that arts and cultural organizations address important social issues, such as systemic racism and "bridging political divisions in the U.S." (27). Older adults expect arts and cultural organizations to be welcoming, accessible, and inclusive (29). The report concludes by acknowledging the necessity of "closing accessibility and equity gaps" associated with aging and affirms the importance of the arts and culture sector in reimagining "the experience of aging today" (32). Given the expectations of older adults for the environments in which they participate in arts and culture activities, it is important to consider what opportunities are afforded by leisure time and to assess barriers that prevent participation by older adults in community arts organizations.

Health and Well-Being Outcomes Associated with Community Arts

Chapter 4 introduced readers to the health and well-being outcomes associated with participation in the arts by older adults. Chapters 5 and 6 argued for person-centered approaches in this regard. Readers are referred to Figures 4.3, 4.5, and 4.7 as illustrations of how these factors work together in linking the sociocultural contexts with domains of well-being that are person-centered toward a continuum of creative aging approaches and outcomes.

Consistent with the evaluative, eudemonic, affective, hedonic, and cultural well-being outcomes discussed in Chapter 4 are studies linking participation in community arts programs with these outcomes. A first example, from 2000, advocates for a stronger relationship between community arts and community development and how the two support social interaction and neighborhood vitality (Lowe 2000). Relatedly, Chapple, and Jackson (2010) posit an integrated epistemology across fields, such as city planning and performance studies, for the purpose of a more unified understanding, with practical applications, of the arts as instrumental. They also address challenges pertaining to audience development, and the vulnerability of artists and neighborhoods associated with advancing and supporting community arts initiatives.

Specific to older adults is a 2006 study demonstrating that older adults participating in cultural programs will experience significant health benefits, including "fewer doctor visits, less medication use, fewer instances of falls, and fewer health problems" than those not participating in such programs (Cohen et al. 2006, 726). Similar findings were associated with Cohen (2009)'s study of participation in arts and music programs. More recently, Edwards and Owen-Booth (2021, 55) corroborate "current literature that outlines creative arts as a positive leisure-based occupation on aging well." Specific recommendations are made to the field of occupational therapy and to "aid clinical reasoning for social prescribing" (55). A study by Bone et al. (2022, 1) concluded that "arts group participation was associated with the positive elements of evaluative, experienced, and eudemonic wellbeing" and that participating "in community arts groups could help promote healthy aging, enabling a growing segment of the population to lead more fulfilling and satisfying lives."

Leisure Time Participation in the Arts and Culture Sector Aligns with Health and Well-Being

Implicit to participation in community arts as represented in *Untapped Opportunity: Older Americans and the Arts* (Culture Track 2022) is the relationship between arts and cultural participation with the leisure time available to older adults. Carpenter (2008) links experiencing the arts and culture to the free time available to many older adults.[3] While recognizing that such participation will occur across the lifespan, she observes—based on her review of the literature—that older adults "expect arts and cultural experiences to be available to them during their free time" and "appear to be more engaged in leisure pursuits than previous generations were" (8). Reinforcing that early engagement with the arts is predictive of later engagement, Carpenter emphasizes that the current generation of older adults were fortunate to "have visual arts, music, dance, and theater included in public education" (8). Carpenter also posits that leisure is informed by the availability of time, the activities engaged in, and the state of mind that people bring to using their leisure time, and conceptualizes leisure behaviorally as an opportunity for choice-making, an outcome of motivation, goal setting, and a source of pleasure (16–17). Despite these common characteristics of leisure, people will not experience their leisure time in the same way as others. Carpenter emphasizes that engaging in leisure time activities will be influenced by "background, beliefs, and perceptions regarding arts participation" (McCarthy and Jinnett, cited in Carpenter 2008, 17), including "the importance of sociopsychological factors, family influences, and previous experiences and how they contribute to individuals' perceptions regarding participation" (Carpenter 2008, 17). How one uses their leisure time will also be influenced by economic factors (e.g., cost), knowledge of opportunities, location of offerings, competitive offerings, skill, and time availability (17). This is very much in keeping with the life course perspective introduced in Chapter 5 and that should be considered in the design of arts and cultural programs within which older adults participate.

The importance of engaging in arts and cultural activities—along with other leisure time possibilities—to physical and cognitive health is well documented in the literature and elsewhere in this book. This literature can assist in the design and implementation of arts and cultural programs for older adults with specific health outcomes and/or recognizing that participation in arts and cultural programming may have health benefits. Recently, Fancourt et al. (2021) identify 600 such "mechanisms" or outcomes associated with leisure activities and physical and mental health. According to these researchers, "some mechanisms operate at micro-levels, affecting individuals or very small groups, whereas others operate at meso-levels, affecting larger groups, communities, and institutions, or at macro-levels, affecting societies and cultures as large" (331).

At the micro-level, this includes psychological processes, such as affect, resilience, sense of self, personal transformation, and cognition, among others. At the meso- and macro-levels, psychological processes include the development of "group values and understanding," "group attitudes," and methods of communication (331). Biological processes at the micro-level include brain function, immunity, the cardiovascular system, metabolism, and overall physical functioning. At the meso- and macro-levels, positive and negative environmental "exposures" are revealed (331–332). Social processes at the micro-level include greater "social contact," the enhancement of "social engagement," "learning traits," and "building social capital," among others. At the meso- and macro-levels, this includes "supporting group cohesion" and "improved equality," among others (332). "Behavioural processes"—such as the "formation of new habits," choice-making, and motivation—will occur at the micro-level. At the meso- and macro-levels, "group learning," "increasing social responsibility," and "increasing health promotion" will occur (332). "Health behaviours" at the micro-level include the development of preventive health measures as well as the management of ill health, among others. At the meso- and macro-levels, the healthcare "delivery," "performance," and "barriers to health care" may be removed (332). This mechanistic framework is posited to support future research related to leisure and physical and mental health by linking "leisure engagement to health outcomes" (335).

Numerous health and well-being benefits derived from older adults' participation in the arts are emphasized in a report released in late 2022, titled *The Next Wave in Creative Aging: Creative Aging Innovation Forums Cross-Industry Report* (Saunders et al. 2022). This report advocates for the integration of arts participation into an interdisciplinary model for providing healthcare to older adults with a focus on "growth and rehabilitation across the life course" rather than on "deficit and loss" (15). Promising pathways for doing so include looking at *social prescribing* arts participation. Within such models, already being used in the United Kingdom, physicians can prescribe for their patients' community involvement, including arts and cultural participation, to support mental and physical health. In the United States, a quickly growing community of healthcare professionals is organizing to advance *social prescribing* (see socialprescribingusa.com).

The Effects of COVID-19 on Arts Participation by Older Adults

The COVID-19 pandemic potentially compromised older adults' ability to garner the benefits of community-based arts participation during leisure time. The full effects of this pandemic on the lives of children, youth, and adults are only beginning to be understood. For older adults, due to their risk of serious illness and death from the virus, the necessity of sheltering in place undoubtedly challenged their use of leisure time with the accompanying risks of social isolation. While still amid the pandemic, an early study of the effects of COVID-19 on the leisure time of older adults was conducted by Wonock et al. (2021). Recognizing the potentially damaging effects of the virus, as well as the constraints posed by the virus on the lives of older adults, they examined the compensatory strategies used by older adults to maintain leisure time activities. Evidence suggests that "older adults have reported finding joy and comfort by maintaining valued relationships, online interaction, and increased engagement in hobbies" and that "having different life experiences led to various ways of coping among older adults" (Whitehead and Torossian, cited in Wonock et al. 2021, 303). This longitudinal qualitative study "aims to explore baby boomers' (born between 1945 and 1965) adaption in times when their leisure opportunities may be impacted" (302). Twenty-eight Canadian older adults participated in the study by posting comments and photos on a multi-author blog. Participants included sixteen men and twelve women. "Income ranged from less than $30,000 to more than $1,000,000 per year." Twenty-three of the participants identified themselves as "Caucasian" (304).

Blog posts, collected over a one-year period, were analyzed "thematically" and were "closely aligned with the Selective Optimization with Compensation (SOC) model" (302). This model "offers a conceptualization of aging well that is not outcome dependent . . . it focuses on older adults' abilities to adjust to declines and losses with their remaining capacities and resources" (302). Results of this study indicate that "participants made choices that maximized their resources to achieve well-being in the context of adversity" (305). Important to this study is that the data collected revealed adjustments made in the early days of the pandemic, challenges associated with social isolation, and how leisure time activities were selected and optimized along with the types of compensatory strategies used. Based on their research, the authors concluded that their "findings demonstrated that older adults successfully adapted to the pandemic utilizing SOC strategies" (312). In addition, "participants in the study demonstrated their ability to make adequate choices, refine their skill sets and knowledge, and acquire new ways to maintain their well-being if necessary" (312).

Important to the focus of this book and chapter is that some participants in the study concentrated on arts and cultural activities during their leisure time. Significant to their coping with social isolation was their "proficiency" in using technology to maintain their social relationships and participate in leisure time activities. The authors posit that the use of technology "may explain why some older adults benefit from its use and adapt well in adverse situations more than others" (312). This speculative statement regarding the use of technology and findings associated with participation in arts and cultural activities is consistent with the Culture Track (2022) research cited above. This statement is also supported by a 2019 Pew Research Center analysis of Bureau of Labor Statistics data demonstrating that Americans over the age of 60 are spending more time "on their TVs, computers, tablets or other electronic devices" (Livingston 2019, 1). In fact, this analysis shows that "across genders and education levels," older adults are spending "more than half of their daily leisure time, four hours and 16 minutes, in front of screens, mostly watching TV or videos" (1). Important to the analysis is the finding that at the time of this research, 73% of older adults are adopting digital technology, including 53% with access to smartphones (1).

Ageism and Ableism as Barriers to Participation

Despite the compensatory strategies used by older adults during the pandemic, such as attending online arts and cultural programs, the COVID-19 toll on older adults in the US was staggering and brought to the fore the degree to which age discrimination is a fact of life for older adults. This barrier to full participation compromises the benefits available through community-based arts participation. On December 13, 2021, *The New York Times* ran a story under the startling headline "As U. S. Nears 800,000 Deaths, 1 of Every 100 Older Americans Has Perished" (Bosman, Harmon, and Sun 2021). This story ran close to the end of the second year of the pandemic. Tragically, as the journalists attest, this death toll was despite the recognized vulnerability of older adults to COVID-19 and its variants. Of these 800,000 deaths, approximately 600,000 were among adults aged 65 years and older. As indicated in the headline, this amounted to 1 in 100 older adults aged 65 years and older dying of the disease as opposed to 1 in 1,400 for those younger than 65. The authors of this story concluded that "the pandemic has amplified an existing divide between older and younger Americans" leading to isolation and loneliness of this segment of the US population. Louise Aronson, a geriatrician at the University of California San Francisco, is quoted in the article as saying "There's all these ways—subtle, overt, direct, indirect—that we are not taking the needs of older people in this pandemic into account."

In their reporting, Bosman, Harmon, and Sun (2021) describe how COVID-19 was virulent by spring 2020 within nursing homes and assisted living facilities. COVID-19 was identified as the third leading cause of death among those sixty-five and older with heart disease and cancer being the first and second causes. Bowman, Harmon, and Sun reported that some of those older adults interviewed felt that because of their age they were perceived as being of less importance than the effects of the virus on the economy. Elizabeth Dugan, an associate professor of gerontology at the University of Massachusetts Boston, is quoted in the article as stating that "the fact that we're so concerned about school and school kids and childcare, and older people have dropped to the side, it's just more evidence of our pervasive ageism in our society."

The American Psychological Association Committee on Aging (2020/2021) released a fact sheet on ageism and COVID-19, bringing public attention to the disproportionate effects of the virus on older adults, particularly older adults of color. In their fact sheet, the Committee on Aging linked COVID-19 with ageism "in a variety of disturbing ways," including age discrimination associated with the allocation of healthcare resources. Alarmingly, the committee referenced medical ethicists who "encouraged use of likelihood of survival in allocation of ventilators (simplifying to younger ages), whereas the prevailing ethical approach focused on underlying conditions." In addition, the committee speculated that the "implementation of federal policy to vaccinate those in long term care and CDC guidelines for prioritizing older adults may have generated and perpetuated resentment and ageist assumptions among younger adults who were later in the queue." However, the committee concluded, despite some public resistance, that, "this approach appears to have been effective with regard to public health; hospitalization rates decreased rapidly, allowing better use of health care resources to address non-COVID health problems among younger and older adults."

In a recent interview, Margaret Morganroth Gullette, a resident scholar at the Women's Studies Research Center at Brandeis University and author of *Ending Ageism: How Not to Shoot Old People*, is known for stating, "fear ageism, not aging" (Daniel 2022). She succinctly describes ageism as associating aging with bodily or economic decline, as well as "hating or shunning older people" (1). Gullette credits former President Trump's rhetoric for bringing ageism to the fore by "linking dementia and disability and expendability and old people" (1). In doing so, Gullette concludes that "ageism rather than incompetence or any other reason that has been ascribed to Trump can explain why his first policy decision about COVID was to do nothing for nursing home residents. That was disastrous" (1). Gullette recognizes ageism as "ageisms plural," meaning that ageism results in

> a spectrum of damages—including internalized shame and job discrimination at early ages.... and "compound ageism,"... what some people felt toward nursing facility residents. A particular form of intersectionality. It was a compound of they're old, they're sick, they're poor, they're women, they have cognitive impairments, they have mental health issues. (1)

It is also important to acknowledge that older adults may internalize negative stereotypes associated with aging and that such internalization will have a negative impact on health and well-being. A positive view of aging by older adults contributes to longevity (Levy et al. 2002).

Gullette's recognition of ageism as intersectional is significant to the person-centered orientation of this book. Her interview implies the intersection of ageism with "ableism." Rabheru and Gillis (2021) identify ageism as intersecting with ableism and "mentalism." They define *ableism* as "stereotyping, prejudice, discrimination, and social oppression toward people with disabilities including physical, sensory, and intellectual disabilities, invisible disabilities, chronic health conditions, psychiatric conditions and others" (1059). They conclude that "ageism ubiquitously and stealthily impacts organizations, laws, and policies across the world" (1059). Those organizations, laws, and policies inherent to the participation of older adults in the arts and culture sector should not be considered immune and must, given the negative consequences of ageism for older adults and society, be considered in relationship to explicit and implicit ableist and mentalist biases.

Rabheru and Gillis (2021)'s definition of *ableism* captures *mentalism* with its inclusion of psychiatric conditions resulting in "placing persons with mental health conditions and psychosocial disabilities in positions of dependence" (1059). Rabheru and Gillis describe the negative impacts of this intersection of ageism and ableism as "enormous" with significant impact on the human rights of older adults (1059). Fortunately, their review of the literature[4] confirms "the efficacy of educational and intergenerational contact in mitigating these biases" (1059). They call for older adults to be perceived as "experts and partners" in any decisions regarding support and care within healthcare systems (1060). As we have argued elsewhere in this book, this recognition of older adults as experts and partners should be extended to all those contexts in which older adults are being served, including within the arts and cultural sector generally and community arts specifically.

Important to participation by older adults in the arts and culture sector is the fact that many of those participating will be experiencing disabilities. Berridge and Martinson (2017) argue that successful and healthy aging cannot assume "the avoidance of disease and disability, and the maintenance of physical and cognitive function, prove to be particularly rare occurrences among American older adults" (84). Their research shows that while the overall health and longevity of older adults continues to improve, older adults living free of any health impairment are in the minority. Berridge and Martinson found that "among the more than 43 million Americans older than age 64, approximately 80 percent have at least one chronic condition and 68 percent have at least two" (National Council on Aging, cited in Berridge and Martinson 2017, 84). In addition, approximately half of older adults are "expected to experience severe cognitive impairment or require long-term care for support with two activities of daily living" (Faveault and Dey, cited in Berridge and Martinson 2017, 84). Berridge and Martinson conclude that "setting criteria for 'success' in aging based primarily on the avoidance of disease, disability, and functional losses sets up the vast majority of the older adult population for failure—a majority of whom are women, and in particular, women of color" (85). Consistent with the discussion of "universal design" in Chapters 5 and 6, these researchers argue for a social model of disability within which social and physical environments can be modified to mitigate disability (86). The emphasis here is on social and environmental supports, such as those possible through universal design and universal design for learning. Important to this process, according to Berridge and Martinson, is permitting older adults to share and define their own experiences, including what successful aging means to them (89). Again, there is congruency here between this orientation to the transformative learning and the arts discussed in Chapter 6. The goal here, as argued by Berridge and Martinson, "is an approach to 'doing old age' that accounts for and prepares for the common experience of aging with disability or chronic illness" (90).

Age-Friendly Communities and Participation in Arts and Culture

This chapter—and this book as a whole—emphasizes the participation of older adults in the arts and cultural sector as one of the many intersecting sectors responding to the needs of older adults. Additional sectors identified include, but are not limited to, healthcare, housing, transportation, commercial, recreation, and spiritual centers. Important to this analysis is that while participation in the arts and culture will primarily occur within the arts and culture sector, other sectors, such as healthcare and congregant housing (assisted living, memory care, hospice, etc.), also provide arts and cultural experiences. Within the arts and cultural sector, participation will occur within museums, community arts centers, libraries, performing arts centers, festivals, cultural centers, and educational institutions, among others. Much of this participation will occur within community arts settings. Box 7.2 provides two examples of strong community-wide arts programs for older adults implemented through strategic partnerships among multiple organizations.

Older adults will choose to participate in arts and culture activities according to individual decisions made within the choice categories listed in Table 2.1. Participation may include specialized programs for older adults or multigenerational programs accessible to older adults. As discussed in Chapter 2, and visualized in Figure 2.2, participation may vary depending on any functional limitations that older adults may be experiencing at any given time. However, when provided with the necessary supports, older adults *can* participate in arts and culture if they are motivated to do so and if they have the support to mitigate any functional limitations, such as through universal design and universal design for learning. Ultimately, what is required is a systemic approach within which the multiple sectors encouraging participation of older adults, including the arts and cultural sector, maximize their *age-friendliness*.

In 2007, the World Health Organization (WHO) published its internationally influential resource titled *Global Age-Friendly Cities: A Guide* (WHO 2007) based on discussions that occurred at the XVIII IAGG World Congress of Gerontology and Geriatrics in Rio de Janeiro, Brazil (WHO 2007, iv). This initiative was motivated by the WHO's recognition of an international aging population and urbanization as "global trends shaping the 21st century" (iv). Based on the concept of "active aging[5]," "the purpose of this guide was to engage cities to become more age-friendly to tap the potential that older people represent for humanity" (1). The guide describes the research informing the initiative and recommendations on how the guide can be used to advance age-friendliness elsewhere. Important to the creation of the guide was listening to the concerns of older adults and those who support them, a life course

---

Box 7.2 Examples of community-wide arts programs for older adults

Program Example—*Arts for the Aging*

Since 1988, Arts for the Aging has provided accessible arts participation programs to diverse communities throughout Greater Washington, DC. The social service organization partners with teaching artists, eldercare facilities, and arts organizations to provide intergenerational "healthy aging" programs through harnessing the power of the visual, musical, performing, and literary arts. Intended outcomes are identified as both health improvement and life enhancement.

Source: artsfortheaging.org

Program Example—*Creative Aging Mid-South*

Since 2003, this organization has provided a wide array of community-based music and arts programs to enhance the quality of life of all older adults in the Memphis, Tennessee region. Diverse studio courses and workshops in the arts are offered as lifelong learning opportunities within the organization's facilities and through partnerships with senior living communities and arts organizations.

Source: creativeagingmidsouth.org

perspective acknowledging multiple types of diversity among older adults, and recognizing that the functional decline often experienced by older adults is influenced by environmental factors. Through this process, the guide addresses age-friendliness as related to "outdoor spaces and buildings; transportation; housing; social participation; respect and social inclusion; civic participation and employment; communication and information; and community support and health services" (1). These features of *age-friendly cities* are seen as intersectional in that "changing one aspect of the city can have positive effects on the lives of older people in other areas" (2). Overall, the guide was initiated by the WHO to support an "age-friendly community movement" (2), supporting cities that are friendly to all people across the lifespan.

The Public Health Agency of Canada was a key supporter and early adopter of the WHO age-friendly initiative (WHO 2007, iv). Four years after the publication of the WHO guide to age-friendly cities, an important study was published in the *Canadian Journal on Aging* that examines the WHO age-friendly concept from an ecological perspective for the purposes of bringing attention to "key issues related to the interplay between the person and the environment that are usefully considered in order to advance age-friendliness research or policy purposes" as related to housing, the social environment, opportunities for participation, informal and formal community supports and health services, transportation, and communication and information (Menec et al. 2011, 480). Maintaining that age-friendliness benefits all people, this study expanded the WHO focus on cities toward a continuum from rural to urban noting that across this continuum the issues facing communities will differ (480). These researchers note that, "for example, older persons living in a multi-ethnic poor neighborhood in a city might experience their community differently than older adults living in less ethnically diverse town located in an otherwise sparsely populated rural area" (481).

Menec et al. (2011)'s ecological model of the *age-friendly community* centers the person, with their unique life course, surrounded first by family and friends, followed by the community environment consisting of housing, social participation opportunities, informal and formal community supports and health services, transportation, and communication and information. A third surround is the policy environment. Important to the focus of this chapter on the arts and culture sector is that social connections (affording arts and cultural participation opportunities, among others) are a two-way exchange between person, family and friends, community environment, and policy environment (484). Associated with their ecological model of the age-friendly community are five principles, derived from the literature, promoting social connectivity as follows:

1. Factors in the environment are interrelated and interact with each other to influence social connectivity.
2. Environmental influences can be described in terms of their immediacy to individuals or groups (close versus distal).

3. The fit between the person and the environment is critical in determining social connectivity.
4. Personal characteristics and environmental conditions change over time and their relationship to social connectivity is dynamic [see Figure 2.2 of this book].
5. There are certain "leverage points (within the person or the environment) that are particularly key in determining social connectivity" (484–485).

Each of these principles is discussed in detail within the article as important to the point of view of older adults (485–486).

Within the United States, the most visible advocate for age-friendly communities is the American Association of Retired Persons (AARP). Available on the association's website are six training modules that introduce the concept and implementation of age-friendly communities (AARP n.d.). Module 1 introduces the AARP definition of *age-friendly communities* as

> places that make it easy for people to live their best lives at every age. They offer diverse housing and transportation choices, safe and accessible public spaces, and ways for people of all ages and abilities to participate in their community.... [They] also promote health, access to information for all, and opportunities for increased social engagement. (AARP n.d.)

The importance and prevalence of age-friendly community initiatives[6] motivated a special 2022 issue of *The Gerontologist*. In the editorial introducing the issue, Meeks (2022) emphasized the field of gerontology's recognition of the relationship of the health and well-being of older adults to the environments that they are inhabiting and shaping. Meeks describes the purpose of this special issue of the journal as "addressing the current progress of age-friendly communities and the relationship between age-friendliness and aging in place" (1). Important to the articles published in this special issue, according to Meek, are the multiple research methods represented and the global perspectives communicated within the issue. Across the research represented in the special issue, Meeks recognized important findings associated with the success and sustainability of the age-friendly models, the relationship of age-friendliness to aging in place, intersectional considerations in the age-friendly models, and strategies for measuring age-friendliness. In concluding the editorial, Meeks, based on her reading of the articles selected for the journal, affirms that "creating and maintaining age-friendly communities" is a complex endeavor (4), the importance and need for additional research to continue to fully understand and respond to this complexity, the need for evaluative strategies, and very importantly "how to incorporate aging into our conceptions of age-friendliness." Also of importance, as has been stressed throughout this chapter and book, is considering "the diversity of communities and whether age-friendly initiatives are inclusive across dimensions including cognitive and physical disability, socioeconomic advantage/disadvantage, ethnicity, and personal/neighborhood historical influences, including trauma" (4).

In all social sectors, including the arts and culture sector, policies and practices for serving older adults continue to evolve. Meeks (2022) concludes that *age-friendliness* as a systemic orientation to serving the needs of older adults, and all people for that matter, must be considered an "incomplete" endeavor. However, despite its incompleteness, it is an orientation that thus far shows promise.[7] To assist readers in responding to that promise, Box 7.3 proposes a series of questions generated from the age-friendly literature cited above, which older adults and arts and cultural organizations should consider when anticipating attending, planning, implementing, and evaluating arts and cultural programs for older adults in community-based settings.

Box 7.3 Questions for community-based arts programs for older adults

Following are a series of questions generated from the age-friendly literature cited above, which older adults and arts and cultural organizations should consider when anticipating attending, planning, implementing, and evaluating arts and cultural programs for older adults in community-based settings. Questions are organized around the larger issues informing age-friendly communities. The questions that follow are suggestive, rather than comprehensive, of all possible questions guiding the implementation of age-friendly arts and cultural programs within formal or informal age-friendly communities.

Social Engagement

- Does the mission of the organization contain language that is inclusive of serving older adults?
- Is an advisory group of older adults and their advocates consulted on a regular basis about program offerings? What other mechanisms exist for collecting the point of views of older adults? Are older adults represented on the board of directors?
- How do the arts and cultural programs assist people of all ages to connect and socialize? Are there opportunities for intergenerational engagement?
- Are barriers to participation, such as ageism and ableism, mitigated within the organization offering arts and cultural programs? If so, how? Does mitigation include staff training around issues of discrimination?
- How is the design and implementation of arts and cultural programs consistent with effective practices for people experiencing memory loss?
- How does the organization offering arts and cultural programs consider the unique life course perspective of participants? How does this consideration of the life course occur? How do the programs cultivate multicultural, multiracial, multiethnic perspectives? How are evolving conceptions of gender and sexual orientation recognized?
- How does the organization offering arts and cultural programs ensure that nobody is excluded based on economic disadvantage? What specific strategies are utilized in this regard?

Has the larger community within which the organization operates engaged in a cultural mapping[8] process to identify the arts and cultural resources available in the community? Does this cultural mapping process include specific attention to arts and cultural resources and opportunities available to older adults and, if applicable, their care partners?

Are programs offered in alternative formats, such as online programs, such that participation is not dependent upon transportation and/or the ability or desire to leave one's place of residence?

Are arts and culture education programs offered supporting a lifelong learning organizational mission?

Communications and Information

Are the communication strategies of the organization disseminated in accessible formats and widely distributed within the community? What are some of the accessible formats utilized? Are these formats consistent with effective practices identified for those experiencing disabilities associated with communication?

Health and Community Supports

In what ways is the organization partnering with health-related institutions and organizations to provide support to those older adults, experiencing significant health concerns, who wish to engage in arts and cultural activities?

Housing

In what ways does the organization participate in community-based conversations around housing within the community?

Transportation

By what means are older adults able to travel to programs?

How does the organization assist people who do not drive to access programs?

How is the organization involved in discussing transportation options in the community in which they are located?

Accessible Public Spaces

Are the outdoor spaces, buildings, and online environments within which programs are offered ADA accessible and safe?

What universal design and universal design for learning strategies are used to promote accessibility?

Civic Engagement and Employment

Does the organization hire or invite volunteerism by older adults? Is there the opportunity for older adult volunteers to engage with younger volunteers?

Is the organization participating in civic forums within which the larger issues of housing, transportation, social engagement, health, and the other attributes associated with age-friendliness are discussed?

Conclusion

Introducing this chapter was reference to artist Perry Johnson and those many people, organizations, and businesses that are associated with his participation in the arts. This included the locations in which his art was created, sold, and exhibited with mention made of housing, the transportation options available to him, healthcare, and safe spaces in which to live, pursue his art, and use his leisure time. Johnson was referenced to bring attention to the larger community that Johnson inhabits; to think of older adults as networked within their communities; to explore the larger networks Johnson's art and artistry are a part of; and to investigate, understand, and appreciate the larger arts and culture sector within which older adults can participate in the arts. Following upon this specific reference to an artist was a more detailed description of the arts and culture sector as defined by organizational and institutional structures, as well as how older adults are defining the sector through the choices they are making on how and where to participate. Emphasis was placed on community arts within the sector. Participation by older adults in this sector was also discussed in relationship to the leisure time available to older adults and how choices associated with leisure can influence health and well-being. *Ageism* and *ableism* were discussed as barriers to participation. Emphasized within this chapter is that the arts and culture sector intersects with several other sectors supporting participation in the arts and culture by older adults. The WHO and AARP age-friendly initiatives along with recent research were cited as supporting a systemic approach to maximizing the engagement by older adults, along with people of all ages, in arts and culture participation in their communities. A list of questions was provided to guide older adults and arts and cultural organizations in considering attendance, planning, implementation, and evaluation of community-based programs for older adults.

This chapter focused on opportunities for older adults to participate independently and autonomously, acknowledging the need for supports as appropriate, in arts programs within a variety of community-based organizations and settings. The next two chapters of this book discuss opportunities for older adults to participate in purposefully designed arts programs to support the specific needs of those in senior living communities and clinical care settings, and at the very end of life.

8
Arts Programs for Older Adults in Residential and Clinical Care Settings

Introduction

The vast majority of older adults are "aging in place" in their communities, and it is generally assumed that people wish to live independently in their own homes as long as possible. When an older adult's health situation demands a higher level of care—whether temporarily or over a long period of time—the older adult can enter into the maze of America's ever-changing eldercare system that encompasses both residential and clinical care settings. This chapter explains this complex system of senior living options, long-term care, subacute care, and hospital care. A full array of such facilities is available to older adults in communities across the country, and the community-based resources described in Chapter 7 may also be provided in these healthcare-focused settings. It is imperative to understand the institutional structures and needs of the residents across these settings when designing and implementing arts programs intended to support specific health and well-being outcomes.

This chapter begins with an overview of America's eldercare and healthcare system and introduces issue areas, such as healthcare quality and healthcare consumerism. Medicare, Medicaid, and long-term care are briefly introduced from the perspective of the range of choices older adults may (or may not) have in choosing their residential setting of care. *Age-friendly healthcare* and *person-centered care* are profiled as two significant movements affecting the full array of healthcare facilities. The second half of the chapter provides a detailed description of the settings of care for older adults in America, as older adults' needs shift from independent living, to assisted living, to clinical care.

Overview of America's Eldercare and Healthcare System

In the natural aging process, older adults frequently require diverse forms of assistance to engage in the activities and relationships that they have reason to value. Older adults also require clinical care to manage chronic diseases, treat a sudden medical emergency, or recover from an injury. Various forms and levels of assistance with daily life activities and medical care can keep older adults fully integrated in the community, but some health conditions require more intensive care that limits an older adult's independence and integration with the community. This chapter discusses opportunities for arts programs and activities for older adults who are housed in institutional settings, such as assisted living facilities, rehabilitation centers, skilled nursing facilities, and hospitals. Hospice and end-of-life care are presented separately, in Chapter 9 of this book.

It is perhaps most useful to think of America's system of providing care to older adults along a healthcare continuum that consists of both residential settings and clinical settings, as depicted in Figure 8.1. When health conditions and lifestyle preferences change, older adults can move across this continuum either rapidly or slowly. For example, a severe stroke may remove an older adult from their home to place them in a hospital for acute care, followed by post-acute care in a rehabilitation center, followed by long-term care in a nursing home or other care setting. Dementia may present as unnoticeable at first, allowing full integration in the community, but over time require support of adult day services and then eventually a 24/7 memory care facility placement. A bad fall may result in a hospitalization with surgery, but then a recovery at home with limited home care support. Couples and roommates may have very different needs throughout the aging process, and may need to make difficult choices regarding the residential care setting that they need.

To engage in a discussion of the healthcare continuum for older adults in America, it is first necessary to profile the changing context of healthcare. Significant trends point toward increasing consumer demands for the healthcare experience, as well as the rise of holistic healthcare and person-centered care that are now central to patients' expectations. For older adults over the age of 65, Medicare and Medicaid play a very important role in determining the choices one has for senior living options and clinical care. And, important steps are being taken to develop "age-friendly" healthcare systems across the nation. Beginning with a big-picture snapshot,

> The U.S. health care system includes a mix of public and private sector financing and is governed by both federal and state laws and regulations. For example, federal laws passed by Congress and administered by the Department of Health and Human Services govern Medicare payment policies and conditions of participation for hospitals and other facilities. States, conversely, regulate which professionals can provide care under specific circumstances. Last, the public–private mix of services, coupled with the fact that the vast majority of publicly financed services are provided by private sector organizations and professionals, has resulted in substantial delegation of authority for oversight of care quality to private entities. For example, medical societies provide oversight for the education, training, and board certification of health care providers; The Joint Commission is responsible for inspecting hospitals; and the National Quality Forum (NQF) provides oversight for care quality measurement for public reporting. (Clancy, Corrigan, and McNeill 2009, 268)

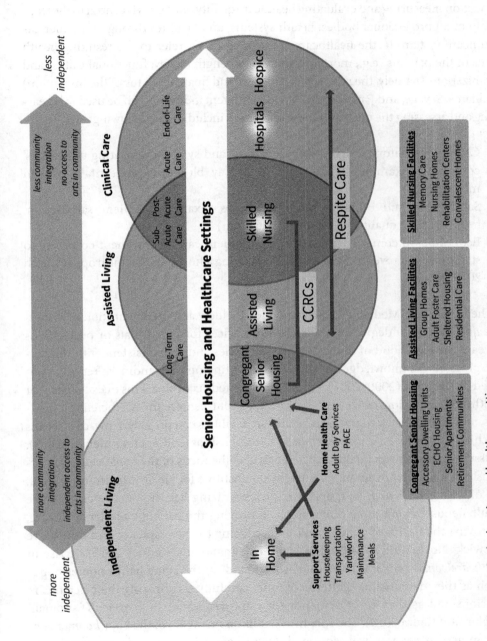

Figure 8.1 Senior housing and healthcare settings
Illustration by Stephanie McCarthy.

Healthcare Quality and Healthcare Consumerism

A focus on measuring and evaluating healthcare quality outcomes is central to the leadership of all professional bodies, health systems, and facilities throughout America's healthcare system. In the healthcare context, *outcomes* refer to the resulting health status of the patients (e.g., mortality, morbidity, length of stay, functional status) and organizations (namely, the rate of staff turnover and financial status of the institution) (Williams, Savage, and Patrician 2017, 146). Different indicators can be used for measuring and assessing the quality of these outcomes, including the following:

- Clinical indicators . . . are observable signs and symptoms relating to patients' conditions (examples: length of hospital stay, blood pressure, intake of pain medication)
- Satisfaction and other reported outcomes (examples: patient satisfaction, health-related quality of life, staff satisfaction)
- Economic outcomes (examples: cost of patient care, recruitment costs due to staff turnover, revenue from patients choosing a hospital, philanthropy) (Ulrich 2009, 130).

The Institute of Medicine (IOM) provides a widely accepted definition of *healthcare quality* as the "degree to which health services for individuals or populations increase the likelihood of desired health outcomes and are consistent with the current professional knowledge" (IOM 1990). Building on two landmark reports published by the IOM (2000; 2001), the IOM promoted six dimensions of excellence for healthcare institutions: effectiveness, safety, patient-centeredness, efficiency, timeliness, and equity. Arts programs in healthcare facilities can provide a low-cost means of achieving improvements in each of these dimensions (Sadler and Ridenour 2009).

Assessing healthcare quality outcomes is also the focus of the *triple aim*, an enormously influential movement initiated by the Institute for Healthcare Improvement. The oft-cited *triple aim* is an approach to optimizing health system performance simultaneously along three dimensions: improving the patient experience of care, improving the health of populations, and reducing the per capita cost of healthcare (Berwick, Nolan, and Whittington 2008; Bisognano and Kenney 2012). A rise in *healthcare consumerism* is largely due to demands of the aging baby boomer population as they demonstrate patterns of more carefully scrutinizing their healthcare decisions and as they exert demands for improved value and service (Esupiñan, Fengler, and Kaura 2014). The roughly 70 million members of the *baby boomer* generation are, in general, well-educated, tech-savvy, and informed consumers who expect to receive full information and insist that their healthcare experience is of the highest possible quality (Sadler and Ridenour 2009, 9). "Today's consumers are demanding more and more from their health care providers on all levels (e.g., physicians, payers, and hospitals), both in terms of the availability of specific service offerings and in the delivery of those services.... In today's world, the *patient* is becoming the central focus of customer service" (Casciani 2017, 111). Healthcare consumerism is also propelling *medical tourism*, which refers to patients traveling to receive medical care. US patients travel to other countries, foreign patients come to the US, and US patients travel domestically to seek out medical care (Keckley and Underwood 2009, 3). Publicly reported patient satisfaction scores, usually collected by hospitals through standardized Press Ganey surveys, are important data points for healthcare consumers in selecting clinical care. As a result, healthcare administrators rely heavily on excellent patient experiences to help support excellent patient satisfaction scores (Sadler and Ridenour 2009, 4).

Healthcare consumerism has driven a patient-centered transformation in healthcare. *Patient-centered care* is essentially "taking an approach to healthcare that consciously adopts the patient's perspective" (Gerteis et al. 1993, 5). Patient-centered care and holistic healthcare go hand in hand, and these concepts are key for artists, arts educators, and arts administrators to understand while developing residential care and clinical care arts programs for older adults. *Holistic healthcare* (also referred to as *whole-person healthcare*) considers the whole person, including mind, body, emotions, and spirit, for optimum health and well-being (Ratini 2020). These models of care have been brought together in what is now referred to as *patient- and family-centered care*, which describes an approach to the planning, delivery, and evaluation of healthcare that is grounded in mutually beneficial partnerships among healthcare providers, patients, and families (Johnson and Abraham 2012). *Patient- and family-centered care* tends to embrace *integrated healthcare*, which brings conventional and complementary approaches to healthcare (such as acupuncture, chiropractic manipulations, naturopathy, massage, meditation, and aromatherapy) together in a coordinated way (National Center for Complementary and Integrative Health 2018). Integrated healthcare, which can also include creative and expressive arts therapies as well as other arts interventions, "emphasizes a holistic, patient-focused approach to health and wellness. The services often include psychological, spiritual, social, functional, and community aspects" (Rollins et al. 2021, 227–228).

Across the United States, hospital CEOs' main concerns have to do with leading their healthcare facilities through financial challenges, healthcare reform implementation, governmental mandates, patient safety, and healthcare quality (Askin and Moore 2014, 22). In addition to managing public policy and financial imperatives, healthcare administrators must develop organizational policies, programs, cultures, and practices that attend to ever-increasing healthcare consumer demands.

"Research, experience, and common sense demonstrate that the arts are appropriate, effective, and cost-efficient strategies" (Sadler and Ridenour 2009, 10) in addressing these healthcare leadership concerns and challenges. For example, empirical studies from around the world convincingly demonstrate how arts programs support the *triple aim* of better health, better care, and lower cost. The arts promote physical and cognitive health and expedite medical recovery for people of all ages. Arts engagement in clinical contexts can alleviate patients' stress and increase their sense of agency and resilience. Arts programs benefit patients at risk of experiencing cognitive decline through a stroke, Alzheimer's disease, or Parkinson's disease. Numerous mental and emotional health benefits derive from the arts in reducing anxiety and depression (Fancourt and Finn 2019). Specific health outcomes and benefits for older adults who participate in arts programs are discussed in detail in Chapter 4 of this book.

The rise of healthcare consumerism along with movements such as *patient- and family-centered care* means that the actual and perceived quality of the healthcare experience must be a significant focus of healthcare administration (Lambert 2016; Sadler and Ridenour 2009). The arts can even contribute to patients' likelihood of recommending a healthcare facility (Slater, Braverman, and Meath 2017). A new healthcare paradigm focused on the whole person and an integrated approach to healing (Serlin 2007) means that the arts have a vital role to play in this emerging humanistic model of healthcare. Longer life spans, increasingly diverse populations, and new models of healthcare access compel a new role for the arts in enhancing a person-centered healthcare experience (Clift and Camic 2016; Fancourt 2017).

The arts also support the quality of care provided by healthcare professionals. The arts are increasingly used in training physicians and nurses through proven educational programs that foster caregivers' self-awareness, empathy, and interpersonal communication abilities. The arts also help medical professionals in developing clinical diagnosis skills. Arts programming in healthcare facilities can help mitigate stress, exhaustion, and "compassion fatigue" so often experienced by healthcare professionals. In fact, the *triple aim* is now being expanded to be the *quadruple aim*, which positions the resilience and well-being of healthcare professionals as essential to healthcare (Bodenheimer and Sinsky 2014). Supporting healthcare staff through the arts can help prevent low productivity, medical errors, and patient perceptions of inadequate care (Abia-Smith 2016; Morgan 2016; Hanna, Rollins, and Lewis 2017; National Organization for Arts in Health 2017; State of the Field Committee 2009).

Healthcare administrators increasingly recognize that the arts are low-cost and highly effective interventions that can improve the financial bottom line. Studies demonstrate that arts programs can shorten the length of hospitalization, reduce the amount of medication prescribed, encourage patient compliance with treatment plans, and prevent healthcare complications that lead to repeated returns to the facility. Integration of the arts in healthcare settings can also boost the morale of medical professionals, which benefits the institution financially by helping to prevent high personnel turnover (National Organization for Arts in Health 2017; State of the Field Committee 2009).

Medicare, Medicaid, and Long-Term Care

America's two largest social health insurance programs—Medicare and Medicaid—play a very important role in determining the set of residential care options and clinical facilities from which older adults and their families may select. In short,

Medicare is a federal program established in 1965 to insure the elderly, although the beneficiaries have broadened over time. "It is the largest insurer in the nation—meaning the policies Medicare sets have an enormous impact on how health care in general is run" (Askin and Moore 2014, 42). In contrast, Medicaid is a joint federal-state program intended to insure the poor. People over the age of 65 who qualify for Medicaid because of their finances are considered "dual eligible." Both of these programs are run by the Centers for Medicare & Medicaid Services (CMS).

> The 1965 Amendments to the Social Security Act of 1935 established the two largest government-sponsored health insurance programs in the history of the U.S., Medicare, Title XVIII of the Act, entitled persons 65 and over to coverage of hospital care under Part A and physicians and other outpatient health services under Part B. Eligibility for Medicare benefits has since been extended to younger people with permanent disabilities, individuals with end-stage renal disease, and persons under hospice care. Medicaid, Title XIX, set up a joint federal-state program entitling financially qualified indigent and low-income persons to basic medical care. This program, too, has undergone numerous iterations at both the state and federal levels as these governments have attempted to strike a balance between equity in coverage for certain services (mandated at the federal level) and states' rights in controlling the use of public funds. (Shanks 2017, 216)

The intricacies of Medicare, Medicaid, and other healthcare insurance policies that older Americans may access go far beyond the scope of this chapter. Medicare Supplement (Medigap) and Medicare Advantage plans make this system even more complex for older adults and their families to navigate. Moreover, older adults' capacity to pay for their healthcare as they age is often stymied by America's healthcare system. One major illness or a long hospital stay can deplete an older adult's savings. Medicare generally covers the needs of relatively healthy older adults. When personal savings are largely exhausted, older adults struggling on small monthly incomes (mainly from Social Security) and shrinking pensions can access their state's Medicaid program for services, such as healthcare, food stamps, medications, mental health treatments, and case management (Rizzo 2016, 77–105). For older adults and their families, the reality of the financial burden associated with residential and clinical care throughout the natural aging process can quickly become overwhelming.

> If medical, nursing, and home care bills are not pouring in now, the prospect that they soon will be lies ominously ahead. Premiums, deductibles, copayments, prescriptions, and other expenses not covered by insurance can quickly consume a nest egg.
> The biggest quandary, even for those with a comfortable savings account, is how to cover the cost of long-term care—the day-to-day help that is needed when someone has a chronic illness or disability. Although families provide much of this care, people often need to pay for some services—home care, day care, or assisted living or nursing home care, and the price tag can be significant. The problem is, Medicare and other health insurance cover very little of these costs.

As a result, people pay out of pocket, and when they use up their funds, they go on Medicaid, government insurance for low-income people, which does cover long-term care. (Morris 2014, 337)

In her outstanding resource titled *How to Care for Aging Parents*, Morris (2014) explains that the scenario of using up most of an older adult's resources in order to become dual-eligible for both Medicare and Medicaid can also have some significant drawbacks. Older adults on Medicaid may need to settle for fewer choices and lower-quality care in the long-term care facilities and healthcare facilities to which they have access in their communities (354). She explains that the most common way that people protect their assets before applying for Medicaid is by "spending down." This term refers to spending one's own money on items that Medicaid does not consider to be an asset, such as one's home, car, personal belongings, payments to home health aides, and prepaid funeral expenses (355–356). Medicaid will cover most long-term care expenses, but the older adults need to use up almost all of their assets in order to be eligible. Also, the Medicaid system generally pays only for long-term care in shared rooms in nursing homes; families cannot rely on having access to private and luxurious assisted living and skilled nursing facility rooms.

An enormous challenge for many older adults and their families is determining how to cover the costs associated with long-term care, which will be a necessity for roughly 70% of older adults at some point in their lives, and for an unknown duration (Osterland 2021, 1). "Long-term care" refers to "a variety of services and supports designed to meet health or personal care needs over an extended period of time" (Rollins 2013, iv). The oldest baby boomers begin turning 80 in 2025, and most long-term care needs begin when older adults reach their mid- to late-80s (Osterland 2021, 2). A crisis in long-term care is on the horizon.

Based on data from the long-running Health and Retirement Study at the University of Michigan, the center estimates that 20% of Americans will need no long-term care services before they die, about 55% will have low to moderate needs and 25% will have "the type of severe needs that most people dread."

It also estimates that 33% of retirees don't have resources to cover even minimal LTC needs, and only a fifth could afford "severe" long-term care needs of four years or more. (Osterland 2021, 2)

According to the information published online by Genworth (see genworth.com/aging-and-you/finances/cost-of-care.html), the annual median national cost for long-term care services in 2021 was as follows:

- In-Home Care
  - Homemaker Services = $59,488
  - Homemaker Health Aide = $61,776

- Community and Assisted Living
  - Adult Day Healthcare = $20,280
  - Assisted Living Facility (private, one-bedroom) = $54,000
- Nursing Home Facility
  - Semi-Private Room = $94,900
  - Private Room = $108,405

The same website provides a tool to forecast long-term care expenses in each of these categories on a monthly basis, and at 10-year intervals extending forward to 2071. The figures are staggering. It can quickly become overwhelming for older adults and their families to try to determine how to best cover these expenses from personal savings and assets, especially when working with fixed incomes. Long-term care insurance exists to fill this gap in insurance coverage, but few older adults either have this kind or insurance or are eligible to purchase it. Roughly 80% of aging baby boomers indicate that they have no plan or savings for paying specifically for long-term care (Geber 2021, 3).

With the impending crisis in American long-term care, many national organizations are scrutinizing the Medicare model of (only) providing nursing home care.

> The National Academy of Medicine, for instance, has launched a major project on the quality of nursing home care. AARP is among the organizations exploring ways to make communities more age friendly. And recently, the Convergence Center for Policy Resolution brought together almost 50 care experts to share ideas for a redesigned system of care.
>
> Some important themes and reform ideas are emerging from this reappraisal. These include making it more feasible for people to age in their own homes and communities, empowering nursing homes to focus on people who really need institutional care, and revamping insurance and the workforce. (Butler 2021, 1)

A report of the Convergence Center for Policy Resolution (2020), titled *Rethinking Care for Older Adults*, provides valuable insight into new program models that may allow older adults to remain much longer in their own homes and communities, as well as specific policy recommendations for changing Medicare and Medicaid to better provide for the long-term care needs of older adults. The impact of COVID-19 on nursing home residents and staff has further prompted calls for rethinking residential care for older Americans. Well-documented issues with infection control and prevention, shared rooms, staff who work with multiple facilities and residents, and inadequate staffing led to this population group being disproportionately impacted by the pandemic (Roubein 2021). As of January 30, 2022, more than 200,000 nursing home facility residents and staff members had died from COVID-19; this population group comprises roughly one-fourth of all COVID deaths in the United States (Chidambaram 2022).

Within this changing context of long-term care, artists and arts administrators have the potential to explore new opportunities. Arts programs specifically designed for health and well-being outcomes in older adults can be a critical component of an emerging landscape of long-term care options throughout America. Adults living in long-term care communities often experience an increased sense of isolation along with the loss of their home, family, and community. Collaborative and intergenerational arts programming can help recreate an improved quality of life for residents by connecting older adults with each other, the facility's staff, and with people and organizations beyond the walls of the facility (Rollins 2013, iv–v).

In long-term residential and clinical care settings, meaningful arts experiences can be designed to achieve both individual and collective outcomes. According to Rollins (2013), the characteristics of meaningful arts experiences in these settings "include being person-centered, focused on healing rather than curing, enabling a change in perception achieved by learning something new, encouraging meaningful engagement, and promoting a sense of being heard and valued" (vii–viii). Moreover, meaningful activities are actually required to be offered by long-term care facilities that are funded by Medicare and Medicaid. This so-called "quality of life" requirement is included in the Federal Nursing Home Reform Act from the Omnibus Budget Reconciliation Act of 1987 (referred to colloquially as "OBRA '87"), which was most recently revised in 2017. OBRA '87 mandates that long-term care facilities provide for an ongoing program of activities designed to meet the interests and the physical, mental, and psychosocial well-being of each resident (Best-Martini, Weeks, and Wirth 2018).

Age-Friendly and Person-Centered Care

The age-friendly movement has taken shape across multiple dimensions (communities, businesses, universities, etc.) to comprise what is now essentially an *age-friendly ecosystem* (Fulmer et al. 2020). Within this ecosystem is a significant movement initiated in 2017 by the John A. Hartford Foundation and the Institute for Healthcare Improvement in partnership with the American Hospital Association and the Catholic Health Association of the United States to advance age-friendly care within clinical settings. Hospitals and post-acute long-term care facilities can now be designated an *Age-Friendly Health System*. Attaining and maintaining this designation requires a healthcare system to assess and document the ways in which the facility addresses the "4Ms Framework of an Age-Friendly Health System," a framework to guide the care of older adults throughout the health system's provision of services (Institute for Healthcare Improvement 2020).

The *4Ms Framework of an Age-Friendly Health System* consists of the following:

- **What Matters**
  Know and align care with each older adult's specific health outcome goals and care preferences including, but not limited to, end-of-life care, and across settings of care.

- **Medication**
  If medication is necessary, use age-friendly medication that does not interfere with "What Matters" to the older adult, "Mobility," or "Mentation" across settings of care.
- **Mentation**
  Prevent, identify, treat, and manage dementia, depression, and delirium across settings of care.
- **Mobility**
  Ensure that older adults move safely every day in order to maintain function and do "What Matters." (Institute for Healthcare Improvement 2020, 5)

These "4Ms" are a good reference point for artists and arts administrators seeking to develop arts programs for health and well-being outcomes of older adult in residential and clinical care settings. At the core of these 4Ms is a commitment to supporting each older adult in achieving the ability to do the things that matter the most to them. This overarching goal of supporting functional ability is discussed throughout the pages of this book. However, older adults will have very diverse sets of health conditions that may require medications, and these medications may interfere with their ability to engage in the activities that they value. Similarly, many older adults have mobility challenges and cognitive challenges that influence their functional ability in the context of participating in arts programs for older adults.

In senior living contexts and in clinical settings, the objectives of arts programs will frequently involve targeting specific health outcomes. Arts programs can be designed to treat specific health challenges and support the management of chronic conditions. In contrast to an *acute condition, chronic conditions* are considered to be health issues that last three or more months. Roughly 80% of older adults have one chronic condition, and 50% have at least two. Artists and arts program administrators in healthcare settings will most frequently encounter older adults with chronic conditions such as arthritis, cardiovascular disease, diabetes, kidney disease, and mental health issues. Although chronic conditions can be controlled and improved, a cure or recovery is often not possible (Williams 2020, 210). As such, treatment of chronic conditions "should be focused on assisting the older adult to function at the highest possible level in the physical, social, psychological, and spiritual arenas of life" (210).

For purposes of considering specific health outcomes that may be addressed through arts programs designed for older adults, it is useful to systematically consider the most common diagnoses that lead to physical and cognitive impairments. Table 8.1 outlines common physiological diagnoses that lead to common physical impairments. Table 8.2 presents a summary of chronic neurological, cognitive, and psychological diagnoses that often lead to cognitive impairments. These two tables include a brief overview of diagnoses, typical symptoms, an overview of the condition as experienced by the older adult, and implications for arts program design and implementation. These two tables are provided to introduce an array of health program outcomes that may be included in arts programs designed for older adults.

Table 8.1 Common chronic physical impairments in older adults

Common Physiological Diagnoses	Typical Symptoms and Issues	General Nature of Chronic Challenges as Experienced by the Older Adult	Implications for Arts Program Design
Cardiovascular System Coronary Artery Disease Congestive Heart Failure Hypertension Peripheral Vascular Disease	Decreased endurance, deconditioning, swelling, high (or low) blood pressure, changes in the skin (ulcers, browning, thinning)	Anxiety, fatigue, depression, loss of control	Include breathing exercises, relaxation, slow-paced activities, social interaction, and participants' choices
Pulmonary System Chronic Obstructive Pulmonary Disease (COPD)	Coughing, light-headed, inability to breathe deeply, decreased endurance	Anxiety, fatigue, depression, loss of control	Include breathing exercises, relaxation, slow-paced activities, social interaction, and participants' choices
Musculoskeletal System Osteoarthritis Degenerative Joint Disease Osteoporosis	Bones break easily, painful joints, achy, stiff movement, rounded spine	Mobility challenges, fear of pain and injury, balance and posture problems, risk of falling, fatigue	Include activities that improve posture and balance, low-impact activities, physical activities adapted to the functional level of the individual
Metabolic and Endocrine System Diabetes (Type 2)	Fatigue, weight loss, vision loss, weakness, confusion, incontinence, thirst, sensations of tingling or numbness	Anxiety	Design programs to address vision challenges and endurance challenges
Urinary System Problems	Urinary incontinence	Reluctance to go out	Provide easy access to restroom
Gastrointestinal System Problems	Constipation, indigestion, heartburn, diverticulosis, ulcers, hemorrhoids	Discomfort	Provide easy access to restroom
Blood, Skin, and Mouth Problems	Anemia, hyperthermia, hypothermia, skin irritations, mouth pain	Fatigue, discomfort, confusion	Include activities adapted to the functional level of the individual

Sources: Best-Martini, Weeks, and Wirth (2018); Dahlkemper (2020c); Morris (2014); Rollins (2013)

Table 8.2 Common chronic cognitive impairments in older adults

Common Neurological, Cognitive, and Psychological Diagnoses	Typical Symptoms and Issues	General Nature of Chronic Challenges as Experienced by the Older Adult	Implications for Arts Program Design
Sensory Losses	Vision loss and hearing loss, also loss of touch, taste, and smell	Social isolation, depression related to losses, may be perceived as mentally impaired by others	Protect against falls and injuries; Include sensory stimulation, activities to learn strategies to adapt to sensory losses, and social interaction
Parkinson's Disease (PD)	Tremors, slow movement, softness of voice, unsteady gait, poor coordination	Social isolation, often perceived by others as having dementia, risk of falling	Protect against falls and injuries, focus on social interaction
Stroke	Symptoms differ if the stroke occurs on the left side or right side of the brain. Difficulty speaking, writing, and reading; disorientation, memory loss, and social isolation. Weakness, numbness, and loss of coordination, especially on one side of the body	Social isolation, communications challenges, vision loss, and mobility challenges	Protect against falls and injuries, focus on social interaction, adapt communications and movements to the individual's needs
Depression	Withdrawal, confusion, fatigue, apathy, memory loss, change in appetite, feelings of hopelessness, irritability, poor hygiene	Anxiety, social isolation, sadness	Focus on enjoyable, relaxing activities that include social interaction
Delirium	Inattentiveness and confusion that come on suddenly, disorientation	Anxiety, social isolation	Focus on reality awareness and activities that include social interaction
Dementia	Various forms of dementia as well as Mild Cognitive Impairment (MCI) and Alzheimer's Disease. Confusion, chronic forgetfulness, and other mental lapses get progressively worse	Depression, feelings of helplessness and hopelessness, decreased safety awareness, social isolation	Focus on reality awareness, sensory stimulation, body-awareness activities, compensatory skills training, social interaction, and relaxation

Sources: Best-Martini, Weeks, and Wirth (2018); Dahlkemper (2020c); Morris (2014); Rollins (2013)

In addition to the conditions profiled in Tables 8.1 and 8.2, there are categories of challenges resulting from anxiety disorders, behavioral disorders, sleep disorders, substance abuse, and overmedication. For people leading arts programs in eldercare settings, behavioral problems may be particularly disruptive to program participants. Examples may include agitation, aggressive and violent behaviors, sexual acting out, rapidly changing moods, disorientation, and paranoia (Dahlkemper 2020a, 287–298). Moreover, adapting to highly diverse cultural backgrounds and language barriers may present particular challenges and opportunities to program leaders and participants.

Because of the prevalence of dementia found among older adults located in assisted living and clinical care settings, it is especially important for anyone serving this population group to be familiar with the general contours of this cognitive impairment. According to the data collected by the Centers for Disease Control and Prevention (CDC) (see cdc.gov/nchs/fastats/alzheimers.htm), roughly a third of adult day services participants, residential care community residents, and home health agency patients have a diagnosis of Alzheimer's disease or other dementias. This percentage rises to close to 50% of all hospice patients and nursing home residents. Whereas mild cognitive impairment may be barely noticeable, many conditions progressively worsen as various forms of dementia. The term *dementia* refers to a group of symptoms that indicate the global loss of cognitive and intellectual functioning. Older adults with dementia may exhibit more severe memory loss, the loss of ability to use language to communicate, the loss of ability to recognize objects or people, loss of movement, and difficulty with planning and organizing information. The most common form of dementia is Alzheimer's disease, which progresses along three stages: early, middle, and late (Rollins 2013, 35–37). General understanding of how the disease presents at these distinct stages is imperative for anyone who provides services in senior living and healthcare settings.

No matter the setting and the intended health benefit, arts programs should take the highly individualized challenges, needs, and preferences of participants into account in planning and implementing the activity. The concept of *person-centered care*, used in residential care facilities, is essentially the same concept as *patient-centered care*, which is used in healthcare facilities. Central to both terms is a commitment to personalizing care, which refers to valuing each patient as a unique individual with different preferences and needs. In addition to excellent medical care, each patient is seeking "respect, kindness, privacy, information, autonomy, choices, care coordination, and inclusion" (Frampton 2009, xxix).

> Care that is person-centered is respectful of and responsive to individual preferences, needs, and values, and ensures that the person's preferences and values guide all decisions....
>
> A person-centered approach to care, in which the recipient of services is the driving force in the development of his or her individual plan, is a de facto standard of quality. Increasingly, healthcare leaders are recognizing the importance of choice, empowerment, and engagement as keys to effective care and positive outcomes in social, emotional, and physical health. (Rollins 2013, viii)

Introduction to Settings of Care for Older Adults in America

As depicted in Figure 8.1, older adults have access to a wide array of senior housing and care programs and facilities. Toward the left of this image, older adults are more independent and more fully integrated in their community; toward the right, they are less independent and less fully integrated in their community. Older adults can move in both directions along this continuum as their needs change, as they recover from injuries or medical treatment, and as they and their families determine the housing and healthcare settings that will best support the well-being and quality of life. Married older adults or domestic partners will not necessarily require the identical support services in different stages of the aging process. Older adults and their family caregivers often need to make difficult decisions as they navigate the complex landscape of senior housing and healthcare options.

Chapter 7 of this book focused on arts programs designed to support the health and well-being of older adults through programs of community-based organizations of all kinds. These programs are designed mainly for those who are living independently at home, and do not have health conditions that limit access to these community-based opportunities. In contrast, Chapter 8 focuses on the design of arts programs in senior living communities and in facilities that provide long-term care (i.e., assisted living and skilled nursing facilities), as well as acute care (i.e., hospitals).

Artists and administrators who design and implement arts programs to serve older adults and caregivers in eldercare facilities should begin with understanding the distinct populations and needs of the people who reside in these settings. They also need to understand the diverse types of senior housing and healthcare facilities, and the general configuration of professional, paraprofessional, and informal caregivers they will be working with in each setting.

Independent Living

The vast majority of Americans over the age of 60 live at home, and most retirement-age adults live either alone or with a spouse or partner. With the aging *baby boomer* population group, the share of all US households age 65 and over is projected to increase from 26% in 2018 to 34% in 2038. Households age 80 and over will grow especially rapidly, to account for 12% of all households by 2038. The share of older adults living alone increases sharply among people in their 80s and beyond, and many individuals in this age range that live alone have higher disability rates and lower incomes than same-age couples (Joint Center for Housing Studies of Harvard University 2019, 2).

> Within the next decade, some 18 million adults will be in their 80s—many living alone and on limited incomes. The need for affordable, accessible housing and in-home supportive services is therefore set to soar. For households in this age group that remain in their

current homes, new transportation alternatives and opportunities for engagement in the community will be critical to their continued ability to live independently. (Joint Center for Housing Studies of Harvard University 2019, 11)

Many innovative programs and community initiatives provide resources to older adults and their caregivers to assist with accommodations that need to be made to the home, such as installing grab bars and widening doors. People find that they can stay at home by hiring some additional housekeeping services, such as yard care and housekeeping, securing transportation through services, such as Uber or Lyft, having groceries delivered, or having meals delivered. Older adults living independently at home have access to a wide array of community organizations, including senior centers and gyms, which offer an array of educational and enrichment programs designed specifically for older adults. The *Village Movement* is growing nationally as a sustainable model for aging in one's community (see giaging.org/issues/the-village-movement/).

In addition to single-family homes, independent older adults have access to age-segregated senior apartment buildings (often referred to as "55+" housing communities) and other "retirement homes" that vary in their availability in communities across the country. Some older adults decide to enter into shared housing arrangements with roommates, as well, although this group is small. Less than 2% of older adults lived with nonrelatives in 2017 (Joint Center for Housing Studies of Harvard University 2019, 3). A living arrangement that consists of two roommates to a group of people who receive an array of services is referred to as *shared* or *congregate* housing (Morris 2014, 408). Independent senior living is known by a number of terms, including *retirement communities, 55+ communities, senior apartments, subsidized senior housing, retirement homes, active senior communities, active adult communities*, and *active senior living*. "Independent senior living is generally appropriate for seniors who are fully or mostly independent, but who may enjoy the companionship of others their age, or who may benefit from amenities such as prepared meals and weekly housekeeping" (A Place for Mom 2015, 5).

Older adults frequently decide to relocate to be closer to family members, and multigenerational living is becoming more common. "Between 2007 and 2017, the number of individuals age 65 and over living in households with at least one adult relative of another generation increased from 6.0 million to 9.8 million to reach 20% of the older population" (Joint Center for Housing Studies of Harvard University 2019, 3). If older relatives move in, the family may consider renovating a single-family house to add an *accessory apartment,* either located inside or attached. With Elder Cottage Housing Opportunity (ECHO) homes, a modular unit is placed temporarily on the property of a family home (Morris 2014, 408). Accessory dwelling units (ADUs), often called an "in-law apartment," "accessory apartment," or a "second unit," have a separate living and sleeping area, a place to cook, and a bathroom. Adding an ADU to a family's home can help the older adult keep their independence (Centers for Medicare and Medicaid Services n.d., 19).

Independent Living to Assisted Living

A change in living arrangements is often precipitated by an older adult's need for additional assistance with activities of daily living (ADL) and instrumental activities of daily living (IADL). *Activities of daily living* refer to daily functions, such as bathing, eating, grooming, dressing, toileting, medication management, getting into a bed or chair, or walking from place to place. *Instrumental activities of daily living* refer to life tasks necessary for maintaining a person's immediate environment. Examples include managing one's medications and finances, using the telephone, preparing meals, laundering, shopping, and house cleaning. An older adult may need help with one or more IADLs and not need help with ADLs. Assessments of ADLs and IADLs are used to measure an older adult's ability to care for himself or herself, and to manage home care tasks. This assessment can be used to help identify needed services and to monitor the progress or deterioration of the older adult (Kernisan and Scott 2021; Pioneer Network 2016, 38; Sowerby 2020, 243–244). The amount of help a person needs with ADLs is "often used as a measure to determine whether he or she meets the requirements for long-term care services in a nursing home as well as government subsidized home- and community-based services" (Pioneer Network 2016, 38).

> The health conditions and personal limitations associated with aging naturally accumulate for older retirees. Twenty-five percent of Americans age 75-84 and 46% of those over 85 have common disabilities around mobility, hearing, or cognition. Forty-four percent of those age 75-84 and 70% of those 85+ have limitations performing activities of daily living, ranging from bathing and dressing to making meals and managing their money. With age also comes an increasing need for assistance, most commonly provided by family members. One in five Americans age 85+ lives in an assisted living or long-term care community. (Edward Jones 2022, 21)

The field of geriatric nursing refers to the importance of the *functional assessment*, which includes a holistic approach to evaluating an older adult's physical, cognitive, and social functions.

> Physical function comprises the individual's current health status in addition to how well the person performs ADLs and IADLs. Cognitive function includes the individual's memory, judgment, and thinking abilities.... Social function involves a psychosocial approach to determine how the individual interacts with the environment and with others. Functional assessment involves evaluating the older adult to determine what the person can do (strengths) and cannot do (deficits)....
>
> Functional assessment assists in setting realistic goals. Cure as a goal is inappropriate for an older individual with chronic, irreversible conditions. The goals for such a patient would be to maximize functional strengths and compensate for deficits to achieve and maintain optimal independence in function. (Sowerby 2020, 243)

For many older adults and their families, a strong desire exists to remain at home even when assistance is required for ADLs and IADLs. An ever-growing array of home- and community-based services exists to support older adults and their family caregivers in this arena of the eldercare spectrum. These healthcare options allow older adults to live at home or in a senior congregant housing setting while still providing important healthcare or personal care support in the community. A community's Aging and Disability Resource Center (ADRC), Area Agency on Aging (AAA), or Center for Independent Living (CIL) can provide valuable information on local resources, and both Medicare and Medicaid may cover some of these services. Community sources, such as volunteer groups, may be found to help with activities, such as shopping and transportation. In short, depending on the older adults' needs, the following kinds of support services may be arranged to help keep them at home:

- Home care, such as cooking, cleaning, or help with other daily activities
- Help with shopping
- Meal programs
- Transportation to medical care
- Transportation to senior centers and community organizations
- Friendly visitor programs
- Help with legal questions, paying bills, and other financial matters
- Home health services, such as physical therapy or minor skilled nursing care (Centers for Medicare and Medicaid Services n.d., 17–18).

On a day-to-day basis, older adults who require support with ADLs and IADLs interact with an array of informal (family) caregivers, paraprofessional caregivers, and professional caregivers. Whereas formal, paid care partners are critical to the support of America's aging population, the number of these individuals is dwarfed by the large number of unpaid, informal care partners found among the family and friends of older adults who provide care. According to the website of the Family Caregiver Alliance, the "typical" American caregiver "is a 46-year-old woman who works outside the home and spends more than 20 hours per week providing unpaid care to her mother." Many caregivers for older adults are also, themselves, older adults.

> About 44 million Americans provide 37 billion hours of unpaid, "informal" care each year for adult family members and friends with chronic illnesses or conditions that prevent them from handling daily activities such as bathing, managing medications or preparing meals on their own. Family caregivers, particularly women, provide over 75% of caregiving support in the United States. In 2007, the estimated economic value of family caregivers' unpaid contributions was at least $375 billion, which is how much it would cost to replace that care with paid services. (caregiver.org)

Informal, unpaid caregivers often work with a limited number of formal paraprofessional caregivers to provide the at-home care needed for older adults. The professional titles of these care partners include certified nursing assistants, home care aides, home health aides, companions, elder assistants, nurses' aides, or orderlies. These individuals may work full-time or part-time, and may be hired privately or through an agency. Paraprofessional care partners may also work in long-term care facilities, assisted living, or skilled nursing setting (Kable 2016, 233). The domain of *home healthcare* refers to various services given to patients at home by registered nurses, licensed practical nurses, therapists, home health aides, or other trained workers. Certified home health agencies often provide and coordinate these services. Home health agencies hire *home health aides*, who are people trained and supervised by a registered nurse to provide basic healthcare and support for ADLs and IADLs. A home health aide is frequently a certified nursing assistant (CNA), which is a person trained and certified to assist individuals with ADLs and IADLs. CNAs are also called a *direct care worker*, a *nursing assistant*, a *personal care assistant*, or an *aide* (Pioneer Network 2016, 40). Federal regulations and accreditation standards from the Joint Commission set minimum levels of quality of care for home healthcare, and the Centers for Medicare and Medicaid Services also have specific requirements for home health agencies (Best-Martini, Weeks, and Wirth 2018, 4).

Thus far, this chapter has discussed the kinds of services that can be arranged for in-home care either in a single-family home or in a senior living community. Two types of services exist that can provide additional community-based support allowing an older adult to live at home while providing more intensive personal care support when informal caregivers are not available.

Adult day services, also known as *adult day care centers*, provide a wide range of daytime social and medical services in a group setting when family caregivers are at work or who need the structure and support offered through a formal program. Socially based programs provide a stimulating, structured setting for older adults who would benefit from reduced time spent in isolation. In contrast,

> Medically-based adult day programs tend to be a low-cost, organized day program consisting of health, social, and recreational services for adults with physical and mental disabilities. Under the direct supervision of professional staff, these programs assist in maintaining or restoring, to the fullest extent possible, an individual's capacity for self-care. These programs usually provide assistance in activities of daily living, cognitive stimulation, leisure activities, and at least one meal each day. (Best-Martini, Weeks, and Wirth 2018, 5)

In participating states, Medicare and Medicaid support the Program of All-Inclusive Care for the Elderly (PACE), which is a distinct national program of adult day services.

> The goal of PACE is to keep participants in the community for as long as it is medically, socially, and financially feasible. The system uses a team of healthcare providers who know the patient and caregivers well, and who can provide complete care for the patient in a

variety of settings, such as at home or in the hospital, an alternative living situation, or an institution. It also allows for adult day care, respite care, transportation, medication coverage, rehabilitation (including maintenance physical and occupational therapy), hearing aids, eyeglasses, and a variety of other benefits. (American Geriatrics Society n.d., 4)

In addition to all the community-based programs that can assist older adults with independent living at home and support older adults and caregivers in shared housing situations, many communities also have excellent senior centers. "Recognized by the Older Americans Act (OAA) as a community focal point, senior centers have become one of the most widely used services among America's older adults. Today, almost 10,000 senior centers serve more than 1 million older adults every day" (National Council on Aging 2022, 1). Senior centers were established for relatively healthy older adults, designed to connect people to community services to help them stay healthy and independent. These programs have traditionally focused on recreation, lectures, and social events. However, with America's population growing older and more diverse, senior centers are evolving in unique ways within each community. "Some are still small social clubs that operate out of a church basement, but others are large, publicly funded organizations, housed in freestanding buildings and offering an array of services, including help with chores, volunteer visitors, homemakers, recreational programs, meals, health screenings, counseling, exercise and computer classes, lectures, and field trips" (Morris 2014, 154). Senior centers are often underutilized by older adults and their family caregivers. These community-based centers are free and open to all older adults and can serve as an excellent source of information and referrals to other local services.

Assisted Living

In Figure 8.1, the assisted living sphere begins when an older adult either requires or seeks out a senior living community that can provide long-term care. Although Figure 8.1 positions assisted living and skilled nursing within the same sphere, there are important differences in the services provided by these facilities that will be discussed in this section. The assisted living sphere also extends into independent living when older adults decide to enter into a *continuing care retirement community* (CCRC). CCRCs, also known as *life plan communities* and *life care centers*, offer a full continuum of senior care services on one campus, including independent living, assisted living, skilled nursing, and memory care. As explained by Morris (2014, 412):

CCRCs . . . are the prix fixe meal on the menu of housing options. They offer it all—from independent living to nursing home care—usually for a fairly hefty price. Many communities accept only people who can get around and live independently. Once a resident has been admitted, however, he has access to a spectrum of care for life. These centers usually include houses and apartments for those who are living independently, and offer these residents a variety of activities, such as golf, swimming, tennis, a gym, lectures, movies, and trips. They also have an assisted living floor or complex, which provides care and services for people who need help with daily tasks such as bathing dressing, and eating. And there is a nursing home unit or wing for residents who are very frail or ill.

The appeal of a continuing care retirement community lies in the fact that older adults are able to remain in a familiar environment regardless of their changing health status. However, CCRCs are neither affordable nor desirable for many older adults, and many other assisted living and skilled nursing facilities exist that support older adults who require support with ADLs and IADLs. Various senior living communities provide *long-term care*, which is a term to describe the kind of care needed to help people with chronic health problems or dementia live as independently as possible (Pioneer Network 2016, 47). Box 8.1 lists several national models of arts-based programs intended to support older adults in diverse settings of long-term care.

"Assisted living facilities provide long-term services and supports (LTSS) to people with functional or cognitive impairments who do not need the level of skilled nursing care provided in nursing homes but cannot live independently" (National Health Policy Forum 2013, 1). Assisted living facilities are currently the fastest-growing long-term care option in the United States, as they provide an important intermediate step for mostly independent older adults with activities of daily living, meals, and housekeeping. Many of these residential settings have a recreation, activities, or programs specialist on staff. Facilities range from large private homes to tall buildings that have several hundred units. Diverse forms of assisted living are provided in *group homes, adult foster care, sheltered housing,* and *residential care.* Unlike

---

Box 8.1 Examples of creative aging programs intended to support older adults in long-term care settings

Program Example—*TimeSlips*
TimeSlips is an evidence-based and award-winning community-based program that "brings joy to elders and their care partners by infusing creativity and meaning-making into care relationships and systems." Certified facilitators use tools of creative expression to develop and lead diverse eldercare communities throughout the world.

Source: timeslips.org

Program Example—*Opening Minds through Art*
Opening Minds through Art is "an award-winning, evidence-based, intergenerational art-making program for people with Alzheimer's disease and other forms of neurocognitive disorders." Trained facilitators and volunteers enable people with dementia to "assume new roles as artists and teachers and leave a legacy of beautiful artwork."

Source: scrippsoma.org

nursing homes, assisted living facilities are not regulated by the federal government. Each state has its own licensing and regulation requirements for assisted living providers, which means that the services provided and quality controls vary by state (American Geriatrics Society n.d., 1–3; A Place for Mom 2015, 8–9).

There is not general consensus on the distinction between assisted living facilities and skilled nursing facilities. Figure 8.1 separates these two categories of senior housing by a shift in the older adult's level of independence. A temporary decrease in functional ability (for example, when recovering from a fall or from a surgery), or a worsening of a chronic illness, or a change in memory care needs may all lead to the need for more medical care by trained medical staff, 24 hours a day. Figure 8.1 places *memory care* facilities, *nursing homes, convalescent homes*, and *rehabilitation centers* all within the skilled nursing group, although there are important differences found among these facilities. The term *skilled nursing* refers to the needs of people who require full-time care, or assistance with most, if not all, activities of daily living (American Seniors Housing Association n.d., 15). The common term used for many different kinds of facilities that provide skilled nursing is *nursing homes*. According to Morris (2014, 415), "about 40 percent of people over the age of 65 will spend at least some time in a nursing home. Most stay for just a few months, recuperating after an injury or illness."

With the ever-increasing number of older adults diagnosed with Alzheimer's disease and dementia, the demand for memory care facilities is growing rapidly. Memory care is often provided in a secure area of an assisted living community or a nursing home, usually on a separate floor or in its own wing. Structured group activities and events are provided by staff specifically trained to care for those with dementia, and most memory care programs include interventions that can decrease the anxieties and support the well-being and safety of people with dementia or other cognitive impairments (American Seniors Housing Association n.d., 12; A Place for Mom 2015, 10–11). Cognitive impairments are common among older adults living in assisted living facilities and nursing homes. In fact, dementia affects at least 50% of nursing home residents (American Geriatrics Society n.d., 11).

Skilled nursing facilities and nursing homes are residential care facilities that provide 24-hour care to people who are unable to care for themselves in other settings or need extensive medical care (Pioneer Network 2016). All such facilities must be licensed by the state in which they operate and must meet additional federal requirements and be certified by the federal government in order to receive reimbursement from Medicare or Medicaid. Facilities that receive federal funds are required to offer the services of a dietetic consultant, a social worker, and an activity director (Dahlkemper 2020b, 160–161). Skilled professionals support a distinct population group within nursing homes. About half of all people who live in nursing homes are age 85 or older, and 72% of residents are women. Around 70% of these residents are single (widowed, divorced, or never married), and many have only a small group of family members and friends for support. More than 80% of nursing home residents need help with three or more ADLs, more than a third have difficulty with hearing or seeing, and about 90% need assistance or supervision with walking. Conditions such as difficulty in being understood and understanding others, incontinence, depression, and inappropriate behaviors are also commonly found in nursing home residents. Roughly 25% of people admitted to skilled nursing facilities remain for three months or less, usually due to completion of rehabilitation or end of life. A little over 20% of residents remain in the facility for an average of 5 years, and about half of all residents spend at least one year in the nursing home (American Geriatrics Society n.d., 10–11).

Nursing homes and skilled nursing facilities are increasingly offering medical services that are similar to those offered in hospitals after acute care has been completed. Medical care provided in these facilities is referred to as *subacute care* (or *transitional care*), which is "a level of medical or rehabilitation care that is less intense than what would be provided in a hospital unit but more than would normally be provided for a resident admitted to a nursing home for long-term placement" (Best-Martini, Weeks, and Wirth 2018, 7–8). Medical care in these facilities includes breathing treatments, support after surgery, wound care, orthopedic care, intravenous therapy, and physical, occupational, and speech therapy. Nursing homes also provide a setting for hospice care and end-of-life care (American Geriatrics Society n.d., 12).

Most assisted living facilities, memory care communities, and nursing homes also offer respite care. *Respite care* typically refers to a short-term stay for the older adult in the senior living community to provide family caregivers with temporary relief. Respite services are typically used by families when the caregiver needs to travel, or just needs a break from caregiving, and when a family is assessing whether a community is right for them or gradually easing their loved one into life at a senior community (A Place for Mom 2015, 21). This service can be particularly valuable for family members caring for people with dementia.

Clinical Care

People of all ages access clinical care throughout their lifetimes, but with the prevalence of chronic diseases as well as sudden changes in health, older adults are likely to receive acute care in clinical settings in a more routine manner. The term *acute care* is used to describe short-term medical care in a doctor's office, a clinic, or a hospital to attend to health problems that are new, quickly worsening, or that result from an accident. A patient's recovery is the primary goal of acute care (Pioneer Network 2016, 38).

In America's healthcare system, most patients experience a continuum of healthcare settings. When a serious illness or accident occurs, most people go to their local hospital. Hospitals differ in their size, location, ownership, and function. The most common type is a general service hospital, but there are additional categories, such as academic centers, for-profit hospitals, children's hospitals, federal hospitals, and psychiatric hospitals. Many additional kinds of hospitals and rehabilitation centers exist to support patients when they require *post-acute care*; that is, when they still require prolonged medical care but no longer need to be an acute care setting in a hospital. These facilities are classified as long-term acute care hospitals, acute rehabilitation hospitals, and traumatic brain injury rehabilitation centers (Rollins et al. 2021, 209–214). In the recovery process, when patients do not require hospital-level medical care but still require services, such as wound care, IV medications, and rehabilitative therapies, patients are located to *subacute care* facilities, such as skilled nursing facilities and nursing homes. The healthcare continuum is complex and often challenging to navigate, as older adult patients move between acute care, post-acute care, and subacute care facilities. Long-term care that may be provided in a patient's home or an assisted living facility also enters into planning for each patient's healthcare needs. Throughout all of these settings, *palliative care* can also be provided. A term that is often incorrectly conflated with hospice care, *palliative care* correctly refers to specialized care for people living with serious illness. It focuses on providing relief from the symptoms and stress of the illness with the goal to improve quality of life for both the patient and the family (National Hospice and Palliative Care Organization n.d.).

A patient enters *hospice care* when cure and recovery are no longer the goals of the healthcare team. This setting of end-of-life care, which provides comprehensive comfort care and support for the family, is discussed in detail in Chapter 9 of this book. With reference to Figure 8.1, however, it is important to include a basic understanding of hospice care here. The term *hospice* refers to both a philosophy of care and to a set of facilities and services. Hospice care may be provided in distinct hospice facilities, but it is most likely provided across the entire range of senior housing settings, including in hospitals, subacute care settings, assisted living facilities, or in the home.

Throughout the healthcare continuum, older adults and their families will encounter a wide array of healthcare professionals. Licensed medical professionals at all levels are regulated by law in their *scope of practice*, which refers to the diagnoses, treatments, and procedures a healthcare provider may perform in each state. Teams of interdisciplinary professionals are in place to meet the needs of older adults in all senior housing and healthcare settings. In acute, post-acute, and subacute clinical settings, older adults and their families interact with a wide array of professionals who are members of the medical team, the nursing team, the rehabilitation team, the administrative team, and the support team (Wiese and Arce 2021, 195–200). With so-called *interprofessional care teams*, healthcare delivery is provided by teams comprising members from several different health professions who bring specialized knowledge, experience, and skills to an older adult's healthcare needs (Askin and Moore 2014, 192–193). In hospitals and clinics, this interprofessional care team comprises physicians, nurses, nurse aides, midlevel practitioners, and allied health professionals (Buchbinder and Buchbinder 2017). The interprofessional team may also include social workers, chaplains, child life specialists, and creative arts therapists. Artists working in the general healthcare

> **Box 8.2 Example of a comprehensive hospital arts program**
>
> **Program Example—*Gifts of Art***
> Gifts of Art at the University of Michigan Medical System (Michigan Medicine) is recognized as one of the first and most comprehensive hospital arts programs in America. A wide array of visual arts and music programs "use the arts to assist and enhance the healing process, reduce stress, support human dignity, and renew the spirit."
> Source: med.umich.edu/goa/

setting to support the environment of care and patient experience may also be members of this interprofessional support team. An example of one of America's largest hospital arts programs is provided in Box 8.2.

Conclusion

This chapter has discussed opportunities for arts programs to be offered throughout the full landscape of residential and clinical care settings for older adults in America. The chapter began with an overview of America's eldercare and healthcare system, a discussion of trends pertaining to healthcare quality and healthcare consumerism, and an introduction to Medicare, Medicaid, and long-term care. Next, the chapter introduced what is meant by *age-friendly* and *person-centered/patient-centered* care. The second half of the chapter systematically discussed the diverse settings of care for older adults in America, as individuals' needs shift from independent living to assisted living to clinical care.

Throughout the community settings discussed in this chapter, arts program leaders will need to work with interprofessional teams to identify challenges and supports for older adults' functional ability. Throughout diverse residential and clinical care settings, specific outcome goals will likely focus on specific physical, cognitive, social, and emotional health outcomes. The evidence base supporting the use of arts to support health goals (see Chapter 4) will likely be very helpful to program leaders in designing, implementing, and evaluating arts programs provided in America's eldercare facilities.

9
Arts Programs in Hospice and End-of-Life Care

Introduction

This chapter extends Chapter 8 with a focus on the specific needs and healthcare settings of patients in hospice and end-of-life care. In this final stage of life, the focus on health and well-being shifts from being patient-centered to being family-centered, where the term *family* refers to the people who are most closely attached to the patient, no matter whether or not they are related. We recognize that personal relationships and family histories are complex and that the nature of any specific family ties will vary. This chapter assumes reasonably healthy family interpersonal dynamics.

The chapter begins with describing what is currently generally understood as a "good death" in the United States within the context of our curative medical model that often disregards the most important needs and developmental tasks of older adults as they near the end of life. This leads to a detailed description of the American hospice system. The focus on spiritual care is a distinct emphasis of hospice, and numerous opportunities exist for the arts to support the spiritual well-being of patients and their families in end-of-life settings. The chapter concludes with emphasizing the use of the arts in programs designed to support reminiscence, legacy, and ritual.

A "Good Death" in America

> Today, advanced medicine wards off death far better than it helps us prepare for peaceful ones. We feel the loss. Many of us hunger to restore a sense of ceremony, community, dignity, and yes, even beauty, to our final passage.... We hope to die well. (Butler 2019, 3)

Technological advances in medicine have dramatically changed the options available to people in the final years, months, and days of life. It is generally understood that most Americans want to spend their final days at home, including being comfortable and surrounded by people who love them. However, many Americans diagnosed with a terminal illness confront a never-ending series of medical technologies that delay death without restoring their health and well-being. The dire situation of medical care for the terminally ill is harshly described by renowned physicians Atul Gawande and Ira Byock:

> You don't have to spend much time with the elderly or those with terminal illness to see how often medicine fails the people it is supposed to help. The waning days of our lives are given over to treatments that adle our brains and sap our bodies for a sliver's chance of benefit. They are spent in institutions—nursing homes and intensive care units—where regimented, anonymous routines cut us off from all the things that matter to us in life. (Gawande 2014, 9)

> At present, just over one-fifth of Americans are at home when they die. Instead, over 30 percent die in nursing homes, where, according to opinion polls, virtually no one says they want to be. Hospitals remain the site of over 50 percent of deaths in most parts of the country, and nearly 30 percent people who die in a hospital spend their last days in an ICU (intensive care unit), where they will likely be sedated or have their arms tied down so they will not pull out breathing tubes, intravenous lines, or catheters. (Byock 2012, 3)

All Americans want a "good death," but our medical system that is focused on treating injuries and diseases often fails older adults and their families at the end of life. The curative model of medicine is deeply entrenched in the United States, with aspects of care focused on physical comfort, dignity, and quality of life often disregarded in healthcare institutions. Older adults correctly fear becoming undignified in how they look and smell, experiencing pain and discomfort, being alone in a sterile and unfamiliar setting, exhausting all of their financial resources, and becoming a burden on their families (Byock 1997, 241–242). People fear the process of dying and the loss of control that it entails, the difficulty that their death presents to their loved ones, and the final transition into the unknown (Koff 1980). Most people envision a "bad death" to be one in which there is no opportunity for advance planning, arranging personal affairs, decreasing the family burden, and saying goodbye. Common concerns of the terminally ill involve regrets, unfinished business, life review, and spiritual matters (Jeffers and Kenny 2009, 107).

The process of dying is unique to each person and is one of the most intimate and vulnerable parts of life (Duncan 2021). In the final months, weeks, and days of life, a person needs information and a sense of control, as well the ability to share their feelings and have a sense of meaning and hope (Wankier 2020). There is no uniform concept of what a "good death" entails; however, there are common factors, such as being free from pain and discomfort, having family present in familiar surroundings, having reconciled relationships, and having a sense of having made a difference in life (Baldwin and Woodhouse 2011; Jeffers and Kenny 2009, 107). It is noteworthy that these aspects of a "good death" have very little to do with medical interventions that may be used to treat physical or cognitive conditions.

For most people today, "death comes only after long medical struggle with an ultimately unstoppable condition—advanced cancer, dementia, Parkinson's disease, progressive organ failure (most commonly the heart, followed in frequency by lungs, kidneys, liver), or else just the accumulating debilities of very old age" (Gawande 2014, 156–157). This final stage of life unfolds in a way that is unique to each person. "Sometimes dying is gentle all the way to the end, and sometimes not. Moments of fear, agitation, confusion, breathlessness, irritability, anger and pain are normal, and although they can often be soothed medically, dying can be wrenching for the dying, and exhausting and distressing to those who are with them" (Butler 2019, 169).

The American healthcare system does an excellent job at prolonging life, but it does not necessarily provide comfort and quality of life for people who are terminally ill. With a curative focus on sustaining life, physicians order new tests and treatments that "can leave someone who is living with an advanced disease physically uncomfortable, feeling lost and confused, not knowing how to get through each day or how to plan for the future" (Byock 2012, 3). As Gawande (2014) explains, our medical system has come to disregard the very important tasks that people seek to take care of as they near the end of life.

> People want to share memories, pass on wisdoms and keepsakes, settle relationships, establish their legacies, make peace with God, and ensure that those who are left behind will be okay. They want to end their stories on their own terms. This role is, observers argue, among life's most important, for both the dying and those left behind. And if it is, the way we deny people this role, out of obtuseness and neglect, is cause for everlasting shame. (Gawande 2014, 249)

As discussed throughout the chapters of this book, the focus of arts programs for older adults should be on supporting individuals' functional ability, i.e., supporting older adults to be able to do the things that matter most to them. "What Matters" is also the foremost "M" of the *4Ms* of age-friendly healthcare systems, discussed in Chapter 8. Person-centered and patient-centered care positions the individual's values, desires, and relationships at the center of healthcare provided to older adults. When a person enters into the final weeks and days of life, "What Matters" to that person and their family must come to the center of all decision-making regarding treatments, medications, and support.

Autonomy manifests in a new way at the end of life. Gawande (2014, 140) contends that there are two concepts of autonomy. The first concept has to do with being able to act independently, free of coercion and limitation. The second concept is autonomy that, Gawande argues, becomes much more important at the end of life. As he puts it, "Whatever the limits and travails we face, we want to retain the autonomy—the freedom—to be the authors of our lives. This is the very marrow of being human." As people become increasingly frail and require more assistance, they still seek to make choices and engage in relationships that are important to them. Supporting autonomy and person-centered care at the end of life suggests the need for specific tasks to be completed in support of quality of life at the end of one's existence. One of America's leading palliative care physicians, Ira Byock, who has

Table 9.1 Developmental landmarks and task work for the end of life

Landmarks	Task Work
Sense of completion with worldly affairs	Transfer of fiscal, legal, and formal social responsibilities
Sense of completion in relationships with community	Closure of multiple social relationships (employment, commerce, organizational, and congregational) Components include: expressions of regret, expressions of forgiveness, acceptance of gratitude and appreciation, leave-taking, and the saying of good-bye
Sense of meaning about one's individual life	Life review The telling of "one's stories" Transmission of knowledge and wisdom
Experienced love of self	Self-acknowledgement Self-forgiveness
Experienced love of others	Acceptance of worthiness
Sense of completion in relationships with family and friends	Reconciliation, fullness of communication, and closure in each of one's important relationships Component tasks include: expressions of regret, expressions of forgiveness and acceptance, expressions of gratitude and appreciation, and expressions of affection. Leave-taking; the saying of good-bye
Acceptance of the finality of life—of one's existence as an individual	Acknowledgement of the totality of personal loss represented by one's dying and experience of personal pain of existential loss Expression of the depth of personal tragedy that dying represents *Decathexis* (emotional withdrawal) from worldly affairs and *cathexis* (emotional connection) with an enduring construct Acceptance of dependency
Sense of a new self (personhood) beyond personal loss	Developing self-awareness in the present
Sense of meaning about life in general	Achieving a sense of awe Recognition of a transcendent realm Developing/achieving a sense of comfort with chaos
Surrender to the transcendent, to the unknown—"letting go"	Note: in pursuit of this landmark, the doer and the task work are one Here, little remains of the ego except the volition to surrender

Source: Byock (2022). "Human Development and Personal Well-Being in Life-Threatening Conditions: Therapeutic Insights and Strategies Derived from Positive Experiences of Individuals and Families." In *Handbook of Psychiatry in Palliative Medicine: Psychosocial Care of the Terminally Ill*, 3rd edition, edited by Harvey Max Chochinov and William Breitbart, 641–667. New York: Oxford University Press. Material from Table 43.1, page 648 reproduced by permission of Ira Byock.

published extensively on end-of-life medical care issues, proposes a framework for various developmental landmarks and task work for the end of life. This table (see Table 9.1) might be best considered as building on the developmental psychology work of Erikson (1982; 1986) and Cohen (2000; 2005), discussed in Chapter 4 of this book.

In America, a "good death" might be most usefully thought of as a process decided upon by a patient and their loved ones, focused on the dying person's sense of comfort and autonomy in attending to these developmental tasks at the end of life (Webb 1997). A patient's ability to "make meaning" of death and dying is suggested to be the key attribute of a good death (Block 2001; Brendel 2007; Daaleman and VandeCreek 2000; Lynn 2001). A sudden death is possible, but increasingly rare. In most cases, older adults will have a considerable period of time in which to focus on what matters most to them at the end and to make meaning of death and dying. The dying person and their loved ones will experience a full range of emotions associated with grief, ranging from denial to anger, bargaining, depression, and acceptance (Kübler-Ross 1969). Anticipatory grief is a common form of grief felt by dying persons and their loved ones before the death occurs (Cascade Health 2019, 192; Reynolds and Botha 2006). A person's loved ones and caregivers also face tremendous challenges in coping with grief after the person's death. The people surrounding the dying person are an important participant group for those designing arts programs in end-of-life settings. "A 'good death' is judged not only by the peace and comfort of the dying person, but by the memories that inhabit, or later haunt, those who survive it" (Butler 2019, 205).

Byock (1997) frames his view of a "good death" to be largely focused on dignity. *Dignity*, as a term, is concerned with how individuals feel, think, and behave in relation to the worth or value of themselves and others (Royal College of Nursing 2008). When dignity is present, people feel autonomous, in control, and comfortable. Byock (1997) explains that we derive dignity from our vigor, our competencies, our accomplishments, and our strengths. Our society reinforces the belief that the loss of our capacities and independence makes us undignified. "The physical signs of disease or advanced age are considered personally degrading, and the body's deterioration, rather than being regarded as an unavoidable human progress, becomes a source of embarrassment" (86). For Byock, dignity can be reconceptualized as the opportunities for personal growth that can still take place through the developmental tasks listed in Table 9.1. He argues, "The waning phase of a person's life deserves to be a time of satisfaction and to stir feelings of self-esteem and self-worth" (86).

Death with Dignity is the name of a state law—first enacted in Oregon in 1994—that legalizes physician-assisted death. The *Death with Dignity Act* "legalizes physician-assisted dying, but specifically prohibits euthanasia, where a physician or other person directly administers the medication to end another's life" (Norman-Eady 2002, 1). Numerous safeguards exist to ensure that terminally ill patients are competent to make the decision and are doing so voluntarily. The Oregon Health Authority regularly publishes reports on data collected pertaining to implementation of this law, including a list of reasons that patients give for wanting to end their lives. The most highly ranked reasons given by terminally ill patients electing physician-assisted death are "loss of dignity," "loss of autonomy," and "the decreasing ability to participate in activities that make life enjoyable" (Weber-Guskar 2019).

As of 2019, nine US states—Oregon, California, Washington, Montana, Colorado, Vermont, Maine, New Jersey, and Hawaii, as well as the District of Columbia—had legal provisions in place that allowed for physician-assisted death. Globally, several other)countries, such as Canada, New Zealand, Spain, Italy, Germany, and the Netherlands, have similar policies in place. Many more countries allow passive euthanasia (i.e., withholding artificial life support, such as a feeding tube or a ventilator). This rise of laws that give individual patients the right to not prolong pain and suffering at the end of life speaks to very human desires for lifelong autonomy, dignity, and control.

The American Hospice System

"Hospice, the philosophy and practice of caring for people who are approaching death, is based on the belief that death is a natural and inevitable part of life and that at some point, rather than battling illness and fighting death at any cost, all efforts should be focused on enhancing what life remains" (Morris 2014, 544). Supporting patients and their families in having a "good death" is at the heart of the global hospice movement,[1] which began in the United Kingdom in the 1960s and came to the United States in the 1970s. *Hospice* is a healthcare movement, an approach to care, a set of interdisciplinary practices, and a compilation of community-based facilities all focused on providing care to people facing death. An excellent description of hospice is quoted by Connor (2009) from the National Hospice and Palliative Care Organization:

> Hospice provides support and care for persons in the last phases of an incurable disease so that they may live as fully and as comfortably as possible. Hospice recognizes that the dying process is part of the normal process of living and focuses on enhancing the quality of remaining life. Hospice affirms life and neither hastens nor postpones death. Hospice exists in the hope and belief that through appropriate care, and the promotion of a caring community sensitive to their needs, that individuals and their families may be free to attain a degree of satisfaction in preparation for death. Hospice recognizes that human growth and development can be a lifelong process. Hospice seeks to preserve and promote the inherent potential for growth within individuals and families during the last phase of life. (Connor 2009, 1–2)

At its core, hospice is a philosophy of care for the terminally ill. An interdisciplinary team provides care in response to the physical, social, spiritual, and emotional needs of individuals and their families as they move through the final stages of an illness, the dying process, and the bereavement period. In hospice, curative medical care is replaced by holistic healthcare designed to address all aspects of a dying person's health and well-being. A patient is eligible for Medicare-supported hospice services when they are diagnosed as having a terminal illness and an expected lifespan of six months. Healthcare experts note that referrals to hospice care often come too late for a person to benefit the most from the end-of-life care provided by these programs, although this is improving. Currently, at least 50% of dying patients are referred to hospice, but most often not for the full period of time when they and their families would have benefited the most (Wankier 2020, 149). As Butler (2019, 143–144) explains, "People who get hospice care early in their disease often continue to work, see friends, and do what matters to them. Paradoxically, their well-being often immediately improves once they get good pain management, and less stressful, better-coordinated medical care at home."

The hospice movement has taken root in communities across the United States as a new ideal for how we and our loved ones can experience a "good death." Hospice programs, services, facilities, and personnel vary from one community to the next, but the ten characteristics listed in Table 9.2 are considered to be essential components of every hospice program. Together, these characteristics reflect basic principles of hospice, such as the patient and the family jointly being the "unit of care," the interdisciplinary and coordinated model of family-centered care, and the focus on controlling pain and symptoms rather than any heroic curative efforts.

In Table 9.2 and in much of the literature and professional practice pertaining to end-of-life care, terms such as *hospice*, *palliative*, and *comfort care* tend to become conflated. These terms actually have distinct meanings; for example, all hospice care is palliative in nature, but not all palliative care is hospice care. Clarification of the distinctions among these terms is available online from the National Hospice and Palliative Care Organization (see caringinfo.org) and summarized in Table 9.3. Similar to other areas of the healthcare continuum, these diverse arenas of care may be most useful to consider along the progression of a serious illness. When a diagnosis is given, people want to pursue treatment options and the potential for a cure with curative medical interventions. As treatment continues and symptoms become more severe, palliative care can be introduced. When the diagnosis arrives that a cure is no longer possible, hospice care is provided for the final period of life. Hospice care includes bereavement support, which continues for the family after a loved one's death.

All areas of end-of-life care listed in Table 9.3 have the potential for enhancement through carefully designed arts programs and activities, as noted in the table. Throughout this continuum of care, creative arts therapists and expressive arts therapists have the opportunity to provide mental health services as part of the clinical team. In all areas of care, artists working in healthcare facilities and community health settings can also provide a range of arts programs and activities that support the patient, family, and caregivers. Artists working in end-of-life settings should

Table 9.2 Ten characteristics of hospice programs in America

	Characteristic of Hospice Care
The patient and family are the unit of care.	Hospices do not admit a patient in isolation. They see each patient as part of a family system. Often the family's needs are equal to or greater than the dying person's. *Family* means those bonded to the patient by blood or emotional ties, i.e., the patient's most immediate attachment network.
Care is provided in the home and in inpatient facilities.	The philosophy of palliative care is to allow people to die where they want. Most people prefer to be cared for in their homes; others need or choose to be in a facility. Hospice and palliative care should be available to patients in all settings.
Symptom management is the focus of treatment.	Hospice patients understand at some level that there is no definitive cure for their illnesses. They seek relief from pain and other symptoms of terminal illness. Palliative care is directed at treating the symptoms, not curing the disease.
Palliative care treats the whole person.	People are not just physical. Palliative care is designed to address physical social, psychological, spiritual, and practical needs of patients with life-limiting illness.
Services are available 24 hours a day, 7 days a week.	People die and have problems at all hours of the day and night. Services must be available 24 hours a day, 7 days a week, including weekends and at 2:00 a.m., if needed.
Palliative care is interdisciplinary.	The hospice team draws on the skills of people in a variety of disciplines who work collaboratively in meeting the patients' various needs. The hospice and palliative care team includes physicians, nurses, social workers and other mental health professionals, chaplains, therapists, pharmacists, and volunteers.
Palliative care is physician directed.	The patient's attending physician must determine that the patient has an incurable condition with a limited life expectancy and must order all palliative care delivered. The hospice medical director oversees the care of all hospice patients and supplements the services of the attending physician. Palliative care specialists can provide consultative services valuable to the attending physician.
Volunteers are an integral part of hospice and palliative care.	Those at the end of life respond uniquely to volunteers. Volunteers work with people facing death out of human concern. Often, they have experienced death in their lives and can appreciate how hard it is for families to handle difficult situations.
Palliative care is community-based care and is provided without regard to ability to pay.	Hospice and palliative care services meet the needs of people with life-limiting illness within their communities and do not deny services on the basis of inability to pay. When reimbursement is exhausted, care to the patient is not diminished.
Bereavement services are provided to families on the basis of need.	Hospice provides a program of bereavement support to all families for at least a year following a patient's death. Palliative care programs also need to provide bereavement services. Grief counseling is begun before a patient's death. Bereavement support may also be extended to those grieving in the community at large, and all bereavement support should be based on need and expressed desire for help.

Source: Reproduced from pages 7–8 of *Hospice and Palliative Care: The Essential Guide*, 2nd edition, edited by Stephen R. Connor, published by Routledge. © Taylor & Francis Group, 2009. Reproduced by arrangement with Taylor & Francis Group.

Table 9.3 Different types of care provided in end-of-life settings

Type of Care	Description	Implications for Arts Programs
Curative care	*Curative or therapeutic care* refers to treatments and therapies provided to a patient with the main intent of fully resolving an illness or condition	*Purpose:* support physical, cognitive, social, and emotional health outcomes *Place:* treatment and recovery in acute, post-acute, and subacute healthcare facilities, and at home *People:* the patient, caregivers, artists, creative arts therapists, and expressive arts therapists *Participation:* active, inventive, and interpretive
Palliative care	*Palliative care* focuses on easing pain and discomfort, reducing stress, and helping people have the highest quality of life possible. Palliative care is appropriate at any stage of a serious illness and can be provided alongside curative care	*Purpose:* support all dimensions of health and well-being *Place:* any residential or healthcare facility and at home *People:* the patient, family, caregivers, artists, creative arts therapists, and expressive arts therapists *Participation:* active, receptive, inventive, interpretive, curatorial, and observational
Hospice care	*Hospice care* focuses on quality of life when a cure is no longer possible, or the burdens of treatment outweigh the benefits Hospice care is an interdisciplinary, team-oriented approach to expert medical care, pain management, and emotional and spiritual support expressly tailored to the patient's and family's wishes and needs	*Purpose:* focus on support of social and emotional health and the five dimensions of well-being (evaluative, eudemonic, affective, hedonic, and cultural) for both the patient and the family *Place:* any residential or healthcare facility and at home *People:* the patient, family, caregivers, hospice interprofessional team, hospice volunteers, artists, creative arts therapists, and expressive arts therapists *Participation:* active, receptive, inventive, interpretive, curatorial, observational, and ambient. A focus on reminiscence, legacy, and ritual
Comfort care	*Comfort care* is a term commonly used to mean end-of-life care Comfort care is the designation given by physician when a patient moves away from life-prolonging or curative therapies; and comfort-focused therapies, symptom management, and pain management are provided. Comfort care is only one part of hospice care	*Purpose:* focus on the patient's symptom management (such as pain reduction) *Place:* any residential or healthcare facility and at home *People:* the patient, family, caregivers, hospice interprofessional team, hospice volunteers, artists, creative arts therapists, and expressive arts therapists *Participation:* receptive, interpretive, curatorial, observational, and ambient. A focus on reminiscence, legacy, and ritual

Table 9.3 Continued

Type of Care	Description	Implications for Arts Programs
Bereavement care	As part of the Medicare hospice benefit, family of a hospice patient has access to bereavement care for 13 months following the death of the patient. Services can range from support groups, memorial services, informational and educational resources, counseling, and referrals to appropriate therapeutic and community resources. Hospice bereavement programs facilitate healthy grieving and aim to prevent grief-related health and mental health problems	*Purpose:* psychosocial and spiritual support of family, focusing on grief counseling and well-being *Place:* community-based groups and at home *People:* the deceased person's family and friends, caregivers, hospice team members (especially chaplains, mental health, and social work professionals), artists, creative arts therapists, and expressive arts therapists *Participation:* active, inventive, interpretive, and curatorial. A focus on reminiscence, legacy, and ritual

Source of definitions: National Hospice and Palliative Care Organization (caringinfo.org)

be trained specifically in providing programs, services, and care for this vulnerable population group (Albright and Carytsas 2021; Lee, McIlfatrick, and Fitzpatrick 2021a; 2021b).

When an older adult is in the phase of life when curative medical interventions are no longer desired—a period of time that can last for days, weeks, months, or years—there are still numerous ways to support their health and well-being. The patient and their family still have the opportunity for considerable growth in attending to the tasks listed in Table 9.1. However, the first task of end-of-life care must be to control physical pain and other symptoms of illness. "Without relief from pain or other distressing physical symptoms, the patient cannot attend to other concerns. Once freed from physical distress, the patient is able to attend to psychological, emotional, interpersonal, social, and transcendent or spiritual matters" (Connor 2009, 177).

It is in the domains of psychosocial and spiritual care that the arts have the opportunity to offer the most benefit to dying people and their families. As introduced in Chapter 4 of this book, the arts can support four areas of health outcomes (physical, cognitive, social, and emotional) and five dimensions of well-being outcomes (evaluative, eudemonic, affective, hedonic, and cultural). At the end of life, desired outcomes for arts programs suggested by Byock's list of developmental landmarks (see Table 9.1) are social and emotional health, as well as both evaluative and eudemonic well-being. Older adults who are dying focus mainly on their relationships and the meaning of their lives. Assuming that physical symptoms have been controlled, the dying person is driven to address these important needs of the mind and the spirit.

Arts in Spiritual Care

In the whole-person care provided by hospice, arts programs have a special role to perform as part of spiritual care. "Spiritual care is for many patients the most important aspect of care, as it is focused on their most important fears and opportunities for growth" (Connor 2009, 176). In 1990, a Spiritual Care Work Group of an International Work Group on Death, Dying and Bereavement developed a useful set of assumptions and principles of spiritual care at the end of life. This work group defined *spirituality* as "concerned with the transcendental, inspirational, and existential way to live one's life, as well as in a fundamental and profound sense, with the person as a human being" (Cascade Health 2019, 169). "The word spirituality, while often thought of as interchangeable with religion, actually encompasses religion itself as just one of several forms of meaning making" (Brendel 2007, 38). A more expansive definition of *spirituality* is offered by Jeffers and Kenny (2009, 100):

> Spirituality, often expressed in a cultural or religious tradition, is the constituent of people's being that provides the framework for their understanding of life's purpose and meaning, their sense of well-being, and their relationships with humanity and the divine. It is a determining factor in how individuals explain and react to life events. Spirituality is an important element in patients' and families' ability to find answers to questions of meaning and purpose in life as well as enable them to cope with illness, dying and death. Spirituality is an indispensable component of quality, holistic healthcare.

Hospice professionals consider spirituality very broadly, based on five major assumptions:

1. Each person has a spiritual dimension.
2. A spiritual orientation influences mental, emotional, and physical responses to dying and bereavement.
3. Facing a terminal illness, death, or bereavement can be a stimulus for spiritual growth.
4. In a multicultural society, a person's spiritual nature is expressed in religious and philosophical beliefs and practices that differ widely, depending upon one's race, gender, class, ethnic heritage, and experience.
5. Spirituality has many faces and can be expressed and enhanced in a variety of ways formal and informal, religious and secular. (Cascade Health 2019, 169)

When providing care to the terminally ill, it is common to encounter spiritual pain. Extreme sadness, loneliness, and fear can manifest as a variety of intense emotions, such as the sense of hopelessness, isolation, vulnerability, unfairness, unworthiness, abandonment, punishment, confusion, and meaninglessness. Indeed, there is no question that the process of dying is a terribly stressful part of life for the dying person and their family, even in situations that are seen as providing relief from suffering and peace. Effective spiritual care acknowledges this deep spiritual anguish, but also puts forward that a "good death" can be something else for the family, too. In hospice, the spiritual care team can support the dying person in achieving their final growth tasks at the end of life and the family in their grief throughout this period and after the death.

The end-of-life developmental landmarks that might be best targeted by arts programs will focus on facilitating the completion of relationships; reinforcing a sense of life satisfaction; providing opportunities for the expression of love, forgiveness, and gratitude; and supporting the dying person in "letting go" at the very end. Many of these end-of-life care needs will be led by interprofessional team members who are specially trained chaplains and mental health providers, but all of the developmental landmarks listed in Table 9.1 can include the expressive arts. In this way, these programs will support evaluative, eudemonic, and cultural well-being in end-of-life settings. The arts offer an effective tool for locating a person in the present moment to foster joy, discovery, and social connections—all of which can provide deep satisfaction and have profound spiritual impacts. The arts also offer unique methods of reviewing one's life, of telling stories, of leaving legacies, and of commemorating important life transitions. In the context of spiritual care provided in hospice settings, the arts can provide programs of reminiscence, legacy, and ritual that are tremendously effective in helping families find meaning and purpose, a sense of well-being, and a connection with the divine. These three types of programs support the dying person at the end of life and can provide enormous support to the family throughout the bereavement process.

As a terminal illness progresses, the physical and psychosocial losses may intensify for both the patient and their family. *Grief* is the natural response to loss; anticipatory grief begins during a protracted illness and continues for the family beyond the death of the patient. *Grief* is defined as "a multifaceted response to death and losses of all kinds, including emotional (affective), psychological (cognitive and behavioural), social and physical reactions" (Waldrop 2007, 198). Within end-of-life settings, the main focus of psychospiritual care for the patient's loved ones is *bereavement*, which refers to the grief process associated with losing a significant person to death (Woodhouse 2011).

Extensive literature on grief and bereavement is available in the fields of counseling and psychology (for example, see Bonnano 2009; Bartocci 2000; Elison and McGonigle 2003; Grollman 1995), many of which build upon Kübler-Ross's landmark study on the stages of grief, *On Death and Dying*, published in 1969. Most Americans are generally aware of what is considered to be a "normal" progression through these stages, beginning with denial and ending with acceptance and hope. However, there is tremendous variation in the emotions and responses that we have to a loved one's death, including anger, relief, regret, guilt, disorientation, and loneliness (Morris 2014, 568–575). Americans also tend to minimize the impact of grief on family members' capacity to fully function in everyday life, and there are few cultural rituals or community ties that can be relied upon to support people in their bereavement process. "People are expected to be back to work or school and ready to function within a few days of the death. The average person thinks it should only take days or weeks to get over a death. The reality is that the first days or weeks are a period of shock. It is only after this time passes that a person is able to begin to deal with the loss" (Conner 2009, 76).

Spiritual care provided within hospice programs provides tremendous community-based support to family members throughout the phases of grief in the year following the death. To be able to recover from losing a loved one, people need to accept the fact of the loss, experience the pain of grief, adjust to life without the deceased, and reinvest in one's own interests in life (Cascade Health 2019, 196–197). Those providing psychospiritual care to dying people and their families can enable people experiencing the pain of grief to do the following:

- Connect with their wholeness
- Make peace with, discover, and respect the coherence of their life's story
- Seek reconciliation with alienated family, friends
- Give and receive love, forgiveness, appreciation, and expressions of affection
- Say good-byes (or, if you prefer, *au revoir*)
- Complete relationships with others
- Assure continuity, relationship, and meaning beyond death (Pastan 1999, 14).

From this discussion, it follows that arts practitioners who seek to develop supportive programs for end-of-life care would be wise to focus on activities that help family and friends meaningfully connect with each other, communicate feelings with each other, say good-bye, and contribute to an individualized sense of holistic well-being. Three distinct and powerful ways that the arts can contribute to end-of-life care are through programs that focus on reminiscence, legacy, and ritual.

Arts for Reminiscence, Legacy, and Ritual

In hospice care, a focus on quality of life is paramount. The patient will likely need support for pain reduction, personal expression, and increased family interactions, all of which can be addressed through arts interventions and activities. Through their scoping survey of existing research on the role of the arts in palliative and end-of-life care, Lee, McIlfatrick, and Fitzpatrick (2021a) conclude that the arts can be effectively used to address quality of life and meaning making, as well as to provide nonpharmacological symptom management. "Arts engagement aligns with palliative care aims by engaging creativity and expression thereby enhancing well-being through discovery, agency, meaning, connection with others, and a sense of self beyond illness" (2). Perhaps most significantly, the arts provide myriad ways in which patients, as well as their families, friends, and caregivers, can find their voice to express a life story and its significance. Through words, images, movements, and sounds, it is possible to share our stories and transform our way of experiencing events surrounding us. The arts can offer a way for people to discover meaning and purpose in what is happening to them through creating legacies and staying connected to others (Hartley 2014; Jarrett 2007).

> Arts practitioners in palliative care are present at a crucial transition in the lives of most families, shaped by powerful emotions and new personal, relationship and social experiences for patients and their families. . . . Using the creative arts with people facing death, dying and all that this brings is not just about offering them a "nice time" or about "taking their minds off their illness." The arts bring with them possibilities: possibilities for motivation and growth, for coping and change, for self-actualisation and self-realisation. They also offer possibilities to make sense of situations, to create something of value and to leave something behind which says "this was me, this is what my life has meant." (Hartley and Payne 2008, 13–14)

Hartley and Payne (2008, 187) suggest that artists providing care to patients approaching the end of life and their families focus on a few basic principles, such as offering choice in the nature of arts participation, encouraging shared arts experiences, focusing on patients' motivations for specific arts projects, and giving objects created through the arts activity to friends and family. Creative writing, visual arts, musical expression, and other arts activities offer myriad ways in which dying people and their families can achieve an array of uses and benefits listed in Box 9.1. All of these arts-based approaches to care also support the list of developmental tasks for the end of life listed in Table 9.1, clearly buoying the well-being of the patient, family, and caregivers.

One main cluster of arts-based activities that provide support to terminally ill patients and their families consists of activities that focus on life review and reminiscence. "As patients grapple with end-of-life issues, the wish to sum up one's life as meaningful often asserts itself" (Safrai 2013, 123). People have a pressing need to evaluate the meaning and purpose of their lives and to tell their life story to family and friends. Patients may choose to tell their stories in languages that are verbal, artistic, or even embodied. Words, photographs, creative works of visual arts, and music are all common ways in which terminally ill people seek to articulate their personal identity, share memories, and communicate their stories with others (Walter 2012). Narrative approaches to facilitating the telling, hearing, and honoring of a life story offer excellent opportunities for interpersonal connections. "Patients facing illness at the end of a long life may engage in a retrospective reappraisal and seek to maintain connection with others; there is often a sense of acceptance and spiritual well-being. These are powerful, poignant, and compelling stories, and patients can be helped to author a meaningful final chapter consistent with their life goals" (Romanoff and Thompson 2006, 310).

Box 9.1 Uses and benefits of psychosocial support programs in hospice and end-of-life care

Vulnerable people at the end of life, who also include family members, [caregivers], those who are bereaved, and communities that are afraid of death and dying, need access to services that can:

- Support them to articulate themselves both to themselves and to others
- Enable them to know that they do still matter
- Bring them together with others outside of sometimes suffocating and controlling networks of families and friends
- Challenge the experience of "social death," which can accompany a terminal diagnosis
- Engage with others outside of the "numbness" of illness and symptoms
- Develop and sustain confident and compassionate communities
- Enable them to create products and legacy and support "remembering"
- Give people the opportunity to surprise themselves and to develop empowerment and self-efficacy
- Help to redress the balance of taking and giving
- Offer people a variety of frameworks and contexts to understand and confront difficult things
- Enable people to create order out of chaos
- Support people to put relationships right—to discover ways of saying "I am sorry" or "I love you" and so forth.

Source: Hartley (2014, 258–259)

The telling of life stories and the expression of one's identity often lead to a second cluster of arts-based care in end-of-life settings, which focuses on legacy. The creation and gifting of legacy art can meaningfully connect the dying person with loved ones through bonds that continue past death. *Legacy art* may best be understood as an artwork created for a specific person, either by or of the person who is dying. The work is intended to serve as a reminder of a person who died. Creative activities at the end of life often result in objects—such as crafts, poems, memoirs, and music recordings—that serve as legacy gifts to family and friends. In addition to supporting relationships between the terminally ill patient and his/her family, the art project also provides the opportunity for the patient to reimagine their individual role as a creative agent (Gray 2022, 123–124). Perhaps most importantly, the creation and gifting of legacy art can provide a tremendous support to patients and their families in the completion of their relationships and in communicating complex emotions, such as love, forgiveness, regret, appreciation, and gratitude.

The third cluster of arts activities and programs that can support those in hospice care focuses on ritual. There is, of course, nothing new in the human need for rituals associated with death, burial, and bereavement. In the mid-1400s, a booklet titled *Ars Moriendi* was first published on the art of dying in the Christian faith, which provided rituals and procedures for dying a good death. The publication was subsequently translated into all the major languages of Europe and remained enormously influential for centuries. Many other religious groups created their own "death manuals" in the four centuries that followed; however, the modern, industrial era has largely forgotten our ancestors' approaches to the rituals of death (Butler 2019, 3–5). That said, even though there is no present-day cultural script to death and dying (Green 2008), a range of rituals, customs, and traditions exist in diverse social groups, families, and faith-based communities.

Many dying people and their families find it helpful to hold one or more ceremonies as they come to terms with the loss they are experiencing, and these ceremonies may take form in a wide spectrum of rituals involving the arts.

> The ceremonies of death are for everyone present, not only the dying. Consider setting up an informal altar or table with flowers, photographs, music and candles and, if you wish, religious images. Bring in beauty. Consider the senses: sight touch, smell, and sound.
> (Butler 2019, 181)

The ceremonies can be cocurated with the patient and, when the patient is actively dying, arts-based support should emphasize passive reception on the part of the patient. It is generally understood that hearing is the last sense to go; therefore, the human voice and music can play a particularly important role at the very end of life. Box 9.2 provides an example of a music program intended specifically for end-of-life care. All rituals and ceremonies held by families in end-of-life settings will be highly individualized and best facilitated through partnerships with social work, mental health, and spiritual care professionals on the interprofessional hospice care team.

No matter what the form is, ceremonies are a social ritual that can provide immense psychospiritual benefit to the dying patient and their family. The death of a loved one is almost always a period of instability and transition in family life, during which rituals can provide meaningful structures of stability and order. Rituals are a potent means of symbolic expression that can affirm continuity and connection for families across space and time, serve as vehicles for transformation of meaning,

---

Box 9.2 Example of an arts program intended for end-of-life care

Program Example—*Music Thanatology*
Music thanatology is a subspecialty of palliative care in which specially trained and certified professionals use "the harp and voice at the bedside to lovingly serve the physical, emotional and spiritual needs of the dying and their loved ones with prescriptive music."

Source: mtai.org

and create bridges for transition to the unknown (Romanoff and Thompson 2006, 312–313). Ceremonies and rituals at the end of life provide comfort, support well-being, and allow patients to face their final stage of existence with dignity (Clements-Cortés 2016). As presented in Table 9.1, the very last task in life is spiritual in nature. At the time of death, a person needs to "let go" and "surrender to the transcendent."

> At the edge of the transcendent—in the midst of "letting go"—a person who has completed the work of development does not disintegrate in dying. Rather, she *dissolves* out of life, becoming increasing ephemeral—less dense or corporeal—but no less integrated, in the passage from life. Personhood becomes gauzy and translucent. Having completed and released the various realms and spheres of his or her previous self, the person who is surrendering to the transcendent is little more than the process itself. "Letting go" is all that is left. (Byock 1997, 238)

The arts as a whole, and music in particular, have been deeply embedded in spiritual traditions, ceremonies, and rituals for centuries. As Byock (1997, 237) explains, "Art is a natural expression and evocation of the deeper self that for many people provides another important source of guidance within the transcendent or spiritual aspects of life." The most meaningful use of the arts at the very end of life is likely found in the integration of music, photographs, and other artwork in the solemn rituals and ceremonies that support the entire family before, at, and after the death.

Conclusion

This chapter provided an overview of the American hospice system and offered strategies for integrating the arts in end-of-life care to support patients and families in attending to the final developmental tasks of life. In particular, this chapter emphasized a potential role for the arts in supporting spiritual care through programs focused on reminiscence, legacy, and ritual.

The final chapter of this book (Chapter 10) builds on all of the information provided in Chapters 1–9 to articulate main findings from our research and recommendations for activating the *arts in healthy aging* ecosystem and the *8Ps Framework for Arts in Healthy Aging*.

10
Advancing Public Policy and Professional Practice for the *Arts in Healthy Aging*

Introduction

Arts in Healthy Aging addresses *why* and *how* purposefully designed arts programs can support the health and well-being of older adults throughout the natural aging process. This final chapter builds on all the material presented in the preceding nine chapters to articulate strategies for mobilizing and advancing the *arts in healthy aging* field across the United States and by extension internationally as appropriate to context.

The first four chapters of this book introduced key concepts that are essential to the field of *creative aging* policy and practice. Chapter 1 opened with a demographic profile of older adults in America and identified the urgent need for programs and services that are designed to support healthy aging. The chapter introduced America's arts and culture sector as an instrument that can be used to support the health and well-being of older adults throughout the aging process. The chapter also introduced the current state of *creative aging* policy and practice, as well as the interdisciplinary domains of knowledge that intersect across arts policy and management, health policy and management, and aging policy and management.

Chapter 2 built on this introduction with a systems-thinking approach to offer foundational concepts in how the creative aging field "works" to provide individual and societal benefits. The chapter positioned *arts in healthy aging* as a subfield of *arts in health* and unpacked the distinct needs of older adults as a targeted population group for arts in health services. Engaging in arts and culture was addressed as a basic human need, and a detailed framework for understanding *choice-based arts participation* was provided. This in-depth discussion of arts participation led to an introduction to logic model thinking, where the inputs of *arts infrastructure* and *education* can be activated, leading to the potential for positive outcomes for both individuals and communities. These benefits accrue as distinct societal impacts, best understood as *public purposes of the arts*. Chapter 2 concluded with an introduction to the elements of our *8Ps Framework for Arts in Healthy Aging*.

Chapters 3–9 alternated in their foci on either big-picture systems and institutional structures or on the individual experiences of older adults. They also alternated in their analytical focus on the arts infrastructure or education as essential inputs in the creative aging logic model. Chapters 3 and 4 expanded on elements introduced in the first two chapters to provide essential history, policy strategies, foundational concepts, and analytical frames for the creative aging field as a whole.

Chapter 3 presented the evolution of creative aging policy in America across the past 50 years. Reflecting changing conceptions of aging over these five decades, *arts and aging* policy has manifested in four distinct, but overlapping, strategies. The National Endowment for the Arts (NEA) served as a national leader in the first three. The first strategy (from 1973 to 1995) can be characterized as an advocacy movement in the arts that addressed *older adults as a special constituency*. During the second strategy, the *arts actively sought a place on the aging policy agenda* as manifested in the four White House Conferences on Aging (WHCoAs) from 1981 to 2015. The third strategy (from 2000 to 2015) featured a shift in positioning *creative aging as a program asset for health policy*. The national policy landscape changed after 2015, after the last White House Council on Aging, and after the dissolution of the National Center for Creative Aging (NCCA) in 2018. Since 2015, the *creative aging* field across the United States has become increasingly decentralized into a loosely linked network with little leadership at the national level. This historical analysis of *arts and aging* policy strategies and the relevant institutional infrastructure in America laid the foundation for the discussion of our recommendations for activating the *arts in healthy aging* ecosystem, provided in the pages that follow.

Chapter 4 offered analytical models that undergird the mechanics of how the arts support health and well-being outcomes in older adults. The chapter began with discussing the *sociocultural context of older adults' health and well-being* and basic concepts and theories regarding *human development in late life*. This material led to an analysis of diverse motivations that older adults may have to choose to participate in creative aging programs and activities. The focus of the chapter then shifted to an in-depth analysis of *how the arts can support distinct health and well-being outcomes* in all phases of the natural aging process. This section offered crucial information for developing metrics for *outputs* and *outcomes* within any logic model used in the creative aging field. This analysis critiqued the basic logic model framework that leads in a linear direction from inputs to outputs to outcomes as inadequate for addressing the distinct needs of older adults. Chapter 4 concluded with a robust presentation of basic design elements that can be manipulated for developing *arts in healthy aging* programs intended to support diverse health and well-being outcomes.

Chapters 5–7 turned to essential theorization necessary for *reimagining the role of arts-based lifelong learning for older adults* across America's communities. In addressing the dearth of conceptual and theoretical resources that are crucial to advance arts education for older adults, these chapters drew extensively from cognate academic fields, such as folklore, gerontology, and education. Chapter 5 discussed theories supporting creativity, culture, folk groups, and the arts in the life course from an arts educator's perspective. The chapter ended with articulating theoretical foundations that support key recommendations for designing and implementing learner-centered arts education programs. Chapter 6 built on this theoretical foundation to explicate the current state of lifelong learning theory and practice. Professional competencies regarding working with older adults were identified and critiqued. *Transformative learning theory* was introduced in depth in this chapter, leading to a set of recommendations for using this theoretical base in developing arts-based educational programs for older adults.

Chapter 7 brought the concepts, theories, and recommendations from the preceding two chapters to life in discussing community-based organizations' arts programs for healthy aging. In this chapter, arts programs were analyzed within a full array of community-based resources for older adults. The chapter emphasized strategies for developing *person-centered approaches* to participation and for contributing to an *age-friendly community* infrastructure. This chapter focused on developing recommendations for structuring arts-based resources for the health and well-being of older adults that are fully integrated in their community.

The vast majority (roughly 95%) of America's older adults are "aging in place" in their communities. Although many arts-based community resources may be designed to support older adults in achieving their lifelong learning goals and in supporting social and emotional health and well-being, community-based creative aging programs can also provide important health benefits. The emphasis on designing arts programs to support concrete physical, cognitive, and emotional health outcomes becomes even more important when programs are provided to older adults in senior living facilities and clinical settings. Chapter 8 provided a comprehensive overview of ways in which arts programs can be used in diverse eldercare settings and healthcare facilities, supporting both *age-friendly healthcare* and *person-centered care* that are essential to the success of these institutions. Chapter 9 built on this material to offer recommendations for how arts programs can support hospice and end-of-life care.

The preceding nine chapters in this book systematically analyzed and presented why and how arts-based lifelong learning and diverse forms of arts participation can contribute to the health and well-being of older adults in America. We have engaged interdisciplinary bodies of scholarship, evidence from the field, and numerous program examples to support the recommendations made throughout these chapters regarding the intentional design of arts programs for older adults. We have offered a rigorous analysis of the evolution of America's relevant public policies, institutional infrastructure, and arts and culture sector; we have also developed theoretical foundations to help advance this field of policy and professional practice.

Now, Chapter 10 brings this knowledge together to articulate main findings from our research, our ideas for activating *America's arts in healthy aging* ecosystem at the national level, and our recommendations for activating the *8Ps Framework for Arts in Healthy Aging*.

Findings on the Current State of *Creative Aging* Policy and Practice in America

The many research findings identified throughout the chapters of this book can be clustered together in the four major themes explained below: (1) societal trends that are building the demand for healthy aging and quality of life in the retirement years; (2) implications of these trends for *arts in healthy aging* programs; (3) significant gaps in extant scholarship that will need to be addressed to help advance the *arts in healthy aging* movement; and (4) challenges currently being faced within public policy and the institutional infrastructure supporting the field.

1. Societal trends that are building the demand for healthy aging and quality of life in the retirement years

The large wave of aging *baby boomers* is setting new expectations for what the aging process can be and is demanding high-quality programs and services to support their quality of life and well-being. Older adults' expectations and desires change as physical, cognitive, and social challenges shift throughout the three phases of late adulthood: early (age 60–75), middle (age 75–85) and late (age 85+). Importantly, the baby boom generation is only the first of the coming cohorts of retirees who are expected to live much longer and much more active lives, forever changing Americans' conceptions of what it means to be an older adult. People are reimagining the retirement years as a time of growth and development, and as a new chapter in life that involves much more than leisure, rest, and recreation. There is a rapidly growing demand for products, services, and community-based support systems that will allow people to age in place in their homes. Across the United States and internationally, public health initiatives increasingly promote *healthy aging* and *age-friendly communities*. Within this framework of dramatic change in older adults' expectations and demands for their quality of life after the age of 60, artists and arts organizations everywhere have tremendous opportunities to expand services to support lifelong learning, life enrichment activities, and concrete health goals. The *arts in healthy aging* field is well positioned for rapid expansion and growth.

However, while some demographic sectors within America's 60+ population group are experiencing a high quality of life throughout a long lifespan, tremendous inequity is found in the health and longevity of older Americans. The recent reduction in life expectancy has been most severe among historically marginalized racial and ethnic communities. As discussed throughout many chapters of this book, significant inequity exists in access to healthcare, programs, and services that support older adults' health and well-being. Moreover, preliminary research on the COVID-19 pandemic indicates that older adults have learned to identify themselves as part of a high-risk group and as responsible for taking health and social measures to avoid illness as much as possible. There is also evidence that the pandemic has reinforced negative images of aging, as well as revived ageism in the media and internalized it among older adults (Gallistl et al. 2022).

2. Implications of these trends for *arts in healthy aging* programs

To address the changing needs and demands for a healthy longevity among America's older adults, *arts in healthy aging* programs should focus on key program design elements that will support health and well-being outcomes throughout the natural aging process. This book has provided numerous tools for systematically developing arts-based lifelong learning programs and arts participation programs that will support health goals across four dimensions (physical, cognitive, social, and emotional) and well-being outcomes in five domains (evaluative, eudemonic, affective, hedonic, and cultural). With whole-person healthcare consisting of a focus on the body, mind, and spirit, *arts in healthy aging* policy and practice should consider health and well-being outcomes to go far beyond the focus of curative medical care. Purposefully designed arts programs can be used as instruments to support specific, concrete, and measurable outcomes in all of these areas.

Much has been written in this book about *functional ability* being the key variable for older adults to achieve healthy longevity. Older adults will pursue different motivations and have differing capacities in their arts participation throughout late adulthood. The field of *creative aging* has come to be understood as creativity throughout the lifespan, and within a "creative longevity" construct. Older adults demonstrate multi-sector engagement across the arts and culture sector and choose to participate in arts activities in highly variable patterns. As such, the primary focus of any arts program designed to support the health and well-being of older adults must place the individual participant—i.e., the needs, desires, motivations, capacity, and goals of the older adult—at the center. Effective *arts in healthy aging* programs must be person-centered, patient-centered, or family-centered at their core.

3. Significant gaps in extant scholarship that will need to be addressed to help advance the *arts in healthy aging* movement

Given the growth of America's older adult population and the economic strength of this group, it is remarkable how scant the body of existing scholarship is in addressing lifelong learning and arts participation opportunities for those aged 60+. The dearth in scholarship is particularly notable in the field of *arts-based lifelong learning*, where an urgent need and demand exists in the field for reconceptualizing arts-based education for older adults. However, the field of *creative aging* is wide open for research and scholarship across all areas of inquiry.

Because most older adults are "aging in place" in their communities, focusing on the sociocultural context of health and well-being should be central to advancing policy and practice in the *creative aging* field. At present, literature on older adults as both a demand constituency and a resource constituency for their communities is virtually nonexistent. Extraordinary opportunities exist for organizations throughout a community to work with older adults as assets for other programs. However, as nonprofit arts organizations have become increasingly professionalized, volunteer opportunities for meaningful activities have narrowed and faced pressure to become more aware of diversity and equity accessibility. In addition, arts administrators can see older adults as a shrinking audience group that needs to be replaced by younger audiences rather than as valued patrons to be retained across their lifespans with programs tailored to address specific well-being and enrichment goals that have developed among today's older adult population.

In general, recent scholarship on the arts and older adults is splintered across multiple fields where scholars may not read or encounter each other; namely, across the fields of knowledge and practice that inform arts policy and management, health policy and management, aging policy and management, and education policy and management. When researching *arts in healthy aging*, it is imperative to consider theories, concepts, and practices in the context of other scholarship in cognate fields. At present, this is rarely done because of the highly siloed nature of the diverse academic fields and professions that comprise the field. Much of the scholarship associated with the arts, health, and well-being currently emerges from the social sciences. Recognizing that there are multiple ways of knowing, scholarship from the arts and humanities should be encouraged. Additional relevant and important research will emerge from indigenous studies, disability studies, ethnic studies, and women's studies. Partnerships between researchers and older adults as coresearchers must be encouraged. Because the field of *arts and aging* now has a history of roughly 50 years, historical research is important for chronicling the field's history and conceptual frameworks with associated initiatives shaping it. In general, research to date has made significant progress in providing evidence of the efficacy of arts programming to addressing and improving the quality of life—physically, mentally, socially, and emotionally—and established a "proof-of-concept" status. Going forward, research may need to focus more on how to take these ideas and practices to scale, toward sustainability, and how to engage older adults more in determining the range of choices provided throughout the *arts in healthy aging* field.

The past 50 years of research, convenings, and reports focused on connecting the arts with aging services have led to a great deal of activity led by practitioners in the *creative aging* domain. Program models have been readily shared and replicated across the country, but a solid national mapping process on the distribution, scale, and patterns of these programs has not taken place. A major barrier to date has been the lack of analytical models to be used in such a mapping initiative, and we hope that this book will aid future researchers in this regard. The 1985-1996 MacArthur Research Network on Successful Aging (https://www.macfound.org/networks/past-research-network-on-successful-aging) may serve as a good model for developing a well-coordinated national research agenda on *arts in healthy aging*.

A first national mapping effort might be formed as a collaborative research project that resembles the mapping initiatives that have been undertaken to map the creative and cultural industries. The goal of this effort would be to identify the current geographic and organizational location of *arts in healthy aging* program offerings, the general design or type of the programs, and the arts disciplines or content emphasized. Just as mapping of the creative and cultural industries blurs boundaries between the nonprofit arts and the commercial arts, mapping *arts in healthy aging* could attract partnerships not only across the arts but also with the humanities, residential communities, healthcare facilities, lifelong learning organizations, libraries, and community-based organizations, such as senior centers. Such a mapping initiative could enhance the *arts in healthy aging* network; provide evidence of the distribution, availability, and variety of programming available; inform age-friendly community planning efforts; provide a database that could produce local information for residents; and make the presence and value of *arts in healthy aging* more visible to the general public.

4. Challenges currently being faced within public policy and the institutional infrastructure supporting the field

A prime challenge facing the broad issue of *arts and aging* is a need to rethink and reconceive the character of the policy issue. Throughout the long trajectory of *arts and aging* policy over the past five decades, the development of solutions in practice has led to a better understanding of the complexity and interdisciplinary nature of the field, the variety of actors at multiple levels of government and sectors of society, the need for space for customizing programs and services, and attention to contextual factors that are involved.[1] These characteristics match the description of what are called "wicked policy problems." In recent years, policy research concerning wicked policy problems has turned its attention to what is called "second-generation" approaches that focus on the role of leadership, particularly adaptive and collaborative leadership, to the possible effectiveness of networks in managing such problems, and to making better use of public policy concepts, such as problem framing, policy design capacity, and policy contexts (Ferlie et al. 2011; Head and Alford 2015; Head 2019). Such "second-generation" policy analysis concerns seem to be emerging as arts and aging policy challenges. Developing the capacity to employ these concepts in rethinking the implications of the emerging frame of *arts in healthy aging* is a challenge that will impact policy formulation and advocacy, practice, communications, and partnerships.

In the United States, the current national landscape of public policy and institutions supporting the *creative aging* movement is in disarray. Since 1975, the arts have attempted multiple strategies and multiple policy frames to position themselves as a resource for the health of older adults. The arts have done so by attaching themselves to larger policy domains, chasing the ever-changing trends that have emerged over the decades in an attempt to enter into the policy agenda of the aging sector or the health sector. As discussed in Chapter 3, each of these strategies has proven to be inadequate, or took place at the wrong time, or was simply not the right political alignment. Over the past 50 years, none of these policy strategies has led to a major step forward on the national agenda. Also, there has never been a national strategy for consistent training and certification of professionals who will actually design and implement arts programs for older adults. The field is in urgent need of professionalization, entrepreneurial programming, and policy leadership.

This book has introduced various dimensions of complexity involved in the arts and culture sector infrastructure, aging issues and needs of older adults, eldercare and healthcare facilities that can benefit from arts programming, arts-based lifelong learning approaches and practices, and a framework for understanding choice-based arts participation of older adults across a natural aging process. The book has explored the evolution of alternative policy framings of the *arts and aging*, arguing that the network of fields engaged in this arena seems to be expanding—from arts, health, and aging to also include lifelong learning, age-friendly city planning, and higher education, among other fields. Greater coordination efforts will be needed to bring this diffuse network together more effectively.

A second challenge is finding or creating a "focusing event" that allows the *arts in healthy aging* issue to open a policy window of opportunity on the health, the aging, the adult education, and/or the arts policy agendas. Historically, this was the function of the WHCoA, but both congressional and presidential support and attentiveness to the recommendations of the WHCoA have waned and become polarized. Currently, given the divided partisan control of the houses of Congress, President Biden's policy agenda faces uncertain prospects. Indeed, the Biden Presidency seems to have already used the device of a WHCoA to convene the White House Conference on Hunger, Nutrition, and Health on September 28, 2022. This conference touched on related problems of older adults, and the agenda considered the whole of society across generations. Conference results launched a nationwide call to action and a package of new public, business, academic, and philanthropic initiatives to end hunger and reduce diet-related disease (White House Briefing Room 2022). The National Council on Aging (NCOA) submitted a set of recommendations on the needs of older adults, but it made no mention of the arts.

Overall, the *arts and aging* field that has formed over the past five decades lacks a coordinated policy community. An emergent policy community has gradually taken shape as a network of ever-changing "stakeholders" and "thought-leaders" from a wide array of organizations. However, there is no full agreement within this group on the "creative aging" construct for the field, nor is there a set of common values and goals across the policy community. The *arts and aging* field to date has focused on three policy communities (i.e., on arts, health, and aging) that each have their own policy agenda, and there is little incentive within the larger policy domains to focus on the arts. The fourth crucial policy field, that of lifelong learning, has largely been absent from these gatherings. In addition, the large policy fields of health, aging, and adult education each compete within themselves for policy priorities and resources. For example, in the education field, lifelong learning for older adults must compete with the massive K-12 public education emphasis of the field. Although convenings having to do with the role of the arts in supporting older adults have taken place on a frequent basis, reports from these gatherings have rarely translated into public policy on the national agenda. Across the field's four policy domains, *creative aging* has not yet been able to garner policy agenda status, political clout, or adequate resources.

Nationally, the *creative aging* policy initiative began losing steam with the unsuccessful attempt to secure a place on the national aging agenda with the 2015 WHCoA. Subsequently, the field has been in limbo since 2015 and in a heightened state of churn since the dissolution of the NCCA in 2018. In addition, the chaos of COVID-19 throughout 2020, 2021, and 2022 slowed progress in coalition-building and policy advocacy related to *arts in healthy aging*. It also prompted the resurgence of the image of older adults as frail, vulnerable, and needing to take measures to protect themselves from social contact. Coming out of the pandemic, most federal and state agencies and organizations have been trying to reinvent themselves, and across all sectors, there is a major national focus on diversity, equity, and inclusion priorities. In 2023, at the time of writing this book, the field of *arts in healthy aging* policy and practice embraces a broad set of stakeholders trying to provide leadership within specific areas that comprise the field. There is no centralized body coordinating initiatives across the field, and there is no organization at present with the authority to "speak" for the *arts in healthy aging* field as a whole. Through convenings and publications, the field appears to be attempting to refocus itself, but it is not apparent which national entity may be in a position to serve as the lead coordinator of the networked governance structure that is taking shape organically. A significant challenge exists for the field to transform its current weak advocacy alliance with the health and aging policy communities in order to mobilize an effective *arts in healthy aging* advocacy campaign.

It is the right time for the *creative aging* movement to reposition itself as the *arts in healthy aging* advocacy and implementation network. This shift in terminology more appropriately demonstrates the crucial linkages among the four fields of policy and practice that comprise this field: the arts, health, aging, and lifelong learning. Also, with the global focus on *healthy aging* as an explicit priority, positioning the arts as a resource to support public health goals across the United States and internationally would be a wise step for policy and program advocacy. Within this policy frame, *creative aging* is positioned as an implementation mechanism rather than a policy issue and it is likely to be one of many types of *arts in healthy aging* programming tools.

Our four main research findings, discussed above, are congruent with those articulated in reports from the two most recent national convenings of thought-leaders in the creative aging field. These reports summarize discussions from *The Summit on Creativity and Aging in America* in 2015 (NEA 2016a) and from a series of virtual forums in the winter of 2022 (Saunders et al. 2022). The 2015 summit was the last time that the NEA and the NCCA sought to attach the arts to health and aging policy agenda-setting processes within a WHCoA. In 2015, the creative aging field also explicitly emphasized the design professions (in addition to the traditional arts segments) as important to advancing the field. The summit was structured by groups focused on three main topics: age-friendly community design, health and wellness and the arts, and lifelong learning and engagement in the arts. The "needs, issues, and barriers" and the "viable solutions" from the executive summary of the report are provided in Box 10.1. Perhaps most relevant to our focus on advancing the *arts in healthy aging* ecosystem is the list of four "recommendations for the field" provided in this report. These are identified as recommendations (1) to launch a national campaign to reframe arts services for older adults; (2) to build a leadership council of arts, aging, health, and community services organizations; (3) to convene a summit of social entrepreneurs in technology and community services; and (4) to establish a research network to build an evidence base to support development of arts and design products and aging services (NEA 2016a, 36). These action steps would all be important to structuring a national advocacy coalition, and all echo the findings and recommendations articulated in this chapter.

In the winter of 2022, Georgetown University's Aging & Health Program, the Kennedy Center Office of Accessibility and VSA, and Mather jointly hosted a series of virtual forums that convened stakeholders from academic institutions (including one of this book's authors), senior living facilities, government agencies, arts organizations, and philanthropic organizations. These *Creative Aging Innovation Forums* were intended to "reveal themes and ideas for the next stage of development in the world of Creative Aging" (Saunders et al. 2022, 3). The convenings led to "identification of three themes: autonomy, mastery, and belonging; access and inclusion; and redefining care systems through a strengths-based lens" (3). The report outlines potential, ideas, and program examples for "interdisciplinary creative problem-solving" in four areas of focus, namely, "research and innovation, systems-level change, infrastructure and spaces, and intergenerational lifelong learning" (3). The list of participants in these forums included mainly academics and professionals who are already members of the established confederation of individuals and organizations invested in the *creative aging* construct of the field (27–28). These convenings and the resulting report served as a positive step in reactivating the national conversation regarding the potential for the arts to support healthy aging, but the focus of this group did not appear to extend beyond once again sharing ideas and model programs within a core group of people. Similarly, findings from a national survey published by Culture Track in 2022, titled *Untapped Opportunity: Older Americans & the Arts*, are noteworthy in that—after decades of conversations about the important role the

Box 10.1 Findings from the 2015 Summit on Creativity and Aging in America

Needs, Issues, and Barriers
- Negative attitudes toward and perceptions about older adults pose a barrier to ensuring that they enjoy a high quality of life. There is a need for a cultural change to combat agism and call attention to the health and wellness benefits of lifelong arts learning and age-friendly design.
- There is a need to establish leadership within the public, private, and nonprofit sectors, in order to promote, across the aging spectrum, equitable access to life enrichment through the arts, design to improve quality of life, and affordable options that promote social inclusion and choice in how and where to age.
- To support the growing older adult demographic, we need new business models for producing high-quality arts and design products and services for older adults. There needs to be a sustainable infrastructure within the public and private sectors to encourage the development of these new business models and to take them to scale.
- There is a lack of research collaborations that recognize the benefits of the arts and design in supporting the health and well-being of older people and the communities in which they live.

Viable Solutions
- Promote culture change within all federal programs and services, and create incentives for the private sector to help overcome negative attitudes toward older adults. By reframing issues to focus on the opportunities that longevity provides to *all* generations, we can give attention to developing services, with innovative input from the arts and design, in order to form an intentional continuum of service across the lifespan.
- Provide leadership across government agencies and develop incentives for the private sector to advocate for access to arts and design services and activities that are high quality and affordable. Provide social inclusion and options in living environments to lower the risk of people having to receive care in an institution when this is not their setting of choice.
- Encourage partnerships and the leveraging of resources in both the public and private sectors to build infrastructure to support products and services in the arts and design. Help bring these models to scale to meet the growing demand from people living longer and healthier lives in communities of their choice.
- Fund interdisciplinary research and collaborations between artists, biomedical and behavioral researchers, public health policymakers, and social entrepreneurs to expand the evidence base that validates arts and design interventions for older adults. Particular focus should be placed on the effects of arts and design on the health and well-being of older people, brain health, management of chronic diseases, caregiving, and the development of the design of homes and other age-friendly community services.

Source: From the National Endowment for the Arts' Publication *The Summit on Creativity and Aging* (2016a, 7–8)

arts can play in supporting the health and well-being of older adults—the field is still considered to be one of "untapped opportunity."

In summary, we argue that the time is right to break the cycle of repeating the same conversations over and over among the same group of people. The *arts in healthy aging* ecosystem must now restructure itself as an advocacy coalition across the four fields of the arts, health, aging, and adult education if it is to be in position to advance national policy in the future. Furthermore, this advocacy coalition will need to rely less on national officials in Congress, the White House, federal agencies, or interested private foundations acting as patrons of political action. Instead, this advocacy coalition must take the prime responsibility for formulating and advocating for an *arts in healthy aging* policy. A grassroots constituency of older adults must also coalesce into an interest group that needs to have its voice heard and to have a seat at the table. Finally, the general public could benefit from a public education effort to understand the value and impact that a well-designed, organized, funded, and implemented *arts in healthy aging* policy could have across generations.

Activating the *Arts in Healthy Aging* Ecosystem

From roughly 2000 to 2015, the community of policy and practice focused on engaging the arts for the health and well-being of older adults coalesced around a shared concept of *creative aging*. This shared framing of the field was effectively voiced by the NCCA, which served as a national hub, convener, advocate, and advisory council until its dissolution in 2018. Since then, no other organization has replaced the NCCA, although several other entities have developed national roles in advancing certain elements of the field. Figure 10.1 illustrates the American *creative aging* national institutional ecosystem that had taken shape by 2018.

The complex 2018 network illustrated in Figure 10.1 positions a set of key agencies and nonprofits at the top: the NEA, the Institute of Museum and Library Services (IMLS), the United States (US) Administration on Aging, and the NCOA. These entities were linked in their support of *creative aging* and also connected with important national initiatives led by other entities. The NEA had one of the most important roles in linking with *creative aging* initiatives led by other key organizations, including the American Assembly of Museums (AAM), the National Assembly of State Arts Agencies (NASAA), and the National Guild for Community Arts Education. Several specific programs had come to the forefront of national attention in the *creative aging* arena and were "franchised" across the country. These included *EngAGE, TimeSlips, Lifetime Arts*, and *Catalyzing Creative Aging*. By 2018, Aroha Philanthropies had become the main national foundation supporter of *creative aging* programs and services across the nation.

There may have been a missed opportunity when the NCCA was disbanded in 2018. The NCCA was legally an independent nonprofit organization that had been designated as a service organization; it may have been possible to transform the

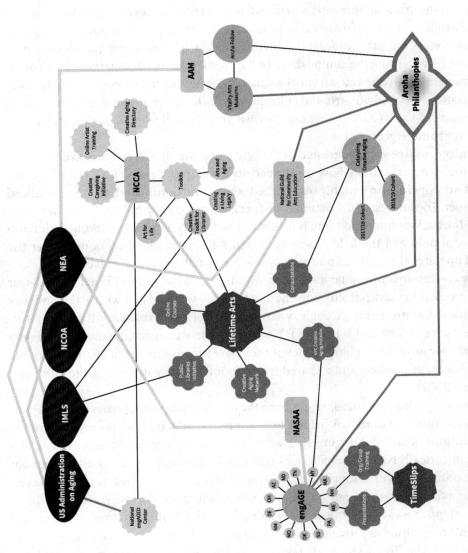

Figure 10.1 America's creative aging institutional infrastructure in 2018
Illustration by Elizabeth Howald and Stephanie McCarthy.

NCCA into a national membership association designed to serve as a peak association that brought together related organizations and individuals concerned with arts, culture, humanities, and lifelong learning services for healthy aging. When mature, such an organization could provide field services, such as public representation and advocacy; convenings, publications, and communications; professional development programs; and other network enhancing activities. There are precedents in the arts and humanities fields where government agencies and foundations have funded professional associations to open their memberships not only to skilled practitioners but also to organizations in a field's infrastructure (as illustrated in Figure 1.3 regarding the composition of the creative sector). Similarly, such an organization might evolve into an entity similar to the NCOA to represent a variety of organizations that provide arts and cultural services for older adults. Perhaps changing the name of the NCCA to *National Council for Arts in Healthy Aging* might signal a different and larger mission.

Indeed, a large gap was created in the field when the NCCA was dissolved in 2018. Although other entities have continued to develop programs and resources, the field now operates in a highly fragmented, siloed, uncoordinated, and decentralized manner. The interest of the national partners listed at the top of Figure 10.1 has faded into the background, and there is no centralized entity at present seeking to develop national policy in the field. There is no centralized coordinating body; rather the field operates at present in mutual autonomy through a division of labor that essentially creates organizational leadership within "fiefdoms" of specific activity. Absent an agreed-upon centralized coordinating body for the field as a whole, the best way to proceed at present is through systems of network governance and collaborative governance (Wang and Ran 2021). However, loosely connected networks can only "work" for advancing public policy if they have a common set of shared goals, assumptions, and beliefs and a shared framing of the policy domain (Goldsmith and Eggers 2004).

In considering options for structuring the *arts in healthy aging* ecosystem as it continues to move forward, it is helpful to assess the distinct roles and constraints of the institutions depicted in Figure 10.1, as well as those of some additional entities that have historically had a national voice in developing the field. As discussed throughout this book, the NEA has long been at the forefront of policy and infrastructure development for the *arts and aging*. However, since the time of the last WHCoA in 2015, it has stepped away from the *arts and aging* field. The Administration on Aging and the IMLS continue to provide national resources only for very specific programs, as does the AAM. The NASAA has taken on a national role in advancing the field, but their work in building and coordinating relevant programs within state arts agencies is largely driven by funding provided by Aroha Philanthropies. NASAA focuses national attention on a specific model of a creative aging program, namely, the distinct Lifetime Arts model of sequential lifelong learning. In 2022, Aroha Philanthropies changed its name to "E.A. Michelson Philanthropy"; the foundation continues to support the same entities and programs. Three major "implementation hubs" currently exist for specific *creative aging* programs across the country: NASAA, Lifetime Arts, and TimeSlips.

There is potential for several national entities not included in Figure 10.1 to play an important national role as the field moves forward. Americans for the Arts has had a distinct focus on advocating for the *arts in health* in the past, but the organization has changed their leadership, health and aging have retreated on their agenda, and they have generally retrenched as an institution. The National Organization for Arts in Health (NOAH), a small membership association established in 2016, is a likely partner for the *arts in healthy aging*, but the organization currently has very limited resources. The NCOA offers the potential to reengage in the *arts in healthy aging* domain, but this well-established national nonprofit has other priority areas regarding aging policy and programs. The John F. Kennedy Center for the Performing Arts has held a role in the field for decades, but *creative aging* is not their central function. The President's Committee on the Arts and the Humanities might offer a short-term locus for coordinating national ecosystem development for the *arts in healthy aging*, but it is important to note that this is not a statutory organization. There are currently no obvious congressional leaders engaging in this field, and there is no longer even a committee focused on aging within the US House of Representatives.

Indeed, the current American landscape for developing *arts in healthy aging* policy and professional practice looks uncertain. For decades, this loosely structured policy community of "thought-leaders," "stakeholders," and "professionals" has been talking among themselves, sharing information and program examples, formulating recommendations, and reinforcing the "creative aging" framing of the field. Notably, these gatherings over the past decades usually lacked participation from experts and groups specifically focused on the needs of older adults (i.e., representatives from the AARP, the NCOA, and other advocates for older adults). Older adults attending meetings, convenings, symposia, and forums routinely state a position of "nothing for us without us." Convenings must offer ample opportunities for older adults to help shape advocacy efforts either as individuals or collectively through organizations representing their interests.

For decades, the *arts and aging* policy community has tried to advance the field nationally, but their strategies for doing so were never successful because this group acted as a confederation of shared but distinct interests rather than a coalition of shared beliefs and policy priorities. Chapter 3 documents the repeated attempts and failures of the arts policy community over the past 50 years to attach itself successfully to either the health policy or the aging policy sector. It is fair to say that, at present, there is no conceivable possibility for *arts in healthy aging* to move onto the national policy agenda. However, there *is* potential for the community of practice that exists in this field to begin to restructure itself so that it has a chance of greater public policy success in the future.

In order to advance the *arts in healthy aging* ecosystem, the field needs to structure itself as an *advocacy coalition*. It is important to remember that public policies "are made by *policy subsystems* consisting of actors dealing with a public problem" (Howlett and Ramesh 1995, 51). Diverse theories and models are used by scholars to analyze the structure and function of these policy subsystems, ranging from *subgovernments* and *iron triangles* to *issue networks, policy networks, policy communities,* and *advocacy coalitions*. The *Advocacy Coalition Framework* (ACF) developed by Paul Sabatier and his colleagues was created to study complex activities of policy actors in policy subsystems. "An advocacy coalition consists of actors from a variety of public and private institutions at all levels of government who share a set of basic beliefs (policy goals plus causal and other perceptions) and who seek to manipulate the rules, budgets, and personnel of government institutions in order to achieve these goals over time" (Jenkins-Smith and Sabatier 1993, 5). In other words, the ACF refers to "collections of actors sharing similar beliefs and coordinating their actions to achieve political goals" (Matti and Sanstrom 2011, 386). An in-depth discussion of the ACF model and how it may be applied to analyze the policy subsystem in the American domain of *arts in healthy aging* extends beyond the scope of this chapter. However, basic theory associated with the ACF can be very helpful in informing our recommendations for structuring the *arts in healthy aging* ecosystem in the coming years.

> An advocacy coalition includes both state and societal actors at the national, sub-national, and local levels of government. It also cleverly combines the role of knowledge and interest in the policy process. The actors come together for reasons of common beliefs, often based on their knowledge of the public problem they share and their common interests. The core of their belief system, consisting of views on the nature of human-kind and some desired state of affairs, is quite stable and holds the coalition together. All those in an advocacy coalition participate in the policy process in order to use the government machinery to pursue their (self-serving) goals. (Howlett and Ramesh 1995, 127)

By thinking of the *arts in healthy aging* policy community as an advocacy coalition, and an advocacy coalition comprising representation from four enormous fields (i.e., arts, health, aging, and adult education) as requisite for advancing national policy, the challenges of structuring a coalition infrastructure come into focus. Kingdon (1984; 2010) argues that a window of opportunity for policy change occurs when the three streams of problems, policy solutions, and politics intersect. Even when the political environment appears inhospitable to the field, there is still much that can be done to "build the window" so that it can be opened when the three streams of problems, policies, and politics do actually align at some point in the future. Building a window that can be opened at the appropriate time requires building an effective advocacy coalition, which in this case must include influential champions who are skilled in forging strategic alliances across the four relevant policy domains. Box 10.2 lists concrete ideas for next steps that might be taken by core agencies, organizations, and associations across the four core constituencies comprising *arts in healthy aging*. Appendix B lists an array of representative organizations that have a relevant national focus and who could be a member of this advocacy coalition.

Box 10.2 Our ideas for specific action steps that might be taken by national organizations to move toward building an advocacy coalition for the *arts in healthy aging*

National Endowment for the Arts (NEA)—support national research and convenings focused on advancing the *arts in healthy aging* field. Support should include developing professionalization in the *arts in healthy aging* field.

President's Committee on the Arts and the Humanities (PCAH)—identify *arts in healthy aging* as an important field requiring national policy development. This body might also be able to strengthen relevant collaboration between public and private stakeholders.

Americans for the Arts (AFTA)—develop national advocacy capacity and network in *arts in healthy aging*, building especially on the organization's long historical focus on arts education. Build advocacy in arts-based lifelong learning, arts in health, and *arts in healthy aging*. Develop an Arts Advocacy Day for *arts in healthy aging* or other focusing event(s).

National Assembly of State Arts Agencies (NASAA)—build on and expand broader *arts in healthy aging* capacity (that is, expand beyond specific types of lifelong learning) at state levels. Work with the regional arts agencies to help facilitate subnational advocacy coalitions.

National Guild for Community Arts Education, Lifetime Arts, and **Teaching Artists Guild**—focus on developing capacity and professionalization in *arts-based lifelong learning*. Partner with NASAA in doing so.

National Council on Aging (NCOA)—reinvest in the arts as an instrument for supporting older adults through Senior Centers programming and as linked to the Aging Mastery Program.

National Organization for Arts in Health (NOAH)—specifically name *arts in healthy aging* as a subfield of *arts in health* and begin to strategize for national engagement and professionalization in this area.

National Arts Service Organizations—The AAM has a major interest in *arts for healthy aging*. We recommend that a coalition be developed to include the other national arts service organizations (League of American Orchestras, Theatre Communications Group, Opera America, Chorus America, Dance USA, etc.). The national service organizations might also establish internal affinity groups focused on *arts for healthy aging* activities among their members. Also, it is well past time for a national survey of arts managers to ask about their perceptions and assumptions about older Americans' needs and priorities for arts programming.

The **John F. Kennedy Center for the Performing Arts** and the **Smithsonian Institution**—as America's national flagship performing arts and visual arts organizations located in Washington, DC, these two organizations might help to convene gatherings of arts organizations interested in developing programming for older adults, and might serve as important repositories of resources and training in the performing arts and museum fields. As nationally focused arts organizations, both the Kennedy Center and the Smithsonian should also model effective practices in program development and program implementation (both intergenerational and more specialized) for older adults.

Professional Associations associated with **Arts Education**, such as the National Art Education Association and the National Association for Music Education, among others. In cooperation with experts and organizations focusing on adult education and lifelong learning, these organizations should begin to systematically address professionalization of the field and curricular initiatives.

Grantmakers in the Arts, Grantmakers In Health, and **Grantmakers In Aging**—we recommend that these three entities collaborate in identifying funding streams and business models to support *arts in healthy aging* programming and advocacy coalition development.

Professional Associations of the Allied Health Professions, such as Recreational Therapy, Occupational Therapy, Disability Studies, Social Work, Creative Arts Therapies, Expressive Arts Therapy, Home Health Care, Senior Living, Nursing, and Healthcare Administration, among others. These domains of scholarship and professional practice should pursue a mutually reinforcing relationship with the other entities in this list. These professionals can align their fields with *arts in healthy aging* in providing services to older adults and serve as champions and advocates of these fields nationally.

Advocates for Older Adults, such as groups within AARP, NCOA, and the Alzheimer's Association—these groups' perspectives are important because they represent the constituency being served and they can inform the *arts in healthy aging* field from the perspective of the needs of older adults. At present, there is no national advocacy group representing older Americans that is focused on advancing *arts in healthy aging*. Advancing the field requires both grasstops and grassroots advocacy at all levels (national, state, and local).

It is clear that America's *arts in healthy aging* ecosystem requires new framing as an advocacy coalition in order to lay the foundation for advancing the field over time. This advocacy coalition must engage partners from across the arts, health, aging, and adult education sectors of society. It is imperative for this advocacy coalition to have a convergence of agreement regarding the problem identification, policy solution options, and the coalition's institutional infrastructure. An effective national advocacy coalition also needs funding, research to inform professional practices, and skilled advocates. In the *arts in healthy aging* field, a strategic coalition of relevant agencies, organizations, and professional associations at all levels (national, state, and local) will need to gradually structure itself through shared goals and beliefs in order to successfully enter onto the national policy agenda. A national entity will need to serve as the coordinating body for this advocacy coalition, and significant resources will be required to transform this coalition into an effective organization. Large investment in this national initiative on the part of major foundations will be required for building the national strategic alliance, and state and local investment in *arts in healthy aging* initiatives will be necessary for developing grassroots advocacy and program development.

An effective structure for the *policy* and *partnerships* "Ps" of the *8Ps Framework for Arts in Healthy Aging* is essential for the field to advance. The role of *policy* and *partnerships* is further clarified by these elements' depiction in the logic model we have developed for activating the field.

Activating the *8Ps Framework for Arts in Healthy Aging*

The chapters of this book have systematically framed what is needed across the United States for the *arts in healthy aging* movement to advance as a field of research and professional practice. The *8Ps Framework for Arts in Healthy Aging*, first introduced in Chapter 2 (see Figure 2.5), has been repeatedly referenced. In this final chapter of the book, we now turn to the issue of what scholars and practitioners can "do" to activate this 8Ps framework. Activating this framework can and should take place nationally, internationally, locally, regionally, and within specific institutions, agencies, and organizations.

Our research findings emphasize the importance of designing and implementing arts programs for older adults that are *person-centered* at their core. Highly individualized programs will take the goals, motivations, and capacity of the participants into account. Older adults will actively determine their own desired program outcomes, select their own forms and styles of arts-based learning and arts participation, and will creatively codesign the program itself.

A participant-driven creative aging program will engage many dimensions in its design. The *program design* will intentionally determine four key elements: *purpose, participation, people,* and *place*. A clear *purpose* of the program should exist regarding an intended support for some aspect of the participant's functional ability. Specific decisions must be made regarding the form and nature of arts *participation* offered by the program. Any combination of *people* (artists, facilitators, older adults, family members, and caregivers) may purposefully come together in the program design. Decisions regarding *place* may also be complex, involving the location, setting, and site of program delivery.

This *program design* set of variables is depicted at the center of the logic model provided in Figure 10.2. We envision this set of program elements to be continually evolving and changing as a process of program codesign takes place between the program providers and participants. With the intersectionality of identities, a person-centered approach to engaging participants' preferences and needs in a *creative aging* program will involve a fluid feedback loop between the inputs and outputs of the logic model. In a participant-driven and process-oriented model of program design, decisions regarding program activities and methods of participation are largely determined on a case-by-case method. In the logic model illustrated in Figure 10.2, a unidirectional approach is now replaced by a cyclical motion that integrates ever-changing decisions made regarding program inputs and outputs.

The logic model depicted in Figure 10.2 draws heavily from conceptual models in literature on community-based participatory research (Wallerstein et al. 2008;

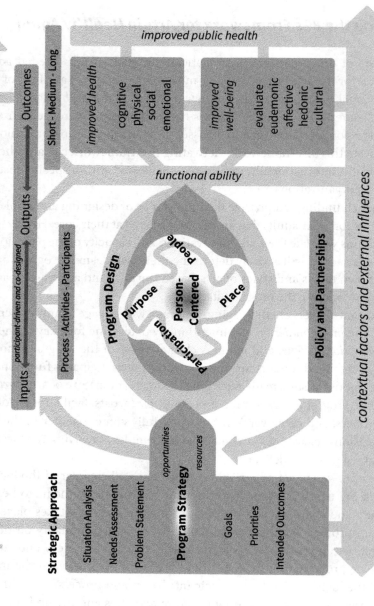

Figure 10.2 Activating the *8Ps Framework for Arts in Healthy Aging*
Illustration by Stephanie McCarthy.

Wallerstein and Duran 2010). In these models, one frequently finds a linear model beginning with *contexts*, leading to *partnerships* and *interventions*, which lead to *outcomes*. Outcomes are understood to be medium-term and long-term in nature, focusing on systems, policies, and social transformations. A feedback loop continually provides evidence from these outcomes back into an analysis of contexts, partnerships, and interventions.

Our logic model embraces this community-engaged model of continuous learning and improvement. We contend that those involved in the design of arts programs intended to support health and well-being outcomes in older adults must constantly focus on assessing needs; monitoring and evaluating program outputs and outcomes; and learning from program successes, challenges, and gaps. Program providers and participants will persistently share their views on the six *Ps* involved in the program design cycle, and the experience gained from program outputs and outcomes has the potential to significantly inform future programs. In addition, the program inputs, outputs, and outcomes must be analyzed within ever-changing contextual factors and external influences. In the *8Ps Framework for Arts in Healthy Aging*, the relevant categories for analysis here are *public policies* in the domains of arts, health, aging, and adult education, as well as the institutional ecology and structuration of the field represented by the term *partnerships*. Please see the prior section of this chapter on our ideas for activating the *arts in healthy aging* ecosystem and for specific recommendations for national *policy* and *partnerships* to advance the field.

The long-term intended outcome of all *arts in healthy aging* programs is clear: to improve public health. The logic model shows how medium-term outcomes measured in older adults will, in time, lead to a collective improvement of health within this population group. As discussed in Chapter 4, evidence of specific outcomes can be measured across the domains of cognitive, physical, social, and emotional health. Specific outcomes can also be assessed in evaluative, eudemonic, affective, hedonic, and cultural well-being.

In this logic model, *functional ability* serves as both an overarching output and the primary focus of short-term outcomes. We understand *functional ability* to be the capacity and motivation of an older adult to do the things that that they have reason to value. The status of an older adult's health and well-being allows them, individually, to determine ever-changing goals that support their subjective quality of life. Therefore, the design of all arts programs for older adults must attend to one or more goals in support of participants' individual functional ability. With lifelong learning programs, functional ability might be best understood as knowledge acquisition and/or skill development. In many health-focused *creative aging* programs, arts-based activities are intentionally used to improve, maintain, or support physical, cognitive, emotional, and social health. In contexts where older adults have less independence and require more support, arts-based programs can still support well-being through a focus on meaning-making, autonomy, dignity, growth, and legacy. Supporting *functional ability*, then, should be understood as the primary goal of all *creative aging* programs, as a specific output of these programs, and as a measure of short-term outcomes.

Chapters 1–4 of this book systematically explain how the *creative aging* movement has evolved to date, and the pressing societal need (namely, supporting the health and well-being of America's rapidly growing cohorts of older adults) that the arts can be employed to address. This analysis attended to manifold opportunities for the arts to support healthy aging, as well as to an array of resources available to policy entrepreneurs and organizational leaders to support advancing this field. This book has thus sought to engage a comprehensive framing process to clearly depict the challenges and opportunities of arts programs as a tool to support the health and well-being of America's older adults and has laid the foundation for pursuing an array of solutions. With reference to Figure 10.2, scholars and practitioners in the *arts in healthy aging* domain of policy and practice will be able to draw on the content of this book for essential knowledge leading to opportunities and resources to strengthen and grow the field. A strategic approach to developing, implementing, and evaluating arts programs for the health and well-being of older adults should always be built on a clear understanding of the contextual situation, articulation of specific needs, and a well-defined problem to be addressed. All program design elements should be informed by distinct goals, priorities, and intended outcomes.

If America's arts organizations, eldercare facilities, healthcare institutions, and older adult advocates are going to activate the model depicted in Figure 10.2, the information provided in Chapters 1–9 of this book should prove beneficial as essential information supporting the *resources*, *opportunities*, and *inputs* necessary for collective action in this field. The time is right for the field of *arts and aging*, which has existed for decades, to pull together in a new national institutional structure and advocacy coalition framed as *arts in healthy aging*. The global focus on the needs of the aging population, advocacy by the AARP, the WHO decade on healthy aging, and the rise of designated age-friendly cities should help provide a sociopolitical context in which action steps targeting older adults will be supported. Grassroots activation of the field will most likely begin at the community level. Mobilizing the *arts in healthy aging* ecosystem will benefit from the promise of partnerships that exist across institutions and organizations at international, national, regional, state, and local levels.

Conclusion

Everyone will grow old, and the demographic shifts long forecasted are now a reality. With our increased longevity, the size and socioeconomic impact of America's aging population will continue to significantly affect communities across the country in decades to come. This dramatic change is not limited to the United States; countries around the world and international organizations are bracing themselves for the challenges and opportunities presented by an aging population. The aging *baby boom* cohort is a harbinger of many large cohorts of older adults that will permanently change the global population by age groups.

In the United States, increasing lifespans urgently require community-based programs and services that support older adults' health and well-being. The arts offer unique opportunities to be part of a system of solutions for supporting healthy lifespans throughout all stages of the aging process. A strong evidence base suggests manifold ways in which the arts contribute to specific health and well-being outcomes, thereby contributing to public health as a whole. Cultural engagement is a basic human need, and opportunities for access to arts and cultural engagement must be provided equitably across societies. *Creativity*—expressed by many people through various modalities of arts participation—is an essential and infinitely renewable human resource throughout the lifespan. Opportunities to engage one's creativity throughout the lifespan require a national expansion of lifelong learning. This concept of "creative longevity" is an essential framework for the health and well-being of older adults. The arts are well proven to be a very effective tool for supporting human growth and development throughout late adulthood, even at the very end of life.

The *arts and aging* field is not new. For roughly 50 years, communities of practitioners and various organizations have been engaged in conversations and information-sharing that has led, most recently, to cohesion around the concept of *creative aging*. In the 2020s, the field is poised to once again reconfigure itself as an advocacy coalition that has been built on these decades of knowledge and expertise, program capacity building, and mobilization efforts. It is the right time to use a systems-thinking approach in developing a new *arts in healthy aging* ecosystem that takes advantage of this collective knowledge and expertise, but repositions the field to be able to become effective in public policy agenda-setting in coming years.

This book has sought to lay a solid foundation for this effort. Our multi-year exploratory research project has led to conceptual frameworks, theoretical analyses, historical perspectives on the evolution of the field, models of professional practice, development of a new logic model for the field, and articulation of specific recommendations to activate and mobilize the *arts in healthy aging* field as a whole. We hope that this comprehensive and interdisciplinary study will serve as a valuable resource to all the policymakers, researchers, students, and practitioners who seek to continue to advance this important field, both nationally and globally.

APPENDIX A

America's *Arts in Healthy Aging* Timeline

This timeline includes representative initiatives, programs, publications, and organizations of national significance in the evolution of the *arts in healthy aging* field in the United States from 1935 to 2022. The timeline references major public policy milestones across the arts, health, and aging sectors. This timeline is suggestive of the overall evolution of the *arts in healthy aging* field, but should not be viewed as comprehensive.

1935–1943 The Federal Art Project (FAP) is initiated as a part of the New Deal Program. Associated with FAP was the opening of community arts programs serving children, youth, and adults across the United States.

1937 The Social Security Act is signed into law.

1939 The United States (US) Department of Health and Human Services is born as the federal agency concerned with health, welfare, and social insurance.

1940s Emergence of Senior Centers.

1947 The National Art Education Association (NAEA) is founded.

1950s Rehabilitation Engineering and Assistive Technology emerges as a field.

1950 The first National Conference on Aging takes place.

The National Council on Aging is established.

The National Association for Music Therapy is founded.

1960s The Kansas Grassroots Art Association is organized. Currently located in Lucas, Kansas, this association preserves, documents, and facilitates the artistry of self-taught artists who typically begin this creative activity during retirement.

1960 Americans for the Arts (then known as American Council for the Arts) is established.

1961 A Senate Special (Temporary) Committee on Aging is established. It acquires permanent status on February 1, 1977.

The first White House Conference on Aging brings together 3,000 advocates, policymakers, and practitioners to debate the construction of an aging policy agenda for the next decade.

1965 The National Endowment for the Arts (NEA) is established.

Medicare and Medicaid are signed into law.

The Older Americans Act is signed into law.

The Administration on Aging is established.

1966 The American Dance Therapy Association is founded.

1967 The Age Discrimination Act is signed into law.

1968 The Architectural Barriers Act requires buildings constructed with federal funds to be accessible.

1969 The American Art Therapy Association is founded.

The National Association for Poetry Therapy is established.

1971 The second White House Conference on Aging takes place.

The John F. Kennedy Center for the Performing Arts opens.

The Kennedy Center for the Performing Arts and the National Council on Aging establish an advisory council to explore cultural programs for older adults. The group convenes from 1971 to 1973, producing the report: *Older Americans and the Arts: A Human Equation* in 1973.

The American Association for Music Therapy is founded.

1973   The NEA awards its first grant to the National Council on Aging to support public and private advocacy building activities, including publications, convenings, and workshops concerning the arts and aging.

The Center on the Arts and Aging becomes a program of the National Council on Aging.

The Older Americans Act is amended to develop Area Agencies on Aging and other expanded services.

Section 504 of the Rehabilitation Act of 1973, a first civil rights law for people with disabilities, is passed. This act made it illegal to discriminate against people with disabilities as applied to any institution or organization receiving federal funding.

1974   The National Assembly of State Arts Agencies (NASAA) is incorporated.

1975   *Elderhostel* (rebranded the *Road Scholar* Program in 2010) is established as a nonprofit educational organization focused on lifelong learning.

1976   The NEA creates an Office of Special Constituencies (OSC) to address needs of four groups: handicapped children and adults; the aging; those institutionalized in hospitals, nursing homes, or prisons; and veterans. The OSC was to provide advocacy with other programs within the NEA and other government agencies, technical assistance, and support for pilot programs.

Older Americans: The Unrealized Audience for the Arts reports on a public opinion poll of arts administrators regarding older audiences. The report was commissioned by the Administration on Aging (at the US Department of Health and Human Services).

1977   The Bernard Osher Foundation is established with the mission to improve quality of life through support for higher education and the arts.

The National Council on Aging publishes *Arts and the Aging: An Agenda for Action*.

1978   Stuart Kandall establishes *Stagebridge Theatre Company* in Oakland, CA.

1979   Susan Perlstein establishes *Elders Share the Arts* in Brooklyn, NY.

The North America Drama Therapy Association is established.

1980s   Architect Ron Mace initiates use of the term "universal design" and principles for universal design. The Center for Universal Design is established at North Carolina State University based in the design for accessibility pioneered by Ronald Mace.

1980   The US House Select Committee on Aging holds a hearing on "The Arts and the Older American," which hears the testimony from the NEA Chair, Livingston Biddle and Deputy Chair for Programs, Mary Ann Tighe, who provide a significant discussion of how the NEA regards arts and aging policy.

1981   Bipartisan House members interested in arts policy form the Congressional Arts Caucus. Membership rapidly grows to nearly 200 members.

The NEA signs an interagency memorandum with the Administration on Aging.

The NEA and the National Council on Aging collaborate in convening the first sanctioned, mini-preconference on the arts and aging for the (third) White House Conference on Aging.

1984   The Center for Applied Technology is created by David Rose and Ann Meyer. They conceived of universal design for learning by applying the principles of universal design to education.

1987   The Omnibus Budget Reconciliation Act ("the Nursing Home Reform Act") mandates significant improvements in eldercare facilities.

1988   Lolo Sarnoff establishes *Arts for the Aging* in Washington, DC.

The Museum of Modern Art in New York City exhibits *Designs for Independent Living*.

1990   The Americans with Disabilities Act is signed into law.

The Committee on Lifelong Learning within the NAEA is established.

1991   The Society for the Arts in Healthcare is established.

1992   *Arts for Older Adults* by Donald H. Hoffman is published.

Thomas R. Cole, Robert Kastenbaum, and Ruth E. Ray (Eds.) publish *Handbook of the Humanities and Aging*.

1994 The International Expressive Arts Therapy Association is established.

The Washington, DC Center on Aging is founded by Gene Cohen. The Societal Education About Aging for Change (SEAChange) initiative is one of the center's signature projects. The focus of the project is on media for children that portray older adults in a positive way. Marsha Weiner is the director.

1995 The NEA OSC is renamed as the Office of AccessAbility to emphasize the agency's concern with improving accessibility to the arts for all.

The NEA survives a congressional threat of elimination but sustains the largest budget cut in its history. This prompts significant staff cuts and a major agency reorganization.

NEA Chair Jane Alexander is one of the twelve featured at the Delegates Banquet for the 1995 (fourth) White House Conference on Aging. She focused on the twin goals of creating more access to the arts and humanities for older adults and increasing sensitivity of aging professionals to the possible benefits of arts to quality of life. An arts and aging mini-preconference takes place, titled "The Arts, the Humanities, and Older Americans."

NEA research report published on *Age and Arts Participation with a Focus on the Baby Boomers*.

1996 Monograph on *The Arts and Older Americans* published by the National Assembly of Local Arts Agencies.

The Telecommunications Act mandates that telecommunications services be accessible to people with disabilities.

1997 The American Assembly publishes *The Arts and the Public Purpose*. Serving older adults is one of the purposes addressed in the report.

1998 Anne Bastings develops *TimeSlips*, a storytelling program for individuals with dementia.

The National Association for Music Therapy and the American Association for Music Therapy merge to form the American Music Therapy Association.

2000 Gene Cohen publishes *The Creative Age: Awakening Human Potential in the Second Half Of Life*.

The Bernard Osher Foundation initiates the *Osher Lifelong Learning Institutes*, which specifically target the development of programs for more mature students who are not necessarily well served by standard continuing education curricula.

2001 The National Center for Creative Aging (NCCA) is established as a program within *Elders Share the Arts*, through a partnership with the National Council on Aging and the NEA. At this time, *Elders Share the Arts* is the "only NEA-funded arts service organization internationally serving older people in their communities with quality programs" (Perlstein 2010, 252).

The Mark Morris Dance Center launches *Dance for PD (Parkinson's Disease)*.

2003 Gary Glazner develops the *Alzheimer's Poetry Project*.

Aging, Creativity, and Art: A Positive Perspective on Late-Life Development by Martin S. Lindauer is published.

2005 The NEA partners with the NCCA, the National Association of Music Manufacturers' International Foundation for Music Research, and the American Association of Retired People (AARP) to convene the mini-conference on "Creativity and Aging in America." This mini-conference focused on the importance and value of professional arts programming for, by, and with older Americans as quality-of-life issues, and highlighted the research of Gene Cohen's NEA-commissioned "Creativity and Aging Study."

Three areas of recommendations were created to cite as recommendations for the subsequent fifth White House Conference on Aging: lifelong learning in community, arts in healthcare, and universal design (Hanna and Perlstein 2008, 11). The fifth White House Conference on Aging theme is "The Booming Dynamics of Aging: From Awareness to Action."

2006   The large *baby boom* generation starts turning 60.

A research team led by Gene Cohen publishes findings from *The Creativity and Aging Study: The Impact of Professionally Conducted Cultural Programs on Older Adults*.

The Museum of Modern Art (MoMA) in New York City launches *"Meet Me,"* the *MoMA Alzheimer's Project*.

The World Health Organization Global Network for Age-Friendly Cities and Communities, an international initiative, is launched. The AARP Network of Age-Friendly States and Communities is the US affiliate.

2007   The World Health Organization publishes *Global Age Friendly Cities: A Guide*.

The NCCA, now led by Gay Hanna, is relocated to Washington, DC as an independent non-profit that is affiliated with the George Washington University Center on the Aging, Health and Humanities, led by Gene Cohen.

The National Guild for Community Arts Education publishes *Creativity Matters: The Arts and Aging Toolkit*.

Encore Creativity for Older Adults, which becomes the largest choral music program for older adults in the United States, is established as a direct result of the Cohen et al. (2006) research publication.

2008   Americans for the Arts publishes a monograph titled *Creativity Matters: Arts and Aging in America*.

Lifetime Arts is founded by Maura O'Malley and Ed Friedman. The organization is "positioned as a service organization to help build an infrastructure for the emerging field of Creative Aging" (McDonough 2013, 31).

The New York City Department of the Aging and the New York City Department of Cultural Affairs collaborate to launch *SM(ART)S: Seniors Meet the Arts*. Funding supports fifty-seven arts organizations to lead programming in more than 150 senior centers.

A *Creativity Matters Symposia Series* is conducted from 2008 to 2011 through a partnership between the National Council on Aging and the MetLife Foundation.

2009   The NCCA research committee, led by Linda Noelker of the Benjamin Rose Institute, conducts a comprehensive literature review of studies that measured the health outcomes of participatory arts programs for older adults (Patterson and Perlstein 2011, 29).

2010   The Patient Protection and Affordable Care Act ("Obamacare") is signed into law.

Creativity and Aging in America Leadership Award given from 2010 to 2014 by the MetLife Foundation.

Grantmakers in the Arts, Grantmakers In Aging, Society for the Arts in Healthcare, and the MetLife Foundation partner in *Grantmakers Partnership Projects* from 2010 to 2014.

Americans for the Arts' Arts Advocacy Day includes "Arts in Health" as an agenda item for policy action.

2011   The NEA and the US Department of Health and Human Services jointly publish a white paper titled *The Arts and Human Development: Framing a National Research Agenda for the Arts, Lifelong Learning, and Individual Wellbeing*.

The Creative Center becomes part of University Settlement in New York, NY and expands their programs to focus on the growing field of Creative Aging.

2013   The *EngAGE* State Arts Agency Professional Development Initiative in Arts, Health, and Aging is designed and launched by the NCCA in partnership with the NEA and the NASAA. *EngAGE* prepares state arts agencies to play leading roles in advancing creative aging, focused specifically on lifelong learning.

The NEA, Aroha Philanthropies, and MetLife Foundation support development of the first *directory of creative aging programs in America*. The same partners support development of *online artist training* to support individual artists everywhere in developing arts programs for older adults.

Appendix A   229

The NEA publishes a report titled *The Arts and Aging, Building the Science.*

The Society for the Arts in Healthcare is renamed the Global Alliance for Arts in Health.

2014 The first national leadership exchange and conference on aging, named *The Creative Age: Exploring the Potential in the Second Half of Life*, takes place as a first-of-its-kind convention for the field of creative aging. More than 500 leaders from the field from 28 states and 6 countries participate.

2015 The NEA holds a *Summit on Creative Aging* as a preconference for the sixth White House Conference on Aging.

A second national leadership exchange and conference on aging takes place, named *The Creative Age: Creativity and Aging in America.*

The NCCA develops a *Distance Learning Series* as a monthly series focusing on an array of topics drawn from the 2015 leadership exchange and conference.

The NEA publishes *How Creativity Works in the Brain.*

The NEA publishes *When Going Gets Tough: Barriers and Motivations Affecting Arts Attendance.*

The Global Alliance for Arts in Health is dissolved.

2016 The third national leadership exchange and conference on aging takes place, named *The Creative Age: Global Perspectives on Creativity and Aging.* Partners include the NCCA, Americans for the Arts, the DC Commission on the Arts and Humanities, Iona Senior Services, Goodwin House, LeadingAGE, the NEA, and other international organizations.

Jennie Smith-Peers replaces Gay Hanna as executive director of the NCCA.

The National Organization for Arts in Health (NOAH) is established, replacing the former Society for the Arts in Healthcare / Global Alliance for Arts in Health.

Folk Art & Aging: Life-Story Objects and Their Makers, by Jon Kay, is published.

Sky Above Clouds: Finding Our Way Through Creativity, Aging, and Illness, by Wendy L. Miller and Gene D. Cohen, is published.

2017 *The Campus for Creative Aging* is opened as a learning community developed by the Region IV Area Agency on Aging.

Catalyzing Creative Aging Programs is launched as a collaborative initiative of Lifetime Arts, Aroha Philanthropies, the National Guild for Community Arts Education, Music Man Foundation, and the Moca Foundation, as well as the first cohort of ten arts organizations.

The NEA publishes *Staying Engaged: Health Patterns of Older Adults Who Participate in the Arts.*

The NOAH publishes *Arts, Health, and Well-Being in America.*

All private members of the President's Committee on the Arts and the Humanities resign in protest after President Trump's comments regarding Charlottesville "Unite the Right" disruption. Trump does not appoint replacements and allows the authorization for the committee to lapse.

2018 The NCCA is restructured and ultimately closes. The 2018 national leadership exchange and conference on aging is canceled.

Elders Share the Arts dismantles its nonprofit organization after 40 years of providing creative aging programming.

The NOAH publishes *Code of Ethics and Standards for Arts in Health Professionals* and *The Future of Arts in Health in America.*

A three-year national initiative titled *Creating Healthy Communities: Arts + Public Health in America* is established. "The initiative sought to expand the intersections of arts, community development and public health through strategic cross-sector collaboration, discovery, translation, and dissemination. The initiative included nine national convenings, a comprehensive research agenda, and the development of an array of resources for driving cross-sector collaboration" (see https://arts.ufl.edu/sites/creating-healthy-communities/creating-healthy-communities-initiative-infographic/).

Appendix A

The Creative Center at University Settlement, in partnership with the NEA and the NYC Department of Cultural Affairs, launches *The Creative Center Training Institute for Artists and Administrators in Creative Aging*.

The *EngAGED National Resource Center for Engaging Older Adults* is established through a partnership of the following: National Association of Area Agencies on Aging, Lifetime Arts, GenerationsUnited, US Administration on Aging, Administration for Community Living, Osher Lifelong Learning Institutes, and the NCCA.

Aroha Philanthropies, American Alliance of Museums, Lifetime Arts, and twenty museums launch a new museum-based national creative aging initiative named *Seeding Vitality Arts in Museums*. *Aroha Fellow for Museums and Creative Aging* program is also launched.

The second round of *Catalyzing Creative Aging Programs* is launched as a collaborative initiative of Lifetime Arts, Aroha Philanthropies, the National Guild for Community Arts Education, NAMM Foundation, and the second cohort of twenty arts organizations.

An annual conference for community arts education, focused on *Ageism and Creative Aging*, hosted by the National Guild for Community Arts Education and Lifetime Arts. A *Catalyzing Creative Aging Institute* takes place as part of the conference.

2019   The NASAA publishes its *Creative Aging Strategy Sampler* and its report on *Leveraging State Investments in Creative Aging: Survey Highlights*.

Various training programs and webinars are developed and offered throughout 2019, such as:

- The Creative Center's *Training Institute for Artists and Administrators in Creative Aging*
- Lifetime Arts' professional development workshops in New York City, Chicago, and Wisconsin
- "Sustaining Creative Aging Programs: Diverse Funding and Partnership Strategies" and "Kick-Start Creative Aging at Your Organization: Lessons Learned from the Field" webinars provided by the National Guild for Community Arts Education

2020   Lifetime Arts launches *Creative Aging 101*, a free online mini-course.

Cross-Cultural Design for Healthy Ageing, edited by Lisa Scharoun, Danny Hills, Carlos Montana-Hoyos, Fanke Peng, and Vivien Sung, is published.

COVID-19 emerges in the United States. Face-to-face community-based arts programs offered for older adults begin to go online. Mass vaccinations begin.

2021   President Biden reauthorizes and reactivates the President's Committee on the Arts and the Humanities.

The NOAH publishes its *Core Curriculum for Arts in Health Professionals*.

Art Therapy and Creative Aging: Reclaiming Elderhood, Health and Wellbeing, by Raquel Chapin Stephenson, is published.

Dementia-Friendly Communities: Why We Need Them and How We Can Create Them, by Susan H. McFadden, is published.

2022   Aroha Philanthropies, the main foundation supporting creative aging programs and initiatives at the national level, changes its name to "E.A. Michelson Philanthropy."

A free, online training resource named *Academy for Creative Aging* is launched by the Pennsylvania Council on the Arts.

Culture Track publishes *Untapped Opportunity: Older Americans and the Arts*.

The Next Wave in Creative Aging: Creative Aging Innovation Forums Cross-Industry Report is published by Georgetown University Aging and Health Program and the Kennedy Center Office of Accessibility and VSA.

COVID-19 vaccinations and boosters continue. While some online arts programs continue, there is a return to face-to-face arts programming for older adults in communities across the United States.

APPENDIX B

National Organizations Advancing the Fields of Arts, Health, Aging, and Lifelong Learning

The list below groups together organizations that have a national focus in the United States on issues pertaining to the arts, health, aging, and lifelong learning sectors. This list mainly includes federal agencies (these usually have websites that end in ".gov") and nonprofit organizations (whose websites usually end in ".org"). Typing the name below into an Internet search engine will quickly lead to each organization. This list of relevant organizations is in constant flux. Moreover, there are other types of organizations that are not included in this list—such as policy think tanks, academic research centers, and international organizations—that can play an important role in advancing the national *arts in healthy aging* field.

Federal Government Entities Focused on Aging

Administration on Aging
Administration for Community Living
Agency for Healthcare Research and Quality
Department of Health and Human Services
Department of Veterans Affairs
Eldercare Locator
Food and Drug Administration
Healthcare Finder
Local Departments of Public Health
National Center on Elder Abuse
National Long-Term Care Information (longtermcare.gov)
National Institute on Aging
NIH Senior Health
National Women's Health
Supplemental Nutrition Assistance Program

National Nonprofits Focused on Aging

American Association of Retired People (AARP)
Adult Protective Services
Advancing States
Aging with Dignity
American Geriatrics Society
American Society on Aging
Alliance for Aging Research
Alliance for Retired Americans
A Place for Mom
Assisted Living Consumer Alliance
Assisted Living Federation of America
ARCH National Respite Network
Caregiver Action Network
Caring
Caring Connections
Center for Medicare Advocacy, Inc.
Center for Workforce Inclusion

Compassion & Choices
ExperienceWorks
Families USA
Family Caregiver Alliance
Gerontological Society of America
Gray Panthers
Hospice Foundation
Justice in Aging
Leading Age
Medicare Rights Center
National Academy of Elder Law Attorneys
National Alliance for Caregiving
National Alliance for Grieving Children
National Adult Day Services Association
National Adult Protective Services Association
National Association for Home Care & Hospice
National Association of Area Agencies on Aging
National Association of County Veteran Service Officers
National Association of Nutrition and Aging Services Programs
National Association of Professional Geriatric Care Managers
National Association of Retired and Senior Volunteer Program Directors
National Association of Social Workers
National Association of State Long-Term Care Ombudsman Programs
National Care Planning Council
National Committee to Preserve Social Security and Medicare
National Consumer Voice for Quality Long-Term Care
National Council on Aging
National Hospice & Palliative Care Organization
National Long-Term Care Ombudsman Resource Center
National Meals on Wheels Association of America
National Senior Corps Association
National Shared Housing Resource Center
National Volunteer Caregiving Network
Older Women's League
Pension Rights Center
Pioneer Network
Points of Light Foundation
Road Scholar
Senior Corps Corporation for National and Community Service
Senior Housing Association of America
Service Corps of Retired Executives
The Society for Post-Acute and Long-Term Care Medicine
USAging
VA Caregiver Support
Village to Village Network
Volunteers of America
Where You Live Matters
Women's Institute for a Secure Retirement

Federal Government Entities Focused on Health

Arthritis Foundation
Centers for Disease Control and Prevention
Centers for Medicaid and Medicare

National Cancer Institute
National Center for Complementary and Alternative Medicine
National Heart, Lung, and Blood Institute
National Institute of Arthritis and Musculoskeletal and Skin Diseases
National Institute of Neurological Disorders and Stroke

National Nonprofits Focused on Health

Alzheimer's Association
Alzheimer's Foundation of America
American Association for Geriatric Psychiatry
American Cancer Society
American Dental Association
American Diabetes Association
American Foundation for the Blind
American Heart Association
American Hospital Association
American Lung Association
American Medical Association
American Podiatric Medical Association
American Society of Consultant Pharmacists
American Stroke Association
Arthritis Foundation
Center for Medicare Advocacy
Center to Advance Palliative Care
Geriatric Mental Health Foundation
Hearing Loss Association of America
Institute for Healthcare Improvement
Institute of Medicine
Medicare Rights Center
National Association for Continence
National Osteoporosis Foundation
National Parkinson Foundation
National State Health Insurance Assistance Resource Center
Parkinson's Disease Foundation
The Joint Commission

Accessibility and Home Modification Federal Agencies and Nonprofits

AARP
ABLEDATA
American Association of People with Disabilities
Disability.gov
Fall Prevention Center of Excellence
Habitat for Humanity
National Rehabilitation Information Center
Paralyzed Veterans of America
This Caring Home

Minority Group Services for Health and Aging

Association of Gay & Lesbian Psychiatrists
Association of Jewish Aging Services of North America

Gay & Lesbian Medical Association
International Association for Indigenous Aging
LGBT Aging Resources Clearinghouse
National Asian Pacific Center on Aging
National Association for Hispanic Elderly
National Caucus and Center on Black Aging
National Hispanic Council on Aging
National Indian Council on Aging
National Resource Center on LGBT Aging
Services and Advocacy for Gay, Lesbian, Bisexual & Transgender Elders (SAGE)

Government Entities and Nonprofits that Provide Financial and Fraud Protection Services for Older Adults

BenefitsCheckUp
GovBenefits
Home Equity Advisor
Internal Revenue Service
National Adult Protective Services Association
National Center of Elder Abuse
National Foundation for Counseling Credit
Pension Rights Center
Social Security Administration

Federal Government Entities Focused on the Arts and Culture

American Folklife Center, Library of Congress
Institute of Museum and Library Services
John F. Kennedy Center for the Performing Arts
National Endowment for the Arts
National Endowment for the Humanities
Smithsonian Institution

National Nonprofits Focused on the Arts

American Alliance of Museums
Americans for the Arts
Chamber Music America
Chorus America
Dance USA
League of American Orchestras
National Assembly of State Arts Agencies
National Association of Music Merchants
National Center for Creative Aging (closed 2018)
Opera America
Theatre Communication Group
VSA: The International Organization for Arts and Disability

Professional Nonprofit Associations Focused on Arts in Health

American Academy of Healthcare Interior Designers
American Art Therapy Association

American College of Healthcare Architects
American Dance Therapy Association
American Horticulture Therapy Association
American Music Therapy Association
American Society of Group Psychotherapy and Psychodrama
American Therapeutic Recreation Association
Association of Professional Art Advisors
Centre for Medical Humanities
The Center for Health Design
Health Humanities Consortium
International Expressive Arts Therapy Association
National Association for Drama Therapy
National Association for Poetry Therapy
National Association of Activity Professionals
National Coalition of Activity Professionals
National Coalition of Creative Arts Therapies Association
National Organization for Arts in Health
North American Drama Therapy Association
Sound Healers Association
Therapeutic Landscapes Network

Professional Nonprofit Associations Focused on Arts and Education

American Association for Adult and Continuing Education
American Folklore Society
Association of Academic Museums and Galleries
The Association of Transformative Learning Theory with the Perspective of Freire
The Bernard Osher Foundation
The Coalition of Lifelong Learning Organizations
College Art Association
Community Arts Association
Community Arts Network
Dance Educators of America
Educational Theatre Association
Imaging America: Artists + Scholars in Public Life
International Transformative Learning Association
Kansas Grassroots Arts Association
Leisure Studies Association
Local Learning: The National Network for Folk Arts in Education
National Art Education Association
National Association for Multicultural Education
National Association for Music Educators
National Association of State Directors of Adult Education
National Guild for Community Arts Education
Society for Disability Studies

Notes

Chapter 2

1. This chapter introduces conceptualization of the *public purposes* of the arts, which is a scholarly topic also referred to as *public benefits, public interest,* and *public value*. Each of these concepts has its own robust body of published research.

Chapter 3

1. Clive Gray defined the phenomenon of *policy attachment* as a "strategy that allows a 'weak' policy sector with limited political clout to attract enough resources to achieve its policy objectives. This is achieved through the sector's attachment to other policy concerns that appear more worthy or that occupy a more central position in the political discourse of the time" (Gray 2002, 81). In the United States, the term "riding the political coattails" refers to a candidate running for a lower office gaining added support from a strong candidate higher on the electoral ballot.
2. Although the NEA has long regarded arts education as a priority, this attention has been focused on children and youth, rather than extending into lifelong learning for adults. Various programs that have historically embedded some attention to older adults include:
    - the theater division and the senior theater movement;
    - activities to support continuing professional development training to artists as a form of lifelong learning;
    - sponsoring research to better document the conditions and challenges facing aging artists;
    - conducting a series of national Surveys of Public Participation in the Arts that include an age variable (see Chapters 2 and 4 for discussion);
    - museum program support for training volunteer docents, many of whom were older adults;
    - folk arts program concern with facilitating the ability of established culture bearers to preserve and transfer their knowledge to next generations of apprentices (see Chapter 5 for discussion of learner-centered arts education for older adults and folklore approaches); and
    - awards to honor the lifetime career accomplishments of folk artists and jazz masters.
3. The Wisconsin study found two explanations for the attitudes regarding the possible development of arts programming designed for older adults (Johnson and Prieve 1976). Nearly half of the arts administrators (46.7%) surveyed regarded senior citizens as having more conservative tastes and as being less willing to try new arts forms or contemporary works (25–26). An almost equal percentage of arts administrators (53.3%) contended that the tastes of older adults were not different from those of the general audience and that this meant there was little need for special senior programming (25–28). Presciently, the report noted the importance of education as a "learning process" that could "be made a part of any artistic experience" in order to deepen understanding and promote greater appreciation (35).
4. Notably, in the 1980s, the NCOA published a series of four informational guides directed to program sponsors (Lewis-Kane, McCutcheon, and McDicken 1986) and to artists seeking to work in aging programs (McCutcheon 1986b), as well as a guide to arts and aging programs (McCutcheon and Wolf 1985) and another guide to aging-related media materials (McCutcheon 1986a). Typically, these publications included examples of program ideas and techniques drawn from a variety of arts disciplines.

238 Notes

5. The conference and pre-events were coordinated by a national advisory committee that included representatives of the executive branch as well as congressional actors with interests and concerns in aging issues and brought together various organized aging constituencies, as well as private agencies and academic experts. Subsequent WHCoAs were separately authorized by independent legislation by Congress, with the 1991 conference included in reauthorization of the Older American Act (Bechill 1990).
6. Notably, former NEA Chair Nancy Hanks was in attendance as a member of the Advisory Committee to the White House Conference and a member of the Conference Technical Committee on Age-Integration within the Media (Waldie 1981, 62–63).
7. Among major items on the arts agenda were internal, administrative issues concerning the peer panel system, the institution of long-term planning, and managing multiple waves of Challenge grants designed to award unusually large grants to major arts institutions in all disciplines that were facing financial difficulties. The NEA also continued to cultivate stronger policy attachments to primary and secondary education policy and with foreign affairs policy through promotion of cultural diplomacy. Also on the agenda was fostering the role of the arts in community development by helping local arts agencies to professionalize, promoting research on the economic impact of the arts in local communities, and supporting a building boom for new arts facilities across the country.
8. The 1994 campaign agenda of the Republican candidates for the US House of Representatives was called the *Contract with America*, which articulated the party's views on needed policy change and dealt primarily with changing the way that Congress worked. It called for congressional term limits, a balanced budget, the line-item veto, tax cuts and reform of Social Security, tax policy, and welfare. As part of the call for a balanced budget, the document included a list of ninety-five programs that it would seek to eliminate. The NEA, the NEH, and the Corporation for Public Broadcasting were on this list. It also called for funding reductions for Medicare, Medicaid, and the Older Americans Act (Blancato 2004, 66). Top priority recommendations of the 1995 WHCoA strongly defended these existing health and aging programs and received considerable media attention. President Clinton vetoed legislation that contained the anti-aging provisions. Similarly, arts and culture policy advocates rallied to protect the three threatened cultural agencies. While not eliminated, the NEA and the NEH suffered severe budget cuts in 1995, which halved the NEA's budget and prompted a dramatic reorganization and significant staff cuts.
9. The meeting, entitled "The Arts, the Humanities and Older Americans," formulated recommendations regarding the promotion and support of universal design; involvement of older adults and scholars in the planning and policymaking processes; and support for increased arts and humanities programs in prevention and healthcare (NEA 1995, 176).
10. While the NEA was the lead sponsor for the *Creativity and Aging Study* (Cohen 2006), there were also additional public and private funders. Funding partners for this study included the Center for Mental Health Services, Substance Abuse and Mental Health Services, DHHS; the National Institute of Mental Health, National Institutes of Health (NIH); AARP/National Retired Teachers Association; Stella and Charles Guttman Foundation, NYC; and the International Foundation for Music Research at NAMM.
11. The 2015 WHCoA was preceded by a series of five regional, invitational forums (coplanned by AARP and the Leadership Council of Aging Organizations and held in Tampa, Seattle, Phoenix, Cleveland, and Boston); five high-profile forums at the White House on select topics (healthy aging, elder justice, caregiving, older women, and retirement security); and over one hundred listening sessions that involved the Administration for Community Living (WHCoA 2015, 2–3, 30).
12. The NEA established the NCCA in 2001 as a grant program of ESTA, a nonprofit arts organization that had pioneered in arts programming for older adults since its founding in 1979 (Jeffri and Hanna 2015, 968). The executive director of ESTA was named the first executive director of the NCCA and she managed the center from her Brooklyn location. Thus, the NCCA was created by an NEA grant awarded to ESTA and was not officially part of the NEA organizational structure.

Notes   239

In 2007, the NCCA was established as an independent nonprofit arts organization and moved to Washington, DC. Its new executive director was Professor Gay Hanna, who held a visiting faculty position at the George Washington University School of Medicine and Health. This appointment affiliated the NCCA with the George Washington Center on Aging, Health and Humanities, led by Professor Gene Cohen, who had launched the idea of *creative aging* in his 2000 book, *The Creative Age: Awakening Human Potential in the Second Half of Life*.

13. These research reports often involved a collaboration with other organizations, such as the NIH, the US Department of Health and Human Services, the Interagency Task Force on the Arts and Human Development, the NCCA, and the Santa Fe Institute working group. The NEA began convening the Interagency Task Force on the Arts and Human Development in 2012. In addition to the NEA, its members included the US DHHS, the NIH, the Swiss National Science Foundation, the NEH, the Institute of Museum and Library Services, and the US Department of Education (Hanna, Noelker, and Bienvenu 2015, 273).

Chapter 4

1. Two good websites for introductory information on the *social determinants of health* are https://health.gov/healthypeople/priority-areas/social-determinants-health and https://www.who.int/health-topics/social-determinants-of-health#tab=tab_1
2. The research database overseen by the University of Florida's Center for Arts in Medicine (see https://www.zotero.org/groups/4516700/center_for_arts_in_medicine_research_database/library) provides a useful current list of peer-reviewed English-language publications in this field. At the time of writing this book, several especially noteworthy research publications on the physiological and cognitive effects of arts participation were recently released by the NeuroArts Blueprint project of Johns Hopkins University's International Arts + Mind Lab (see https://neuroartsblueprint.org) and by the WHO Collaborating Centre for Arts & Health at University College London (see https://artshealthcc.org). The European Union (with partners) released a major report titled *Culture for Health Report* in November 2022, with a subtitle as a "Scoping review of culture, well-being, and health interventions and their evidence, impacts, challenges and policy recommendations for Europe" (see cultureforhealth.eu).

Chapter 5

1. To learn more about Perry Johnson and to see examples of his artistry, go to OSLP Arts and Culture Center (https://www.artsandcultureeugene.org/perry.html).
2. To learn more about Marian Sykes and to see examples of her artistry, go to Fairfield Arts (https://www.youtube.com/watch?v=uWLmWTNlB7k).
3. To Learn more about Aminah Robinson and to see examples of her artistry, go to the Columbus Museum of Art (https://www.columbusmuseum.org/raggin-on-the-art-of-aminah-brenda-lynn-robinsons-house-and-journals/).

Chapter 6

1. For the purposes of this chapter and book, the term "arts educator" refers to a provider that has completed an undergraduate or graduate degree that included significant coursework in one or more of the arts disciplines; coursework in adult education theory and practice; and experience in

working with older adults within their degree programs or postgraduation. Also preferred would be coursework associated with gerontology, particularly the subfields critical and social gerontology. "Arts educator" may also refer to a provider who identifies as an "artist, "teaching artist," and/or "arts therapist." Coupled with this identification can be completion of degree programs associated with the arts and/or significant experience in an arts discipline. In those cases where an educator falls into one of these categorizations and does not have such knowledge and experience, supervision by a professional who does is appropriate. The emphasis here is on providers who are credentialed or experienced in ways like those other professionals working with older adults. Such professionals may include physical therapists, occupational therapists, psychologists, social workers, and medical personnel. However, as Davenport, Lawton, and Manifold (2020, 56) acknowledge, state certification assessments do not at present "evaluate an art educator's potential ability to work with older members of the community."

2. Emerging from the field of creative aging are important documents and publications that do address the creation and implementation of arts programs for older adults and that can be used as a basis for the development and implementation of transformative arts programs. Some examples follow.

- Boyer (2007)'s *Creativity Matters: The Arts and Aging Toolkit* is a comprehensive tool kit that provides an overview of arts and aging programs existing at the time of publication; descriptions of the significant benefits that older adults can experience as a result of participating in the arts; contextual information on the organizational structures through which arts programs are offered to older adults; effective practices that arts educators can emulate; strategies for program planning, design, and implementation; development of the learning community; the competencies that arts educators should possess; and evaluation among other topics discussed. Theoretically, this tool kit is based in andragogy with an emphasis on participation, sequential learning, and mastery through arts skill development.
- *Lifetime Arts: National Leaders in Creative Aging Program Development* (2022) is an excellent resource for designing arts education programs for older adults. With some modification, these resources can contribute to curricular planning with older adults that responds to the aims of transformative learning.
- Rollins (2013)'s *Bringing the Arts to Life: A Guide to the Arts and Long-Term Care*, while not specifically focused on transformative learning, does acknowledge that "aging demonstrates the transformative power of imagination for populations suffering common disabilities of age: frailty, dementia, and depression" (90). Therefore, this guide's emphasis is on arts-based approaches with less emphasis on skill development and with greater emphasis on creativity and process. This guide, with its focus on long-term care communities, is of particular importance to residential and healthcare settings discussed in Chapter 8 of this book.
- Basting (2021a; 2021b)'s *Creative Care: A Revolutionary Approach to Dementia and Elder Care* and *Creative Care: Imagination Kit* are associated with Basting's pioneering work in cultivating transformative arts experiences among older adults experiencing dementia. Designed for family members, care partners, and those others providing services to people experiencing dementia, the emphasis is on imagination rather than memory. These two publications are an outgrowth of *TimeSlips* (timeslips.org), founded by Basting, an international network of those bringing "joy to elders and their care partners by infusing creativity and meaning making into care relationships." Of note is the study of *TimeSlips* published by George and Houser (2014), in which they recommend longitudinal study of transformative learning (682).
- In 2022, the Pennsylvania Council on the Arts launched the online Academy of Creative Aging for the purpose of providing resources to artists, arts educators, and others working with older adults. Participation in the academy is possible by engaging with a series of self-paced multimedia modules, which upon completion results in certification. Engagement in the academy can also occur through the academy's *Lessons on Demand* drawing from the academy's online video library. The goal of the academy "is to prepare professionals to engage older adults in substantive creative aging projects and activities that will positively impact the cognitive functions and wellbeing of seniors" (Pennsylvania Council on the Arts n.d., 1).

3. The European concept *Bildung*, with its emphasis on meaning as combining a "cognitive event" with "a social construct that is produced and changed in social interactions" (Laros, Fuhr, and Taylor

2017, ix) has been compared to transformative learning. Bildung, "refers to processes of interpretation, understanding, or appropriation (*Aneignung*) of knowledge that transforms a learner's personality" (ix). Readers interested in the relationships that exist between transformative learning theory and Bildung will find numerous examples, including some that are arts related, in *Transformative Learning Meets 'Bildung': An International Exchange* (Laros, Fuhr, and Taylor 2017).

Chapter 7

1. This orientation to Perry Johnson, and the network associated with his artistry, is in part informed by Becker (2008)'s sociological concept of "art worlds." For Becker, "all artistic work, like all human activity, involves the joint activity of a number, often a large number, of people. Through their cooperation, the art work we eventually see or hear comes to be and continues to be" (1). Perry Johnson and other art makers are at the center of this activity. "Art worlds," for Becker, "consist of all the people whose activities are necessary to the production of the characteristic works which the world, and perhaps others as well, define art" (34).
2. Arlene Goldbard has written extensively on community arts and community cultural development. We particularly recommend her 2009 book, *New Creative Community: The Art of Cultural Development*.
3. While not specifically focused on the older adult, *Arts and Cultural Programming: A Leisure Perspective* (Carpenter and Blandy 2008) does include chapters relevant to those conceptualizing, planning, implementing, and evaluating arts and cultural programs for older adults. Theoretical perspectives, programming approaches, program management, cultivating audiences, program evaluation, marketing, festivals, and community arts are among the topics discussed by the contributors.
4. For educational initiatives mitigating ageism, see the Washington DC Center on Aging's Societal Education About Aging for Change (SEAChange) project directed by Marsha Weiner (dccenteronaging.org/projects/seachange/) and the Intergenerational Schools initiative at igschools.org. SEAChange, in partnership with the Children's Division of the American Library Association, focuses on media promoting positive portrayals of older adults. The initiative supports the recent "Creating Children's Books Centered on the Adventures of Older Adults" action item included in *The Next Wave in Creative Aging: Creative Aging Innovation Forums Cross-Industry Report* (Saunders et al. 2022). The Intergenerational Schools' mission is to "connect, create, and guide a multigenerational community of lifelong learners and spirited citizens as we strive for academic excellence."
5. *Active aging* as referenced in *Global Age-Friendly Cities: A Guide* (WHO 2007) "is the process of optimizing opportunities for health, participation and security in order to enhance quality of life as people age" (11). In 2015, *active aging* was replaced by *healthy aging* (WHO 2018).
6. See McFadden (2021) for approaches to creating dementia-friendly communities and Scharoun et al. (2020) for cross-cultural design approaches that can be incorporated into age-friendly communities.
7. A promising development in housing for older adults is the "Village Movement." This movement responds to older adults' preference for living independently to the greatest extent possible at home. Villages are nonprofit membership organizations providing support for older adults wishing to remain at home. For more information on the Villages Movement, see https://www.helpfulvillage.com/the-village-movement and see agingactioninitiative.org/resources/the-villages-movement/ for details associated with this movement.
8. Duxbury and Redaelli (2020) define *cultural mapping* "as a mode of inquiry and a methodological tool that aims to make visible the ways local stories, practices, relationships, memories, and

rituals constitute places as meaningful locations" (1). Cultural mapping results in identification of cultural assets within any given community and assists communities in articulating "a 'sense of place,'" people-place meanings, and distinctive elements" (1) associated with any given community. Cultural mapping is widely practiced internationally, including within the United States and Canada. A Cultural Planning Toolkit is available through the Creative City Network of Canada (2010), accessible at https://www2.gov.bc.ca/assets/gov/sports-recreation-arts-and-culture/events-hosting/hosting-toolkit/cultural_planning_toolkit.pdf.

Chapter 9

1. The global hospice movement is largely attributed to its matriarch, Dame Cicely Saunders, who trained first as a nurse, then as a social worker, and finally as a physician. Her philosophy to manage pain and the total needs of dying patients and her approach of using a team to treat the whole person has become the foundation for hospice care everywhere. In 1967, Saunders opened St Christopher's Hospice outside London. St Christopher's Hospice has a long history of integrating arts programs and services in hospice care, with international leaders Nigel Hartley and Malcolm Payne in this specialized field (Hartley and Payne 2008). Hospice first came to North America in 1971, a movement led by Florence Wald, dean of nursing at Yale. The American hospice system has grown dramatically over the past 50 years. In 2020, the National Hospice and Palliative Care Organization reported that roughly 50.7% of Medicare patients were enrolled in hospice at the time of death, with routine home care (i.e., hospice care provided in the patient's own home, an assisted living facility, nursing home, or other congregate living facility) accounting for 98.2% of the care provided. Data collected in 2018 showed that there were 4,639 Medicare-certified hospices in operation across the United States (see https://nhpco.org/hospice-facts-figures/).

Chapter 10

1. The health field is developing interests in similar concerns. A first step toward developing the capacity to understand and adapt planning and practice involves a review of literature on the subject of concern. Examples of such research in healthcare include Brazier (2005); Coles et al. (2022); and Liverani, Hawkins, and Parkhurst (2013).

References

Abia-Smith, Lisa. 2016. "Preparing the Mind and Learning to See: Art Museums as Training Grounds for Medical Students and Residents." In *Managing Arts Programs in Healthcare*, edited by Patricia Dewey Lambert, 255–270. New York, NY: Routledge.

Administration on Aging. 2021. *2020 Profile of Older Americans*. Washington, DC: U.S. Department of Health and Human Services, The Administration for Community Living.

Administration for Community Living. 2021. "Projected Future Growth of Older Population." Accessed June 30, 2021. https://acl.gov/aging-and-disability-in-america/data-and-research/projected-future-growth-older-population

Albright, Ariadne and Ferol P. Carytsas, eds. 2021. *Core Curriculum for Arts in Health Professionals*. San Diego, CA: National Organization for Arts in Health.

Alderfer, Clayton P. 1969. "An Empirical Test of a New Theory of Human Needs." *Organizational Behavior and Human Performance* 4: 142–175.

All-Party Parliamentary Group on Arts, Health and Wellbeing. 2017. *Creative Health: The Arts for Health and Wellbeing*. London, UK: Author.

Alzheimer's Association. 2021. "Alzheimer's Disease Facts and Figures." Accessed September 15, 2021. https://alz.org/alzheimers-dementia/facts-figures

American Assembly. 1997. *The Arts and the Public Purpose*. New York, NY: American Assembly, Columbia University. Accessed January 30, 2023. https://ia800303.us.archive.org/31/items/artspublicpurpos00amer/artspublicpurpos00amer.pdf

American Association for Retired Persons (AARP). n.d. *Age Friendly Training Videos*. Washington, DC: AARP. Accessed January 30, 2023. https://www.aarp.org/livable-communities/network-age-friendly-communities/age-friendly-training-videos/

American Folklore Society. 2022. "What is Folklore?" Accessed January 30, 2022. https://whatisfolklore.org/

American Geriatrics Society. n.d. "Is Assisted Living Right for You?" Accessed January 20, 2020. https://www.healthinaging.org/age-friendly-healthcare-you/care-settings/assisted-living

The American Psychological Association (APA) Committee on Aging. 2020/2021. "Ageism and Covid-10." Accessed on January 30, 2023. https://www.apa.org/topics/covid-19/research-ageism?_ga=2.263035916.1212811041.1673050874-1986364307.1673050873

American Senior Housing Association. n.d. "Where You Live Matters Senior Living Glossary." Accessed January 20, 2020. http://whereyoulivematters.org

Americans for the Arts. 2005. "Recommendations from Mini-Conference on Creativity and Aging in America, May 18–19." Accessed October 1, 2022. http://americansforthearts.org/sites/default/files/creativity%20and20%Aging.pdf

Americans for the Arts. 2013. "Arts in Health: Issue Brief." In *Arts Advocacy Day: Congressional Arts Handbook*. Washington, DC: Americans for the Arts.

A Place for Mom. 2015. "Guide to Senior Housing & Care." Accessed January 20, 2020. https://www.aplaceformom.com

Applewhite, Ashton. 2016. *This Chair Rocks: A Manifesto Against Ageism*. New York, NY: Celadon.

Askin, Elisabeth and Nathan Moore. 2014. *The Health Care Handbook: A Clear and Concise Guide to the United States Health Care System*, 2nd ed. St Louis, Missouri: Washington University in St. Louis.

Bailey-Johnson, Juanita. 2012. "Positionality and Transformative Learning: A Tale of Inclusion and Exclusion." In *The Handbook of Transformative Learning: Theory, Research, and Practice*, edited by Edward W. Taylor and Patricia Cranton, 260–273. Hoboken, NJ; John Wiley and Sons.

Baldwin, Moyra A. and Jan Woodhouse. 2011. "Good Death." In *Key Concepts in Palliative Care*, edited by Moyra A. Baldwin and Jan Woodhouse, 77–81. Thousand Oaks, CA: Sage.

Barnett, Karen, Stewart Mecer, Michael Norbury, Graham Watt, Sally Wyke, and Bruce Guthrie. 2012. "Epidemiology of Multimorbidity and Implications for Health Care, Research, and Medical Education: A Cross-Sectional Study." *Lancet* 380: 37–43. doi: 10.1016/S0140-6736(12)60240-2

Barret, Diane B. 1993. "Art Programming for Older Adults: What's Out There?" *Studies in Art Education* 34 (3): 133–140.

Bartocci, Barbara. 2000. *Nobody's Child Anymore*. Notre Dame, IN: Sorin Books.

Basting, Anne. 2021a. *Creative Care: A Revolutionary Approach to Dementia and Elder Care*. New York, NY: HarperOne.

Basting, Anne. 2021b. *Creative Care Imagination Kit*. New York, NY: Harper Collins.

Baumgartner, Frank R. and Bryan D. Jones. 1993. *Agendas and Instability in American Politics*. Chicago: University of Chicago Press.

Beardsly, Eleonor. 2021. "This French Pianist Has Been Playing for 102 years and Just Released a New Album." *NPR*. Accessed September 20, 2022. https://www.npr.org/sections/deceptivecadence/2021/09/20/1036622670/107-year-old-french-pianist-colette-maze-new-album

Bechill, William. 1990. "White House Conferences on Aging: An Assessment of Their Public Policy Influences." *Journal of Aging and Social Policy* 2 (3/4): 12–25.

Becker, Howard S. 2008. *Art Worlds*. Berkeley, CA: University of California.

Beisgen, Beverly A. and Marilyn Crouch Kraitchman. 2003. *Senior Centers: Opportunities for Successful Aging*. New York, NY: Springer.

Berridge, Clara W. and Marty Martinson. 2017. "Valuing Old Age Without Leveraging Ableism." *Generations: Journal of American Society on Aging* 41 (4): 83–91.

Berwick, Donald M., Thomas W. Nolan, and John Whittington. 2008. "The Triple Aim: Care, Health, and Cost." *Health Affairs* 27 (3): 759–769.

Best-Martini, Elizabeth, Mary Anne Weeks, and Priscilla Wirth. 2018. *Long-Term Care for Activity Professionals, Social Services Professionals, and Recreational Therapists*, 7th ed. Enumclaw, WA: Idyll Arbor, Inc.

Beutell, Nicholas. 2006. "Life Satisfaction." Sloan Network Encyclopedia Entry. Sloan Work and Family Research Network. https://wfrn.org/wp-content/uploads/2018/09/Life-Satisfaction-encyclopedia.pdf

Binstock, Robert H. 2005a. "Old-Age Policies, Politics, and Ageism." *Generations: Journal of the American Society on Aging* 24 (3): 73–78.

Binstock, Robert H. 2005b. "Social Security and Medicare: Present Bush and the Delegates Reject Each Other." *Public Policy and Aging Report* 15 (1): 9–12.

Bisognano, Maureen and Charles Kenney. 2012. *Pursuing the Triple Aim: Seven Innovators Show the Way to Better Care, Better Health, and Lower Costs*. San Francisco: Jossey-Bass.

Black Listed Culture. 2022. "Aminah Brenda Lynn Robinson." *Black Listed Culture* 1 (23). Accessed January 29, 2021. https://blacklistedculture.com/aminah-brenda-lynn-robinson/

Blancato, Robert B. 2004. "Advocacy and Aging Policy." *Generations: Journal of the American Society on Aging* 28 (1): 65–69.

Blanchard, Janice. 2006. "As the Pendulum Swings: A Historical Review of the Politics and Policies of the Arts and Aging." *Generations: Journal of the American Society on Aging* 30 (1): 50–56.

Blandy, Doug. 2008. "Cultural Programming." In *Arts and Cultural Programming: A Leisure Perspective*, edited by Gaylene Carpenter and Doug Blandy, 173–184. Champaign, IL: Human Kinetics.

Block, Susan D. 2001. "Psychological Considerations, Growth and Transcendence at the End of Life: The Arts of the Possible." *JAMA* 285 (22): 2898–2905.

Bodenheimer, Thomas and Christine Sinsky. 2014 "From Triple to Quadruple Aim: Care of the Patient Requires Care of the Provider." *Annals of Family Medicine* 12 (6): 573–576.

Bone, Jessica K., Daisy Fancourt, Meg E. Fluharty, Elise Paul, Jill Sonke, and Feifei Bu. 2022. "Associations Between Participation in Community Arts Groups and Aspects of Wellbeing in Older Adults in the United States: A Propensity Score Mathing Analysis. Aging and Mental Health." Accessed January 30, 2023. https://tandfonline.com/doi/pdf/10.1080/13607863.2022.2068129?needAccess=true

Bonnano, George A. 2009. *The Other Side of Sadness: What the New Science of Bereavement Tells Us About Life After Loss*. New York, NY: Basic Books.

Bosman, Julie, Amy Harmon, and Albert Sun. 2021. "As U. S. Nears 800,000 Virus Deaths, 1 of Every 100 Older Adults Has Perished." *New York Times*. Accessed January 30, 2023. https://www.nytimes.com/2021/12/13/us/covid-deaths-elderly-americans.html?action=click&module=RelatedLinks&pgtype=Article

Boyer, Johanna Misey. 2007. *Creativity Matters: The Arts and Aging Toolkit*. New York, NY: National Guild of Community Schools of the Arts.

Bradley, Robert H. and Robert Corwyn. 2004. "Life Satisfaction among European American, African American, Chinese American, Mexican American, and Dominican American Adolescents." *International Journal of Behavioral Development* 28 (5): 385–400. doi 10.1080/01650250444000072

Brazier, Kay D. 2005. "Influence of Contextual Factors on Healthcare Leadership." *Leadership and Organiation Development Journal* 26 (2): 128–140.

Brendel, William. 2007. "Pedagogy of the Terminally Ill: Exploring Meaning-Making among Hospice Patients through Transformative Learning Theory." In *Conference Proceedings from Transformative Learning: Issues of Difference and Diversity*, edited by Patricia Cranton and Edward Taylor, 36–41. Penn State University-Harrisburg.

Buchbinder, Sharon B. and Dale Buchbinder. 2017. "Managing Health Care Professionals." In *Introduction to Health Care Management*, 3rd ed., edited by Sharon B. Buchbinder and Nancy H. Shanks, 279–320. Burlington, MA: Jones & Bartlett Learning.

Bukaty, Robert F. 2021, June 23. "The Pandemic Led to the Biggest Drop in U.S. Life Expectance Since WWII, Study Find." Accessed October 1, 2021. https://www.npr.org/

Burke, Leann. 2017. "Chesterton Woman Makes Hooked Rugs Based on Memories." *The Times of Northwest Indiana*. https://www.nwitimes.com/news/local/porter/duneland/chesterton/chesterton-woman-makes-hooked-rugs-based-on-memories/article_5d4b8506-34c4-5c47-8d06-3267a77dc91e.amp.html

Burstein, Joyce. 2014. "Integrating Arts: Cultural Anthropology and Expressive Culture in the Social Studies Curriculum." *Social Studies Research and Practice* 9 (2): 132–144.

Butler, Katy. 2019. *The Art of Dying Well*. New York, NY: Scribner.

Butler, Stuart M. 2021. "Time to Rethink Nursing Homes." *The JAMA Forum*, April 13. https://jamanetwork.com/journals/jama/fullarticle/2778504

Byock, Ira. 1997. *Dying Well: Peace and Possibilities at the End of Life*. New York, NY: Riverhead Books.

Byock, Ira. 2012. *The Best Care Possible: A Physician's Quest to Transform Care through the End of Life*. New York, NY: Avery.

Byock, Ira. 2022. "Human Development and Personal Well-Being in Life-Threatening Conditions: Therapeutic Insights and Strategies Derived from Positive Experiences of Individuals and Families." In *Handbook of Psychiatry in Palliative Medicine: Psychosocial Care of the Terminally Ill*, 3rd ed., edited by Harvey Max Chochinov and William Breitbart, 641–667. New York, NY: Oxford University Press.

Callahan, Suzanne and Diane Mataraza. 2011. *Thought Leader Forum on Arts & Aging*. Seattle, WA: Grantmakers in the Arts. Accessed March 1, 2020. https://www.giarts.org/sites/default/files/Thought-Leader-Forum-on-Arts-Aging.pdf

Camfield, Laura, and Suzanne M. Skevington. 2008. "On Subjective Well-Being and Quality of Life." *Journal of Health Psychology* 13: 764–775. doi: 10.1177/1359105308093860.

Carlsen, Mary Baird. 1991. *Creative Aging: A Meaning-Making Perspective*. New York, NY: W. W. Norton & Company.

Carnes, R. 2015. "Shining Like the Sun: A Photographic Memory Infuses the Brilliant Art of Perry Johnson." *The Eugene Weekly*. Accessed February 1, 2022. https://www.eugeneweekly.com/2015/10/01/shining-like-the-sun/

Carpenter, Gaylene. 2008. "Overview of Arts and Cultural Programming." In *Arts and Cultural Programming: A Leisure Perspective*, edited by Gaylene Carpenter and Doug Blandy, 3–22. Champaign, IL: Human Kinetics.

Carpenter, Gaylene and Doug Blandy, eds. 2008. *Arts and Cultural Programming: A Leisure Perspective*. Champaign, IL: Human Kinetics.

Carr, Kelly, Patricia L. Weir, Dory Azar, and Nadia R. Azar. 2013. "Universal Design: A Step Toward Successful Aging." *Journal of Aging Research* 2013: 1–8.

Cascade Health. 2019. *Hospice Volunteer Training Manual*. Eugene, Oregon: Author.

References

Casciani, Susan. 2017. "Strategic Planning." In *Introduction to Health Care Management*, 3rd ed., edited by Sharon B. Buchbinder and Nancy H. Shanks, 107–124. Burlington, MA: Jones & Bartlett Learning.

Centers for Medicare & Medicaid Services. n.d. "Your Guide to Choosing a Nursing Home or Other Long-Term Services & Supports." Accessed January 15, 2020. https://medicare.gov/sites/default/files/2019-10/02174-nursing-home-other-long-term-services.pdf

Chapple, Karen, and Shannon Jackson. 2010. "Commentary: Arts, Neighborhoods, and Social Practices: Towards an Integrated Epistemology of Community Arts." *Journal of Planning Education and Research* 29 (4): 478–490.

Chidambaram, Priya. 2022. "Over 200,000 Residents and Staff in Long-Term Care Facilities Have Died from COVID-19." *Kaiser Family Foundation*, February 3. https://kff.org.policy-watch/over-200000-residents-and-staff-in-long-term-care-facilities-have-died-from-covid-19/

Clancy, Carolyn M., Janet M. Corrigan, and Dwight N. McNeill. 2009. "Patient-Centered Care as Public Policy: The Role of Government, Payers, and the General Public." In *Putting Patients First: Best Practices in Patient-Centered Care*, 2nd ed., edited by Susan B. Frampton and Patrick Charmel, 267–284. San Francisco: Jossey-Bass.

Clements-Cortés, Amy. 2016. "Development and Efficacy of Music Therapy Techniques within Palliative Care." *Complementary Therapies in Clinical Practice* 23: 125–129.

Clift, Stephen, and Paul M. Camic, eds. 2016. *Oxford Textbook of Creative Arts, Health, and Wellbeing: International Perspectives on Practice, Policy, and Research*. Oxford, UK: Oxford University Press.

Cohen, Elias S. 1990. "The White House Conference on Aging: An Anachronism." *Journal of Aging and Social Policy* 2 (3–4): 27–35.

Cohen, Gene. 2000. *The Creative Age: Awakening Human Potential in the Second Half of Life*. New York, NY: HarperCollins.

Cohen, Gene. 2005. *The Mature Mind: The Positive Power of the Aging Brain*. New York, NY: Basic Books.

Cohen, Gene. 2006. "The Creativity and Aging Study: The Impact of Professionally Conducted Cultural Programs on Older Adults." *The Center on Aging, Health & Humanities, The George Washington University (GW)*. Retrieved from http://hscrc.himmelfarb.gwu.edu/son_ncafacpubs/2

Cohen, Gene. 2009. "New Theories and Research Findings on the Positive Influence of Music and Art on Health and Ageing." *Arts & Health* 1 (1): 48–62.

Cohen, Gene D., Susan Perlstein, Jeff Chapline, Jeanne Kelly, Kimberly M. Firth, and Samuel Simmens. 2006. "The Impact of Professionally Conducted Cultural Programs on the Physical Health, Mental Health, and Social Functioning of Older Adults." *The Gerontologist* 46 (6): 726–734.

Coles, Emma, Julie Anderson, Margaret Maxwell, Fiona M. Harris, Nicola M. Gray, Gill Milner, and Stephen MacGillivray. 2022. "The Influence of Contextual Factors on Healthcare Quality Improvement Initiatives: A Realist Review." *Systematic Reviews* 9 (94). doi: 10.1186/e13643-020-01344-3

Columbus Museum of Art. 2021. "Raggin'On: An Aminah Robinson Inspired Activity Journal." Accessed February 15, 2022. https://www.columbusmuseum.org/wp-content/uploads/2021/02/color-Aminah-Journal-small.pdf

Congdon, Kristin and Doug Blandy. 2003. "Community Arts." In *Encyclopedia of Community: From the Village to the Virtual World*, edited by Karen Christensen and David Levinson, 242–245. Thousand Oaks, CA: Sage.

Connor, Stephen R. 2009. *Hospice and Palliative Care: The Essential Guide*, 2nd ed. New York, NY: Routledge.

Convergence Center for Policy Resolution. 2020. *Rethinking Care for Older Adults*. https://convergencepolicy.org/wp-content/uploads/2020/12/Rethinking-Care-for-Older-Adults_12-10-20.pdf

Coughlin, Joseph F. 2017. *The Longevity Economy*. New York, NY: PublicAffairs.

Cranton, Patricia and Chad Hoggan. 2012. "Evaluating Transformative Learning." In *The Handbook of Transformative Learning*, edited by Edward W. Taylor and Patricia Cranton, 520–535. Hoboken, NJ: John Wiley & Sons.

Creative City Network of Canada. 2010. "Cultural Planning Toolkit." Accessed January 30, 2023. https://www2.gov.bc.ca/assets/gov/sports-recreation-arts-and-culture/events-hosting/hosting-toolkit/cultural_planning_toolkit.pdf

Culture Track. 2022. "Untapped Opportunity: Older Americans and the Arts." Accessed January 30, 2023. https://s28475.pcdn.co/wpcontent/uploads/2022/06/CCTTUntappedOpportunity.pdf

Cummings, Jr., Milton C. 1991. "Government and the Arts: An Overview." In *Public Money and the Muse*, edited by Stephen Benedict, 31–79. New York, NY: Norton.

Daaleman, Timothy P. and Larry VandeCreek. 2000. "Placing Religion and Spirituality in End-of-Life Care." *JAMA* 284 (19): 2514–2517.

Dahlkemper, Tamara. 2020a. "Common Clinical Problems: Psychological." In *Caring for Older Adults Holistically*, 7th ed., edited by Tamara R. Dahlkemper, 281–300. Philadelphia: F.A. Davis.

Dahlkemper, Tamara. 2020b. "Environments of Care." In *Caring for Older Adults Holistically*, 7th ed., edited by Tamara R. Dahlkemper, 155–168. Philadelphia: F.A. Davis.

Dahlkemper, Tamara, ed. 2020c. *Caring for Older Adults Holistically*, 7th ed. Philadelphia: F.A. Davis.

Daniel, Mac. 2022. *Ageism's Toll in the Age of COVID*. Harvard Radcliffe Institute. Accessed January 30, 2023. https://www.radcliffe.harvard.edu/news-and-ideas/ageism-s-toll-in-the-age-of-covid

Davenport, Melanie, Pamela Harris Lawton, and Marjorie Manifold. 2020. "Art Education for Older Adults: Rationale, Issues, and Strategies." *International Journal of Lifelong Learning in Art Education* 3: 54–68.

Diener, Ed. 1984. "Subjective Well-Being." *Psychological Bulletin* 95: 542–575.

Diener, Ed. 2006. "Guidelines for National Indicators of Subjective Well-Being and Ill-Being." *Journal of Happiness Studies* 7 (4): 397–404.

Dissanayake, Ellen. 1988. *What is Art For?* Seattle: University of Washington Press.

Dissanayake, Ellen. 2013. "Art as a Human Universal: An Adaptationist View." In *Origins of Religion, Cognition and Culture*, edited by Armin W. Geertz, 121–139. Durham, UK: Acumen.

Duncan, Katie. 2021. *The Dying Process*. Self-published.

Dunn, Dana S. 2021. "Understanding Ableism and Negative Reactions to Disability." *American Psychological Association*. Accessed January 30, 2023. https://www.apa.org/ed/precollege/psychology-teacher-network/introductory-psychology/ableism-negative-reactions-disability

Duxbury, Nancy, and Eleonora Redaelli. 2020. "Cultural Mapping." *Oxford Bibliographies*. Accessed January 30, 2023. https://www.oxfordbibliographies.com/display/document/obo-9780199756841/obo-9780199756841-0249.xml

Ecker, David. 1963. "The Artistic Process as Qualitative Problem Solving." *The Journal of Aesthetics and Art Criticism* 21 (3): 283–290.

Edward Jones. 2022. *Longevity and the New Journey of Retirement*. https://edwardjones.com/sites/default/files/acquiadam/2022-05/AgeWaveReportMay2022.pdf

Edwards, Luned, and Behan Owen-Booth. 2021. "An Exploration of Engagement in Community-Based Creative Activities as an Occupation for Older Adults." *Irish Journal of Occupational Therapy* 49 (1): 51–57.

Elder Jr., Glen H. 1994. "Time, Human Agency, and Social Change: Perspectives on the Life Course." *Social Psychology Quarterly* 57 (1): 4–15.

Elison, Jennifer and Chris McGonigle. 2003. *Liberating Losses: When Death Brings Relief*. Cambridge, MA: Perseus Books Group.

Erikson, Erik. 1961. "The Roots of Virtue." In *The Humanist Frame*, edited by J. Huxley, 147–165. New York, NY: Harper & Brothers.

Erikson, Erik. 1982. *The Life Cycle Completed*. New York, NY: Norton.

Erikson, Erik H., Joan M. Erikson, and Helen Q. Kivnik. 1986. *Vital Involvement in Old Age: The Experience of Old Age in Our Time*. New York, NY: Norton.

Erikson, Joan M. 1988. *Wisdom and the Senses: The Way of Creativity*. New York, NY: Norton.

Estupiñan, Jaime, Keith Fengler, and Ashish Kaura. 2014. *The Birth of the Healthcare Consumer: Growing Demands for Choice, Engagement, and Experience*. New York, NY: Strategy& and PWC.

Fancourt, Daisy. 2017. *Arts in Health: Designing and Researching Interventions*. Oxford, UK: Oxford University Press.

Fancourt, Daisy, and Saoirse Finn. 2019. *What is the Evidence on the Role of the Arts in Improving Health and Well-Being? A Scoping Review*. Copenhagen: WHO Regional Office for Europe (Health Evidence Network (HEN) Synthesis Report 67).

References

Fancourt, Daisy, Henry Aughterson, Soairse Finn, Emma Walker, and Andrew Steptoe. 2021. "How Leisure Activities Affect Health: A Narrative Review and Multi-level Theoretical Framework of Mechanisms in Action." *Lancet Psychiatry* 8: 329–339.

Fareed, Charlyn Green. 2009. "Culture Matters: Developing Culturally Responsive Transformative Learning Experiences in Communities of Color." In *Innovations in Transformative Learning: Space, Culture, & the Arts*, edited by Beth Fisher-Yoshida, Kathy Dee Geller, and Steven A. Schapiro, 117–132. New York, NY: Peter Lang.Federal Interagency Forum on Aging-Related Statistics (FIFARS). 2020. *Older Americans 2020: Key Indicators of Well-Being*. Washington, DC: U.S. Government Printing Office.

Federal Interagency Forum on Aging-Related Statistics (FIFARS). 2021. Accessed June 30. https://www.agingstats.gov

Feintuch, Burt, ed. 2003. "Introduction." In *Eight Words for the Study of Expressive Culture*, 1–6. Urbana, IL: University of Illinois

Ferlie, Ewan, Louise Fitzgerald, Gerry McGivern, Sue Dopson, and Chris Bennett. 2011. "Public Policy Networks and 'Wicket Problems': A Nascent Solution?" *Public Administration* 89 (2): 307–324.

Findsen, Brian, and Marvin Formosa. 2011. *Lifelong Learning in Later Life: A Handbook on Older Adult Learning*. Rotterdam: Sense.

Firman, James, and Susan Stiles. 2018. *Aging Mastery Playbook*. Arlington, VA: National Council on Aging.

Fleige, Marion. 2017. "Transformative Learning, Bildung, and Art Education." In *Transformative Learning Meets Bildung: An International Exchange*, edited by Anna Laros, Thomas Fuhr, and Edward Taylor, 317–330. Rotterdam: Sense.

Fowler, James W. 1984. *Becoming Adults, Becoming Christian: Adult Development and Christian Faith*. San Francisco: Harper & Row.

Frampton, Susan B. 2009. "Introduction: Patient-Centered Care Moves into the Mainstream." In *Putting Patients First: Best Practices in Patient-Centered Care*, 2nd ed., edited by Susan B. Frampton and Patrick A. Charmel, xxvii–xl. San Francisco: Jossey-Bass.

Fraser, Andrew, Hilary Bungay, and Carol Munn-Giddings. 2014. "The Value of the Use of Participatory Arts Activities in Residential Care Settings to Enhance the Well-Being and Quality of Life of Older People: A Rapid Review of the Literature." *Arts & Health* 6 (3): 266–278.

Fulmer, Terry, Pinkey Patel, Nicole Levy, Kedar Mate, Amy Berman, Leslie Pelton, John Beard, Alexandre Kalache, and John Auerbach. 2020. "Moving Toward a Global Age-Friendly Ecosystem." *Journal of the American Geriatrics Society* 68 (9): 1936–1940.

Gallistl, Vera, Lukas Rickter, Theresa Heidinger, Teresa Schutz, Rebeka Rohner, Lisa Hengl, and Frank Kolland. 2022. "Precarious Aging in a Global Pandemic – Older Adults' Experiences of Being at Risk Due to COVID-19." *Ageing and Society*: 1–19. Doi: 10.1017/50144686X220000381

Gardner, Howard. 1983. *Frames of Mind: The Theory of Multiple Intelligences*. New York, NY: Basic Books.

Gawande, Atul. 2014. *Being Mortal: Medicine and What Matters in the End*. New York, NY: Picador.

Geber, Sara Zeff. 2021. "Hey Boomer: Medicare Won't Cover Your Long-Term Care." *Forbes*, July 28. https://forbes.com/sites/sarazeffgeber/2021/07/28/hey-boomer-medicare-wont-cover-your-long-term-care/?sh=45465b3a2074

Genworth. 2021 "Cost of Care." Accessed March 15, 2022. https://genworth.com/aging-and-you/finances/cost-of-care.html

George, Daniel R., and Winona Houser. 2014. "'I'm a Storyteller!': Exploring the Benefits of TimeSlips Creative Expression Program at a Nursing Home." *American Journal of Alzheimer's Disease & Other Dementias*, 28 (8): 678–684.

Gerteis, Margaret, Susan Edgman-Levitan, Jennifer Daley, and Thomas L. Delbanco. 1993. "Introduction: Medicine and Health from the Patient's Perspective." In *Through the Patient's Eyes: Understanding and Promoting Patient-Centered Care*, edited by Margaret Gerteis, Susan Edgman-Levitan, Jennifer Daley, and Thomas L. Delbanco, 1–15. New York, NY: John Wiley & Sons.

Goldbard, Arlene. 2009. *New Creative Community: The Art of Cultural Development*. Oakland, CA: New Village Press.

Goldsmith, Stephen and William D. Eggers. 2004. *Governing by Network: The New Shape of the Public Sector*. Washington, DC: Brookings Institution Press.

Gray, Clive. 2002. "Local Government and the Arts." *Local Government Studies* 29 (1): 77–90.

Gray, Marlaine Figueroa. 2022. *Creating Care: Art and Medicine in US Hospitals*. New York, NY: Lexington Books.

Green, James. 2008. *Beyond the Good Death: The Anthropology of Modern Dying*. Philadelphia: University of Pennsylvania Press.

Greene, Maxine. 1995. *Releasing the Imagination: Essays on Education, the Arts, and Social Change*. San Francisco, CA: Jossey-Bass.

Greene, Maxine. 2001. *Variations on a Blue Guitar: The Lincoln Center Institute Lectures on Aesthetic Education*. New York, NY: Teachers College.

Greenfield, Emily A., Mia Oberlink, Andrew E. Scharlach, Margaret B. Neal, and Phillip B. Stafford. 2015. "Age-Friendly Community Initiatives: Conceptual Issues and Key Questions." *The Gerontologist* 55 (2): 191–198.

Grollman, Earl A. 1995. *Living When a Loved One Has Died*. Boston, MA: Beacon Press.

Guerrero, Lourdes R. and Steven P. Wallace. 2021. "The Impact of COVID-19 on Diverse Older Adults and Health Equity in the United States." *Frontiers in Public Health* 9 (661592): 1–9. doi: 10.3389/fpubh.2021.661592.

Halpin-Healy, Carolyn. 2015. "Report from the Field: Multi-Cultural Dialogue and Transformative Learning in Arts and Minds Programs at The Studio Museum in Harlem." *Museum and Society* 13 (2): 188–194.

Hamer, Lynne and Paddy Bowman. 2011. "Introduction: Through the Schoolhouse Door." In *Through the Schoolhouse Door: Folklore, Community, Curriculum*, edited by Paddy Bowman and Lynne Hamer, 1–18. Logan, UT: Utah State University.

Hanna, Gay Powell. 2013. "The Central Role of Creative Aging." *The Journal of Art for Life*. Accessed June 15, 2020. https://journals.flvc.org/jafl/article/view/84239

Hanna, Gay Powell. 2016. "Arts, Health, and Aging." In *Managing Arts Programs in Healthcare*, edited by Patricia Dewey Lambert, 189–201. New York, NY: Routledge.

Hanna, Gay Powell, Linda S. Noelker, and Beth Bienvenu. 2015. "The Arts, Health, and Aging in America: 2005–2015." *The Gerontologist* 55 (2): 271–277.

Hanna, Gay, Judy Rollins, and Lorie Lewis. 2017. *Arts in Medicine Literature Review*. Seattle, WA: Grantmakers in the Arts. Accessed June 15, 2020. https://www.giarts.org/sites/default/files/2017-02-Arts-Medicine-Literature-Review.pdf

Hanna, Gay, and Susan Perlstein. 2008. *Creativity Matters: Arts and Aging in America*. Washington, DC: Americans for the Arts. Accessed May 1, 2020. https://www.giarts.org/article/creativity-matters-arts-and-aging-america

Hartley, Nigel. 2014. *End of Life Care: A Guide for Therapists, Artists and Arts Therapists*. London, UK: Jessica Kingsley Publishers.

Hartley, Nigel and Malcolm Payne, eds. 2008. *The Creative Arts in Palliative Care*. London, UK: Jessica Kingsley Publishers.

Havighurst, Robert J. 1972. *Developmental Tasks and Education*, 3rd ed. New York, NY: David McKay.

Head, Brian W. 2019. "Forty Years of Wicked Problems Literature: Forging Closer Links to Policy Studies." *Policy and Society* 38 (2): 180–197.

Head, Brian W. and John Alford. 2015. "Wicked Problems: Implications for Public Policy and Management." *Administration & Society* 47 (6): 711–739.

Hogan, Chad, Soni Simpson, and Heather Stuckey, eds. 2009. *Creative Expression in Transformative Learning: Tools and Techniques for Educators of Adults*. Malabar, FL: Krieger.

Howlett, Michael and M. Ramesh. 1995. *Studying Public Policy: Policy Cycles and Policy Subsystems*. New York, NY: Oxford University Press.

Hughes, Anne K., Clare Luz, Dennis Hall, Penny Gardner, Chris Walker Hennessey, and Lynn Lammers. 2016. "Transformative Theatre: A Promising Educational Tool for Improving Health Encounters With LGBT Older Adults." *Gerontology & Geriatrics Education* 37: 292–306.

Hurston, Zora Neale. n.d. "Excerpt from *Dust Tracks on the Road*." *Zora Neale Hurston: The Official Website of Zora Neale Hurston*. Accessed January 30, 2023. https://www.zoranealehurston.com/resource/excerpt-from-dust-tracks-on-a-road/

Institute for Healthcare Improvement. July 2020. *Age-Friendly Health Systems: Guide to Using the 4Ms in the Care of Older Adults.* https://ihi.org/Engage/Initiatives/Age-Friendly-Health-Systems/Docume nts/IHIAgeFriendlyHealthSystems_GuidetoUsing4MsCare.pdfInstitute of Medicine (IOM). 1990. *Medicare: A Strategy for Quality Assurance.* Washington, DC: National Academies Press.

Institute of Medicine (IOM). 2000. *To Err Is Human: Building a Safer Health System.* Washington, DC: National Academies Press.

Institute of Medicine (IOM). 2001. *Crossing the Quality Chasm: Building a New Health System for the 21st Century.* Washington, DC: National Academies Press.

Ivey, Bill. 2008. "Introduction: The Question of Participation." In *Engaging Art: The Next Great Transformation of America's Cultural Life,* edited by Steven J. Tepper and Bill Ivey, 1–16. New York, NY: Routledge.

Jarrett, Lucinda, ed. 2007. *Creative Engagement in Palliative Care.* New York, NY: Radcliffe Publishing Ltd.

Jarvis, Peter. 2008. "Learning from Everyday Life." In *The Routledge International Handbook of Lifelong Learning,* edited by Peter Jarvis, 19–30. London, UK: Taylor & Francis.

Jeffers, Steven L. and Dennis Kenny. 2009. "Spiritual and Cultural Diversity: Inner Resources for Healing." In *Putting Patients First: Best Practices in Patient-Centered Care,* 2nd ed., edited by Susan B. Frampton and Patrick A. Charmel, 95–112. San Francisco: Jossey-Bass.

Jeffri, Joan and Gay Hanna. 2015. "National Center for Creative Aging." In *The Encyclopedia of Adulthood and Aging,* 968–972. Wiley Online Library. Accessed September 30, 2022. https://doi.org/10.1002/9781118521373.wbeaa118

Jenkins-Smith, Hank C. and Paul A. Sabatier. 1993. "The Study of Public Policy Processes." In *Policy Change and Learning: An Advocacy Coalition Approach,* edited by Paul A. Sabatier and Hank C. Jenkins-Smith, 1–12. Boulder: Westview.

Johnson, Alton C. and Arthur Prieve. 1976. *Older Americans: The Unrealized Audience for the Arts.* Monograph commissioned by the Administration on Aging and the U.S. Department of Health, Education, and Welfare. Madison, WI: Center for Arts Administration, University of Wisconsin-Madison Bolz Graduate School of Business.

Johnson, Beverly H. and Marie R. Abraham. 2012. *Partnering with Patients, Residents, and Families: A Resource for Leaders of Hospitals, Ambulatory Care Settings, and Long-Term Care Communities.* Institute for Patient- and Family-Centered Care.

Johnson, Mira. 2021. *Growing Roots: Rewilding, Transformative Learning, and Ecological Consciousness in Nature Connection.* Dissertation in Adult Education. The Pennsylvania State University: The Graduate School.

Joint Center for Housing Studies of Harvard University. 2019. *Housing America's Older Adults 2019.* https://jchs.harvard.edu/sites/default/files/reports/files/Harvard_JCHS_Housing_Americas_Ol der_Adults_2019.pdf

Jost, Lauren. 2022. "Storytelling: I Know a Thing or Two, Brooklyn Public Library Central Branch." *Creative Aging 101: Case Study – Storytelling.* https://www.youtube.com/watch?v=GIeVU05x vo4&list=PLL1N0KwbK1d-zRjWvCe5cSBGTgTccjRwo&index=26

Kable, Lynn. 2016. "Using the Arts to Care for Paraprofessional and Family Caregivers." In *Managing Arts Programs in Healthcare,* edited by Patricia Dewey Lambert, 231–243. New York, NY: Routledge.

Katz, Stephen, ed. 2005. *Cultural Aging: Life Course, Lifestyle, and Senior Worlds.* Peterborough, Ontario: Broadview.

Katz, Stephen and Erin Campbell. 2005. "Creativity Across the Life Course? Titian, Michelangelo, and Older Artist Narratives." In *Cultural Aging: Life Course, Lifestyle, and Senior* Worlds, edited by Stephen Katz, 101–117. Petersborough, Ontario: Broadview.

Kay, Jon. 2016. *Folk Art & Aging: Life-Story Objects and Their Makers.* Bloomington, IN: Indiana University.

Keckley, Paul H. and Howard R. Underwood. 2009. *Medical Tourism: Consumers in Search of Value.* Washington, DC: Deloitte Center for Health Solutions.

Kernisan, Leslie and Paula Spencer Scott. 2021. *When Your Aging Parent Needs Help.* San Francisco, CA: Better Health While Aging.

Kingdon, John W. 1984. *Agendas, Alternatives, and Public Policies.* Boston: Little Brown.

Kingdon, John W. 2010. *Agendas, Alternatives, and Public Policies*, 2nd ed. New York, NY: Longman.
Kirshenblatt-Gimblett, Barbara, Mary Hufford, Marjorie Hunt, and Steve Zeitlin. 2006. "The Grand Generation: Folklore and the Culture of Aging." *Generations* 30 (1): 32–37.
Klein, Sheri R. 2018. "Coming to Our Senses: Everyday Landscapes, Aesthetics, and Transformative Learning." *Journal of Transformative Education* 16 (1): 3–16.
Knowles, Malcolm S., Elwood F. Holton III, and Richard A. Swanson. 1998. *The Adult Learner: The Definitive Classic in Adult Education and Human Resource Development*, 5th ed. New York, NY: Heinemann.
Koff, Theodore H. 1980. *Hospice: A Caring Community*. Cambridge, MA: Winthrop Publishers.
Kroth, Michael and Patricia Cranton. 2014. *Stories of Transformative Learning*. Rotterdam: Sense.
Kübler-Ross, Elisabeth. 1969. *On Death and Dying*. New York, NY: Scribner.
Lambert, Patricia Dewey, ed. 2016. *Managing Arts Programs in Healthcare*. New York, NY: Routledge.
Lambert, Patricia Dewey, Judy Rollins, Jill Sonke, and Randy Cohen. 2016. "Introducing the Arts in Healthcare Field." In *Managing Arts Programs in Healthcare*, edited by Patricia Dewey Lambert, 1–19. New York, NY: Routledge.
Laros, Anna, Thomas Fuhr, and Edward W. Taylor, eds. 2017. *Transformative Learning Meets 'Bildung': An International Exchange*. Rotterdam: Sense.
Larson, Renya T. H., and Susan Perlstein. 2003. "Creative Aging: A New Field for the 21st Century." *Teaching Artist Journal* 1 (3): 144–151.
Lawrence, Randee Lipson. 2005. "Knowledge Construction as Contested Terrain: Adult Learning Through Artistic Expression." In *Artistic Ways of Knowing: Expanded Opportunities for Teaching and Learning*, edited by Randee Lipson Lawrence, 3–12. Hoboken, NJ: Wiley.
Lawrence, Randee Lipson. 2012. "Transformative Learning Through Artistic Expression: Getting Out of Our Heads." In *The Handbook of Transformative Learning: Theory, Research, and Practice*, edited by Edward W. Taylor and Patricia Cranton, 471–485. Hoboken, NJ: John Wiley and Sons.
Lawton, Pamela Harris, and Angela M. LaPorte. 2013. "Beyond Traditional Art Education: Transformative Lifelong Learning in Community-Based Settings with Older Adults." *Studies in Art Education* 54 (4): 310–320.
Lebowitz, Barry, Nancy Miller, Audrey Faulkner, and Mary Harper. 1983. "Observations from the White House Conference: Panel Presentation." *Gerontology and Geriatrics Education* 3 (3): 177–182.
Learning for Justice: Our Multicultural Self. 2021. Accessed November 1, 2022. https://www.learningforjustice.org/classroom-resources/lessons/my-multicultural-self
Lee, Jenny Baxley, Sonja McIlfatrick, and Lisa Fitzpatrick. 2021a. "Examining the Range and Scope of Artists' Professional Practices with Individuals with Palliative Care Needs: An International Cross-Sectional Online Survey." *Frontiers in Psychology* 12: 1–14. doi: 10.3389/fpsyg2021.773451
Lee, Jenny Baxley, Sonja McIlfatrick, and Lisa Fitzpatrick. 2021b. "Arts Engagement Facilitated by Artists with Individuals with Life-Limiting Illness: A Systematic Review of the Literature." *Palliative Medicine* 35 (10): 1815–1831. doi: 10.1177/02692163211045895
Levinson, Daniel J. 1978. *The Seasons of a Man's Life*. New York, NY: Knopf.
Levy, Becca R., Martin D. Slade, Suzanne R. Kunkel, and Stanislav V. Kasi. 2002. "Longevity Increased by Positive Self-Perceptions of Aging." *Journal of Personality and Social Psychology* 83 (2): 261–270.
Lewis-Kane, Melody, Priscilla McCutcheon, and Robert McDicken. 1986. *Arts Mentor Program: A Manual for Sponsors*. National Council on Aging.
Lifetime Arts. 2022. "National Leaders in Creative Aging Program Development." Accessed October 30, 2022. https://www.lifetimearts.org/
Lindauer, Martin S. 2003. *Aging, Creativity, and Art: A Positive Perspective on Late-Life Development*. New York, NY: Kluwer Academic/Plenum Publishers.
Lindland, Eric, Nathaniel Kendall-Taylor, Abigail Haydon, and Marissa Fond. 2016. "Gauging Aging: Expert and Public Understanding of Aging in America." *Communication and the Public* 1 (2): 211–229.
Liverani M, Hawkins B, Parkhurst JO. 2013. "Political and Institutional Influences on the Use of Evidence in Public Health Policy. A Systematic Review." *PLoS One* 8 (10): e77404. doi:10.1371/journal.pone.0077404. PMID: 24204823; PMCID: PMC3813708.

References

Livingston, Gretchen. 2019. "Americans 60 and Older are Spending More Time in Front of Their Screens than a Decade Ago." *Pew Research Center*. Accessed January 30, 2023. https://urldefense.com/v3/__https://www.pewresearch.org/fact-tank/2019/06/18/americans-60-and-older-are-spending-more-time-in-front-of-their-screens-than-a-decade-ago/__;!!C5qS4YX3!Ce5nx4KG3TJ641nI1t_jegJT3TtjydKHd2voYkO9G2iCIZKBiRkEsXN0gUEmb0q830hmuxk__eZ5oAmonpeA-w$

Lloyd, Timothy. 2021. "Introduction." In *What Folklorists Do: Professional Possibilities in Folklore Studies*, edited by Timothy Lloyd, xi-xvii. Bloomington, IN: Indiana University.

Love, Kurt. 2011. "Enacting a Transformative Education." In *Critical Pedagogy in the Twenty-First Century: A New Generation of Scholars*, edited by Curry Stephenson Malott and Bradley Porfilio, 419–453. Information Age.

Lowe, Seana S. 2000. "Creating Community: Art for Community Development." *Journal of Contemporary Ethnography* 29 (3): 357–386.

Lynn, Joanne. 2001. "Serving Patients Who May Die Soon and Their Families: The Role of Hospice and Other Services." *JAMA* 285 (7): 925–932.

Maslow, Abraham H. 1954. *Motivation and Personality*. New York, NY: Harper.

Mayor's Art Show. 2019. "2019 Artist Statements and Information." https://www.eugene-or.gov/DocumentCenter/View/47211/2019-MAS-Artist-Statements

Matti, Simon and Annica Sanstrom. 2011. "The Rationale Determining Advocacy Coalitions: Examining Coordination Networks and Corresponding Beliefs." *Policy Studies Journal* 39 (3): 385–410.

McCarthy, Kevin F., Elizabeth H. Ondaatje, Laura Zakaras, and Arthur Brooks. 2004. *Gifts of the Muse: Reframing the Debate About the Benefits of the Arts*. Santa Monica, CA: The RAND Corporation. https://www.rand.org/content/dam/rand/pubs/monographs/2005/RAND_MG218.pdf

McCutcheon, Priscilla. 1986a. *An Arts and Aging Media Sourcebook: Films, Videos, Slide/Tape Shows*. Washington, DC: National Center on Arts and the Aging, National Council on Aging.

McCutcheon, Priscilla. 1986b. *A Manual for Artists: How to Find Work in the Field of Aging*. Washington, DC: National Council on Aging.

McCutcheon, Priscilla and Cathryn Wolf. 1985. *The Resource Guide to People, Places and Programs in Arts and Aging*. Washington, DC: National Council on Aging.

McDonough, Shannon K. 2013. "Lifetime Arts: Delivering Arts Education Programs for Today's Older Adults." *Public Libraries Online*. http://publiclibrariesonline.org/2013/06/lifetime-arts-delivering-arts-education-programs-for-todays-older-adults/

McFadden, Susan H. 2021. *Dementia-Friendly Communities: Why We Need Them and How We Can Create Them*. London, UK: Jessica Kingsley.

McGarth, Valerie. 2009. "Reviewing the Evidence of How Adult Students Learn: An Examination of Knowles' Model of Andragogy." *Adult Learner: The Irish Journal of Adult and Community Education*: 99–110.

McNeill, Lynne S. 2013. *Folklore Rules: A Fun, Quick, and Useful Introduction to the Field of Academic Folklore Studies*. Logan, UT: Utah State University.

Meeks, Suzanne. 2022. "Age-Friendly Communities: Introduction to the Special Issue." *The Gerontologist* 62 (1): 1–5.

Mehrotra, Chandra M., and Lisa S. Wagner. 2019. *Aging and Diversity: An Active Learning Experience*, 3rd ed. New York, NY: Routledge.

Menec, Verena H., Robin Means, Norah Keating, Graham Parkhurst, and Jacquie Eales. 2011. "Conceptualizing Age-Friendly Communities." *Canadian Journal on Aging / La Revue canadienne du vieillissement* 30 (3): 479–493.

Mezirow, Jack. 1975. *Education for Perspective Transformation: Women's Reentry Programs in Community Colleges*. New York, NY: Center for Adult Education, Columbia University.

Mezirow, Jack. 1991. *Transformative Dimensions of Adult Learning*. San Francisco, CA: Jossey-Bass.

Mezirow, Jack. 2011. "Transformative Learning Theory." In *Transformative Learning in Practice: Insights from Community, Workplace, and Higher Education*, edited by Jack Mezirow and Edward W. Taylor, 18–31. Hoboken, NJ: John Wiley & Sons.

Mezirow, Jack, and Edward W. Taylor, eds. 2011. *Transformative Learning in Practice: Insights from Community, Workplace, and Higher Education*. Hoboken, NJ: John Wiley & Sons.Michelson, Ellen and Teresa Bonner. 2018. "Arts and Aging: Interview with Aroha Philanthropies Founder Ellen Michelson, and Executive Director Teresa Bonner." In Barry's Blog, July 8, 2018. https://blog.westaf.org/2018/07/arts-and-aging-interview-with-aroha.html

Miller, Jennifer Blackburn. 2020. "Transformative Learning and the Arts: A Literature Review." *Journal of Transformative Education* 18 (4): 338–355.

Merriam, Sharon B. 1990. "Reminiscence and Life Review: The Potential for Educational Intervention." In *Introduction to Educational Gerontology*, edited by Ronald H. Sherron and D. Barry Lumsden, 41–58. New York, NY: Hemisphere.

Moody, Harry R. 1988. *Abundance of Life: Human Development Policies for an Aging Population*. New York, NY: Columbia University Press.

Morgan, Nancy. 2016. "Arts Programs for Medical Staff." In *Managing Arts Programs in Healthcare*, edited by Patricia Dewey Lambert, 244–254. New York, NY: Routledge.

Morris, Virginia. 2014. *How to Care for Aging Parents*, 3rd ed. New York, NY: Workman Publishing.

Napier, A. David. (2017). "Culture Matters: Using a Cultural Contexts of Health Approach to Enhance Policy-Making." *Cultural Contexts of Health and Well-Being. Policy Brief, No. 1.* World Health Organization Regional Office for Europe. https://www.euro.who.int/__data/assets/pdf_file/0009/334269/14780_World-Health-Organisation_Context-of-Health_TEXT-AW-WEB.pdf

National Assembly of State Arts Agencies and National Endowment for the Arts. 1994. *Design for Accessibility: A Cultural Administrator's Handbook*. Washington, DC: National Assembly of State Arts Agencies and National Endowment for the Arts.

National Assembly of State Arts Agencies (NASAA). 2019a. "Strategy Sampler: Creative Aging." Accessed February 1, 2020. https://nasaa-arts.org/nasaa_research/creative-aging-strategy-sampler/

National Assembly of State Arts Agencies (NASAA). 2019b. *Survey Highlights: Leveraging State Investments in Creative Aging*. Washington, DC: NASAA. https://nasaa-arts.org/nasaa_research/survey-highlights-leveraging-state-investments-in-creative-aging/

National Center for Complementary and Integrative Health (NCCIH). 2018. "Complementary, Alternative, or Integrative Health. What's in a Name?" Accessed June 30, 2021. https://nccih.nih.gov/health/integrative-health

National Center for Creative Aging (NCCA). n.d. *Designing and Delivering Arts Programs for Older Adult Learners: Instructor's Curriculum Manual for Classroom Education of Professional Artists*. Washington, DC: Author.

National Council on Aging (NCOA). 2021a. "Aging Mastery Program." Accessed June 30, 2022. https://ncoa.org/AMP

National Council on Aging (NCOA). 2021b. "Get the Facts on Healthy Aging." Accessed June 30, 2022. https://www.ncoa.org/article/get-the-facts-on-healthy-aging

National Council on Aging (NCOA). 2022. "Get the Facts on Senior Centers." Accessed July 19, 2022. https://ncoa.org/article/get-the-facts-on-senior-centers

National Endowment for the Arts (NEA). 1978. *Annual Report, 1978*. Washington, DC: NEA.

National Endowment for the Arts (NEA). 1995. *Annual Report, 1995*. Washington, DC: NEA.

National Endowment of the Arts (NEA), with National Center for Creative Aging (NCCA), NAMM, and AARP. 2005. "Recommendations for the Mini-Conference on Creativity and Aging in America." May 18–19, 2005. Accessed November 1, 2022. Retrieved from http://blog.afta.org/sites/default/foels/creativity%29and29%Aging.pdf

National Endowment for the Arts (NEA). 2011. *The Arts and Human Development: Framing a National Research Agenda for the Arts, Lifelong Learning, and Individual Well-Being*. Washington, DC: NEA Office of Research & Analysis.

National Endowment for the Arts (NEA). 2012. *How Art Works: The National Endowment for the Arts' Five-Year Research Agenda, with a System Map and Measurement Model*. Washington, DC: National Endowment for the Arts Office of Research & Analysis.

National Endowment for the Arts (NEA). 2013. *The Arts and Aging: Building the Science*. Washington, DC: NEA Office of Research & Analysis.

National Endowment for the Arts (NEA). 2015a. *How Creativity Works in the Brain*. Washington, DC: NEA Office of Research & Analysis.

National Endowment for the Arts (NEA). 2015b. *When Going Gets Tough: Barriers and Motivations Affecting Arts Attendance*. Washington DC: NEA Office of Research & Analysis.

National Endowment for the Arts (NEA). 2016a. *The Summit on Creativity and Aging in America*. Washington, DC: Author.

National Endowment for the Arts (NEA). 2016b. *The National Endowment for the Arts Guide to Community-Engaged Research in the Arts and Health*. Washington, DC: NEA Office of Research & Analysis.

National Foundation on the Arts and the Humanities, U.S. Code 20 (1965), § 952.

National Health Policy Forum of The George Washington University. 2013. "Assisted Living: Facilities, Financing, and Oversight." January 29. https://www.nhpf.org

National Hospice and Palliative Care Organization. n.d. Assessed June 10, 2022. http://caringinfo.org

National Organization for Arts in Health (NOAH). 2017. *Arts, Health, and Well-Being in America*. San Diego, CA: Author.

Noice, Tony, Helga Noice, and Arthur F. Kramer. 2013. "Participatory Arts for Older Adults: A Review of Benefits and Challenges." *The Gerontologist* 54 (5): 741–753.

NORC at the University of Chicago. 2021. "Executive Summary: Maintaining Physical and Mental Well-Being of Older Adults and their Caregivers During Public Health Emergencies." https://www.norc.org/PDFs/Maintaining%20Physical%20and%20Mental%20Well/OACExecutiveSummary.pdf

Norman-Eady, Sandra. 2002. "Oregon's Assisted Suicide Law." Accessed April 15, 2022. https://www.gcga.ct.gov/2002/rpt/2002-R-0077.htm

Novak-Leonard, Jennifer L., and Alan S. Brown. 2011. *Beyond Attendance: A Multi-Modal Understanding of Arts Participation*. Washington, DC: National Endowment for the Arts.

Oakman, Rosemarie and Doug Blandy. 2021. "'I See History and the Future:' Memory Loss, Art Education, and Online Learning." *Art Education* 74 (4): 13–15.

Older Americans Act of 1965. Public Law 89–131 as amended through Public Law 116–131, enacted March 25, 2020.

Opam, Kwame. 2021, February 26. "Overlooked No More: Aminah Brenda Lynn Robinson, Whose Art Chronicled Black Life." *The New York Times*. Updated May 2, 2021. https://www.nytimes.com/2021/02/26/obituaries/aminah-brenda-lynn-robinson-overlooked.html

O'Rand, Angela. 1996. "The Precious and the Precocious: Understanding Cumulative Disadvantage Over the Life Course." *The Gerontologist*. 36: 230–238.

Osterland, Andrew. 2021. "Aging Baby Boomers Raise the Risk of a Long-Term-Care Crisis in the United States." *CNBC*, November 8, 2021. https://www.cnbc.com/2021/11/08/aging-baby-boomers-raise-the-risk-of-a-long-term-care-crisis-in-the-us.html

O'Sullivan, Edmund. 2002. "The Project and Vision of Transformative Education: Integral Transformative Learning." In *Expanding the Boundaries of Transformative Learning: Essays on Theory and Praxis*, edited by Edmund O'Sullivan, Amish Morrell, and Mary Ann O'Connor, 1–12. New York, NY: Palgrave.

Pankratz, David. 1989. "Arts Policy and Older Adults." *Journal of Arts Management and Law* 19 (4): 13–64.

Pastan, Linda. 1999. "The Five Stages of Grief." In *Grief and the Healing Arts: Creativity as Therapy*, edited by Sandra L. Bertman, 2–20. New York, NY: Baywood Publishing Company, Inc.

Patterson, Michael C., and Susan Perlstein. 2011. "Good for the Heart, Good for the Soul: The Creative Arts and Brain Health in Later Life." *Generations* 35: 27–36.

Pennsylvania Council on the Arts. n.d. "Arts Training for Working with Older Adults." *The Academy for Creative Aging*. Accessed January 30, 2023. https://www.academyforcreativeaging.org/

Peck, Robert. 1956. "Psychological Developments in the Second Half of Life." In *Psychological Aspects of Aging*, edited by J. E. Anderson, 42–53. Washington, DC: American Psychological Association.

Pierce, Molly. 2019. *Designing Spaces that Support Health for the Whole Person: A Sensory Processing Perspective of Healthcare Design in Community-Based Settings*. University of Oregon Master's Project. https://scholarsbank.uoregon.edu/xmlui/bitstream/handle/1794/24739/final_masters_research_project_pierce.pdf?sequence=1&isAllowed=y

Pioneer Network. 2016. "Definitions of Common Terms Used in Long-Term Care and Culture Change." Accessed February 10, 2021. https://www.pioneernetwork.net/wp-content/uploads/2016/10/Definitions-of-Common-Terms-Used-in-Long-Term-Care-and-Culture-Change.pdf

Pocius, Gerald L. 2003. "Art." In *Eight Words for the Study of Expressive Culture*, edited by Burt Feintuch, 42–68. Urbana, IL: University of Illinois.

Population Reference Bureau. 2016. "Longevity Research: Unraveling the Determinants of Healthy Aging and Longer Life Spans." *Today's Research on Aging* (34). Accessed June 30, 2021. https://prb.org/resources/longevity-research-unraveling-the-determinants-of-healthy-aging-and-longer-life-spans

Population Reference Bureau. 2019. "America's Changing Population." *Population Bulletin* 74 (1). Accessed June 30, 2021. https://prb.org/wp-content/uploads/2020/10/2019-74-1-Pop-Bulletin-Census.pdf

Population Reference Bureau. 2021. "Fact Sheet Aging in the United States." Accessed June 30, 2021. https://www.prb.org/resources/fact-sheet-aging-in-the-united-states/

Prasoon, Rituparna and K. R. Chaturvedi. 2016. "Life Satisfaction: A Literature Review." *The Researcher – International Journal of Management, Humanities, and Social Sciences* 1 (2): 24–31.

Puner, Morton. 1974. *To the Good Long Life: What We Know About Growing Old*. New York, NY: Universe Books.

Quadagno, Jill 2005. *Aging and Life Course: An Introduction to Social Gerontology*. Boston: McGraw.

Rabheru, Kiran and Margaret Gillis. 2021. "Navigating the Perfect Storm of Ageism, Mentalism, and Ableism: A Prevention Model." *American Journal of Geriatric Psychiatry* 29 (10): 1058–1061.

Rajan, Kumar B., and Rekha S. Rajan. 2017. *Staying Engaged: Health Patterns of Older Adults Who Participate in the Arts*. Washington, DC: National Endowment for the Arts.

Ratini, Melinda. 2020. "Holistic Medicine: What It Is, Treatments, Philosophy, and More." *Web MD*. https://webmd.com/balance/guide/what-is-holistic-medicine

Reynolds, Linda and Derek Botha. 2006. "Anticipatory Grief: Its Nature, Impact, and Reasons for Contradictory Findings." *Counselling, Psychotherapy, and Health* 2 (2): 15–26.

Riley, Matilda White and Joan Waring Foner. 1988. "Sociology of Age." In *Handbook of Aging and the Social Sciences*, edited by Robert H. Binstock and Linda K. George, 243–290. Newbury Park, CA: Sage.

Riley, Matilda White, and John W. Riley Jr. 1994. "Structural Lag: Past and Future." In *Age and Structural Lag: Society's Failure to Provide Meaningful Opportunities in Work, Family, and Leisure*, edited by Matilda White Riley, Robert L. Kahn, and Anne Foner, 15–36. Hoboken, NJ: John Wiley & Sons.

Rizzo, Karyn. 2016. *Aging in America: Navigating our Healthcare System*. Self-published.

Rollins, Judy. 2013. *Bringing the Arts to Life: A Guide to the Arts and Long-Term Care*. Washington, DC: Global Alliance for Arts & Health.

Rollins, Judy, Cam Busch, Mukta Panda, and Nancy Tilson-Mallett. 2021. "Care Delivery." In *Core Curriculum for Arts in Health Professionals*, edited by Ariadne Albright and Ferol P. Carytsas, 208–247. San Diego, CA: National Organization for Arts in Health.

Romanoff, Bronna D. and Barbara E. Thompson. 2006. "Meaning Construction in Palliative Care: The Use of Narrative, Ritual, and the Expressive Arts." *American Journal of Hospice & Palliative Medicine* 23 (4): 309–316.

Roubein, Rachel. 2021. "Will the Nursing Home of the Future be an Actual Home?" *Politico*, April 30, 2021. https://www.politico.com/news/agenda/2021/04/30/nursing-home-future-483460

Royal College of Nursing. 2008. *Defending Dignity – Challenges and Opportunities for Nursing*. https://www.dignityincare.org.uk/_assets/RCN_Digntiy_at_the_heart_of_everything_we_do.pdf

Ryder, Norman. 1965. "The Cohort as a Concept in the Study of Social Change." *American Sociological Review* 30 (3): 843–86.

Sadler, Blair L. and Annette Ridenour. 2009. *Transforming the Healthcare Experience through the Arts*. San Diego, CA: Aesthetics, Inc.

Safrai, Mary B. 2013. "Art Therapy in Hospice: A Catalyst for Insight and Healing." *Art Therapy: Journal of the American Art Therapy Association* 30 (3): 122–129.

Saunders, Pamela A., Caroline Edasis, Gay Hanna, Betty Siegel, and Adam Hansen. 2022. *The Next Wave in Creative Aging: Creative Innovation Forums Cross Industry Report*. Washington, DC: Georgetown University Aging and Health Program, Kennedy Center Office of Accessibility, and Mather.

Scharoun, Lisa, Danny Hills, Carlos Montana-Hoyes, Fanke Peng, and Vivien Sung. 2020. *Cross-Cultural Design for Healthy Aging*. Chicago and Bristol, UK: Intellect.

Searle, Michelle, Claire Ahn, Lynn Fels, and Katrina Carbone. 2021. "Illuminating Transformative Learning / Assessment: Infusing Creativity, Reciprocity, and Care into Higher Education." *Journal of Transformative Education*, 19 (4): 339–365.

Serlin, Ilene Ava 2007. *Whole Person Healthcare Volume 3: The Arts & Health*. Westport, CT: Praeger.

Shanks Nancy H. 2017. "Financing Health Care and Health Insurance." In *Introduction to Health Care Management*, 3rd ed., edited by Sharon B. Buchbinder and Nancy H. Shanks, 203–246. Burlington, MA: Jones & Bartlett Learning.

Slater, Jana Kay. 2016. "Evaluating the Arts in Healthcare Program: Building a Story About the Program's Activities, Paths to Improvement, and Achievements." In *Managing Arts Programs in Healthcare*, edited by Patricia Dewey Lambert, 139–154. New York, NY: Routledge.

Slater, Jana Kay, Marc T. Braverman, and Thomas Meath. 2017. "Patient Satisfaction with a Hospital's Arts-Enhanced Environment as a Predictor of the Likelihood of Recommending the Hospital." *Arts & Health*, 9 (2), 97–110. doi: 10/1080/17533-15.2016.1185448

The Smithsonian Center for Folklife and Cultural Heritage. 2021. "Education: A Glossary of Key Terms." Accessed January 30, 2023. https://folklife.si.edu/the-smithsonian-folklife-and-oral-history-interviewing-guide/a-glossary-of-key-terms/smithsonian

Sonke, Jill, Judy Rollins, Randi Brandman, and John Graham-Pole. 2009. "The State of the Arts in Healthcare in the United States." *Arts & Health* 1 (2): 107–135.

Sonke, Jill, Tasha Golden, Samantha Francois, Jamie Hand, Anita Chandra, Lydia Clemmons, David Fakunle, Maria Rosario Jackson, Susan Magsamen, Victor Rubin, Kelley Sams, and Stacey Springs. 2019. *Creating healthy communities through cross-sector collaboration* [White paper]. Gainesville, FL: University of Florida Center for Arts in Medicine / ArtPlace America.

Sowerby, Holli. 2020. "Physiological Assessment." In *Caring for Older Adults Holistically*, 7th ed., edited by Tamara R. Dahlkemper, 229–247. Philadelphia: F.A. Davis.

State of the Field Committee. 2009. *State of the Field Report: Arts in Healthcare 2009*. Washington, DC: Society for the Arts in Healthcare.

Statista. 2022. "Share of Old Age Population (65 Years and Older) in the Total U.S. Population from 1950 to 2050." Accessed November 1, 2022. https://statista.com/statistics/457922/share-of-old-age-population-in-the-total-US-population/

Stein, Michael. 1998. *The Prosperous Retirement: Guide to the New Reality*. Boulder, CO: Emstco Press.

Steinmetz, Margery Pabst. 2015. "The Creative Caregiving Initiative: Arts at the Intersection of Wellness." *GIA Reader* 26 (2). Accessed March 2, 2022. https://giarts.org/article/creative-caregiving-initative

Stern, Mark J. 2011. *Age and Arts Participation: A Case Against Demographic Destiny*. Washington, DC: National Endowment for the Arts.

Storey, Keith. 2022. *Systematic Instruction of Functional Skills for Students and Adults with Disabilities*. Springfield, IL: Charles C. Thomas.

Sunderland, Jacqueline T. 1973. *Older Americans and the Arts: The Human Equation*. Washington, DC: John F. Kennedy Center for the Performing Arts: National Center on the Arts and Aging.

Sunderland, Jacqueline T. 1982. "The Arts and the Aging Advocacy Movement in the United States: A Historic Perspective." *Educational Gerontology: An International Quarterly* 8 (2): 195–205.

Tam, Maureen. 2014. "A Distinctive Theory of Teaching and Learning for Older Learners: Why and Why Not?" *International Journal of Lifelong Education*, 33 (6): 811–820.

Taylor, Edward W. 2011. "Fostering Transformative Learning." In *Transformative Learning in Practice: Insights from Community, Workplace, and Higher Education*, edited by Jack Mezirow and Edward W. Taylor, 3–17. Hoboken, NJ: John Wiley & Sons.

Taylor, Edward W., and Anna Laros. 2014. "Researching the Practice of Fostering Transformative Learning: Lessons from the Study of Andragogy." *Journal of Transformative Education* 12 (2): 134–147.

Tepper, Steven J., and Yang Gao. 2008. "Engaging Art: What Counts?" In *Engaging Art: The Next Great Transformation of America's Cultural Life*, edited by Steven J. Tepper and Bill Ivey, 17–48. New York, NY: Routledge.

Thornton, Lucia. 2013. *Whole Person Caring: An Interprofessional Model for Healing and Wellness*. Indianapolis, IN: Sigma Theta Tau International.

Throsby, David. 2001. *Economics and Culture*. Cambridge, UK: Cambridge University Press.

Throsby, David. 2010. *The Economics of Cultural Policy*. New York, NY: Cambridge University Press.

Toelken, Barre. 1996. *The Dynamics of Folklore*. Logan, UT: Utah State University.

Tuttle, Cody, Jill Tanem, Megan Lahr, Jonathan Schroeder, Mariana Tuttle, and Carrie Henning-Smith. 2020 *Chartbook 2020: Rural-Urban Differences Among Older Adults*. Minneapolis, MN: University of Minnesota Rural Health Research Center.

Uhlenberg, Peter, and Sonia Miner. 1996. "Life Course and Aging: A Cohort Perspective." In *Handbook of Aging and Social Sciences*, edited by Richard H. Binstock and Linda K. George, 208–228. San Diego, CA: Academic Press.

Ulrich, Roger S. 2009. "Effects of Viewing Art on Health Outcomes." In *Putting Patients First: Best Practices in Patient-Centered Care*, 2nd ed., edited by Susan B. Frampton and Patrick A. Charmel, 129–150. San Francisco: Jossey-Bass.

United Nations. 1948. "Universal Declaration of Human Rights." Accessed April 1, 2022. https://www.un.org/en/about-us/universal-declaration-of-human-rights

United Nations Economic, Social and Cultural Organization (UNESCO). 2014. *UNESCO Culture for Development Indicators Methodology Manual*. www.unesco.org/creativity/cdis

United Nations Economic, Social and Cultural Organization (UNESCO). 2001, November. "Universal Declaration on Cultural Diversity." Accessed April 1, 2022. https://adsdatabase.ohchr.org/IssueLibrary/UNESCO%20Universal%20Declaration%20on%20Cultural%20Diversity.pdf

United Nations Human Rights: Office of the High Commissioner. n.d. "A Cultural Rights Approach to Heritage: Special Rapporteur in the Field of Cultural Rights." Accessed January 30, 2023. https://www.ohchr.org/en/special-procedures/sr-cultural-rights/cultural-rights-approach-heritage

U.S. Congress. 1981, February 7. Hearing on "The Arts and the Older American." Select Committee on Aging, 96th Congress, Second Session. Comm. Pub. No. 96-222.

Ventegodt, Soren, Joav Merrick, and Niels Jorgen Andersen. 2003. "Quality of Life Theory I. The IQOL: An Integrative Theory of the Global Quality of Life Concept." *The Scientific World Journal* 3: 1030–1040. Doi: 10.1100/tsw.2003.82

Wacker, Robbyn R. and Karen A. Roberto. 2014. *Community Resources for Older Adults: Programs and Services in an Era of Change*. Los Angeles: SAGE.

Waldie, Jerome. 1981. Reports from the White House Conference on Aging, 1981, Numbers 1–13. April 11, 1980–November 1981. Washington, DC: White House Conference on Aging.

Waldrop, Deborah P. 2007. "Caregiver Grief in Terminal Illness and Bereavement: A Mixed-Methods Study." *Health & Social Work* 32 (3): 197–206.

Wallerstein, Nina and Bonnie Duran. 2010, April. "Community-Based Participatory Research Contributions to Intervention Research: The Intersection of Science and Practice to Improve Health Equity." *American Journal of Public Health* 100 (Supp 1): S40–S46. doi: 10.2105/AJPH.2009.184036

Wallerstein, Nina, John G. Oetzel, Bonnie Duran, Greg Tafoya, Lorenda Belone, and Rebecca Rae. 2008. "CBPR: What Predicts Outcomes?" In *Community-Based Participatory Research for Health*, 2nd ed, edited by Meredith Minkler and Nina Wallerstein, 371–392. San Francisco: Jossey-Bass.

Walter, Tony. 2012. "How People Who Are Dying or Mourning Engage with the Arts." *Music and Arts in Action* 4 (1): 73–98. Accessed November 1, 2018. http://musicandartsinaction.net/index/php/maia/article/view/dyingmourning

Wang, Huanming, and Bing Ran. 2021. "Network Governance and Collaborative Governance: A Thematic Analysis on their Similarities, Differences, and Entanglements." *Public Management Review* 25 (6): 1187–1211. doi: 10.1080/14719037.2021.2011389

Wankier, Jamie. 2020. "End-of-Life Issues." In *Caring for Older Adults Holistically*, 7th ed., edited by Tamara R. Dahlkemper, 142–154. Philadelphia: F.A. Davis.

Washburn, Allyson. 2021. "Wither Transformative Education? Taking Stock into the Twenty-First Century." *Journal of Transformative Education* 19 (4): 306–338.

Webb, Marilyn. 1997. *The Good Death: The New American Search to Reshape the End of Life*. New York, NY: Bantam Books.

Weber-Guskar, Eva. 2019. "Deciding with Dignity: The Account of Human Dignity as an Attitude and its Implications for Assisted Suicide." *Bioethics* 34 (1): 135–141. doi: 10.1111/bioe.12637

White House Briefing Room. 2015. "Fact Sheet: The White House Conference on Aging." Office of the Press Secretary, July 13, 2015. https://whitehouse.gov/briefing-room-statements-releases

White House Briefing Room. 2022. "Fact Sheet: The Biden-Harris Administration Announces More Than $8 Billion in New Commitments as Part of Call to Action for White House Conference on Hunger, Nutrition, and Health." September 28, 2022. https://whitehouse.gov/biefing-room-statements-releases

White House Conference on Aging (WHCoA). 1981. Reports 1–13. Washington, DC: Department of Health and Human Services.

White House Conference on Aging (WHCoA). 1996, February. *The Road to an Aging Policy for the 21st Century: Final Report.* Washington, DC: President of the United States.

White House Conference on Aging (WHCoA). 2015. *Final Report.* Washington, DC: President of the United States.

Wiese, Kim and Lauren Arce. 2021. "Healthcare Culture." In *Core Curriculum for Arts in Health Professionals*, edited by Ariadne Albright and Ferol P. Carytsas, 194–206. San Diego, CA: National Organization for Arts in Health.

Williams, Kristiann. 2020. "Common Medical Diagnoses." In *Caring for Older Adults Holistically*, 7th ed., edited by Tamara R. Dahlkemper, 209–228. Philadelphia: F.A. Davis.

Williams, Eric S., Grant T. Savage, and Patricia A. Patrician. 2017. "Quality Improvement Basics." In *Introduction to Health Care Management*, 3rd ed., edited by Sharon B. Buchbinder and Nancy H. Shanks, 145–168. Burlington, MA: Jones & Bartlett Learning.Wilson, Arthur L. 2008. "Lifelong Learning in the United States." In *The Routledge International Handbook of Lifelong Learning*, edited by Peter Jarvis, 512–520. London, UK: Taylor & Francis.

Wolf, Mary Alice. 2008. "Older Adulthood." In *The Routledge International Handbook of Lifelong Learning*, edited by Peter Jarvis, 56–64. London, UK: Taylor & Francis.

Wonock, Chung, Rebecca M. Genoe, Pattara Tavilsup, Samara Sternes, and Toni Liechty. 2021. "The Ups and Downs of Older Adults' Leisure During the Pandemic." *World Leisure Journal* 63 (3): 301–315.

Woodhouse, Jan. 2011. "Loss, Grief, and Bereavement." In *Key Concepts in Palliative Care*, edited by Moyra A. Baldwin and Jan Woodhouse, 107–112. Thousand Oaks, CA: Sage.World Health Organization (WHO). 2007. *Global Age-Friendly Cities: A Guide.* Geneva, Switzerland: WHO.

World Health Organization (WHO). 2015. *World Report on Ageing and Health.* World Health Organization. https://apps.who.int/iris/handle/10665/186463

World Health Organization (WHO). 2018. "The Global Network for Age-Friendly Cities and Communities: Looking Back Over the Last Decade, Looking Forward to the Next." Accessed January 30, 2023. https://www.who.int/publications/i/item/WHO-FWC-ALC-18.4

World Health Organization (WHO). 2020. "Ageing: Healthy Ageing and Functional Ability." Accessed June 30, 2021. https://www.who.int/westernpacific/news/q-a-detail/ageing-healthy-ageing-and-functional-ability

World Health Organization (WHO). 2021. *Decade of Healthy Aging 2021–2030.* https://who.int/initiatives/decade-of-healthy-aging

World Health Organization (WHO). 2022. *Constitution.* https://www.int/about/governance/constitution

Wyszomirski, Margaret Jane. 1995. "The Politics of Arts Policy: Subgovernment to Issue Network." In *America's Commitment to Culture: Public Policy and the Arts*, edited by Kevin V. Mulcahy and Margaret Jane Wyszomirski, 47–76. Boulder, Colorado: Westview.

Wyszomirski, Margaret Jane. 2000. "Raison d'Etat, Raisons des Arts: Thinking about Public Purposes." In *The Public Life of the Arts in America*, edited by Joni M. Cherbo and Margaret J. Wyszomirski, 50–78. Piscataway, NJ: Rutgers University Press.

Wyszomirski, Margaret Jane. 2008. "The Local Creative Economy in the United States of America." In *The Cultural Economy*, edited by Helmut Anheier and Yudhishthir Raj Isar, 199–212. Thousand Oaks, CA: Sage Publications.

Wyszomirski, Margaret Jane. 2013. "Shaping a Triple-Bottom-Line for Nonprofit Arts Organizations: Micro-, Macro-, and Meta-Policy Influences." *Cultural Trends* 22 (3–4): 156–66.

Index

For the benefit of digital users, indexed terms that span two pages (e.g., 52–53) may, on occasion, appear on only one of those pages.
Tables, figures, and boxes are indicated by t, f, and b following the page number

ableism 38, 149–52
Academy of Creative Aging 240n.2
accessory dwelling units 174
active participation in arts 84–85, 97–99
activities of daily living 175
acute care 181
Administration on Aging (AoA) 52, 55–56, 58, 214–15
adult day services (day care centers) 177
adult learning 52–53, 102, 116–17, 121, 122, 124, 125
  see also lifelong learning
advocacy coalition framework
  action steps for advocates for older adults 217b
  advocacy coalition 215–18
  advocacy movement 51–56
aesthetics 114
affective well-being 92
age consciousness 5
age-friendly communities 68, 152–56
age-friendly ecosystem 8–9, 33, 168
age-friendly health system 168–72
ageism 38, 149–52
Aggie's Story (play) 119
aging in place 4, 11, 36–37, 59–60, 155–56, 206
  see also independent living
Aging Mastery Program (NCOA) 10–11, 93, 94f
Alderfer, C. P. 76
Alexander, J. 58
Alzheimer's disease 9, 68, 81, 172, 180
ambient participation 43
American Assembly 45, 141–43
American Alliance of Museums (AAM) 214–15
American Association of Retired Persons (AARP) 57, 59, 155
Americans for the Arts (AFTA)
  action steps 217b
  Arts Advocacy Day 58, 68–69
  Arts in Health briefing paper 68–69
andragogy 115–16, 123

anticipatory grief 188
Aroha Philanthropies, *see* E.A. Michelson Philanthropy
art(s)
  choice-based arts participation 25, 29, 39–43, 144, 201
  culture and 13
  definition 1, 14b
  education, 22, 50, 68, 117
  educator, 120n.1 (*see also* Teaching Artists Guild)
  human development 25
  life course 108–13
  psychobiological view 107
  public health 33
  public purposes of 43–45
  slipperiness of concept 108
  transformative learning 128–31
"Art of Aging: Creativity Matters" campaign 64–65
arts administration 23
Arts Advocacy Day 58, 68–69
arts and culture sector 13–20, 140–45
"Arts and Minds" program, Studio of Museum of Harlem 135–36
"Arts and the Older American", hearing 53
Arts and the Public Purpose, The (American Assembly) 45, 141
arts-based education 22, 63, 94–97, 114–16
Arts for the Aging 153b
arts in community health (and well-being) 30–31, 32
arts in health 23
  Arts In Health briefing paper 68–69
  creative aging 29–33
arts in healthcare 30–31
arts in healthy aging 1, 29
  activating the ecosystem 212–19
  8Ps Framework 45–47, 219–22
  need for research and resources 11–13
  see also creative aging
arts in medicine 30–31
arts in public health 30–31, 32

Index

arts participation 22–23, 39–43
  attending (receptive) participation 84–72, 97–99
  barriers to 38, 97, 149–52
  benefits 40–41
  choice categories 42t
  creative (active) participation 84–85, 97–99
  8Ps Framework 46–47
  healthy aging 84–89
  modes of participation 42–43
  motivations 75–77, 79f, 95, 103–5
The Arts, Humanities, and Older Americans 227
arts policy, *see* policy
assisted living 175–81
attending art 84–85, 97–99
autobiographical memories 103–4
autonomy 97–99, 186–87

baby boomers 5, 34–35, 59, 63–64, 162–63, 204
Bailey-Johnson, J. 127
barriers to arts participation 38, 97, 155
Bastings, A. 63

behavioral problems 172
beholding 129–31
bereavement 192t, 195–96
Berridge, C. W. 151–52
Biddle, L. 53, 54–55
Biden presidency 208
birth cohort 5
Blandy, D. 140
blog posts 148–49
Bone, J. K. 146
Bowman, P. 115
Boyer, J. M. 64–65, 102
Bringing the Arts to Life: A Guide to the Arts and Long-Term Care 240n.2
Brown, A. 42
Bush administration 59
Byock, I. 185, 186–87, 188, 200

Camfield, L. 90
Campbell, E. 112
Canadian Journal on Aging, age-friendly concept article 154
caregivers 68, 176–77
care settings for older adults 173–83
Carpenter, G. 146–47
Catalyzing Creative Aging initiative, National Guild for Community Arts Education 67
ceremonies 199–200
certified nursing assistants 176–77
chronic health conditions 9, 80, 151–52, 169, 170t, 171t

clinical care 181–83
cognitive impairment 9, 80–81, 151–52, 171t, 172, 180
Cohen, G. 59, 64, 74–75, 76, 77, 85, 105–6, 122, 146
cohorts 5, 110, 111–12, 113–14
  see also baby boomers
comfort care 192t
community-based arts 23, 33, 97, 123, 140, 148, 149–50
  age-friendly communities 68, 152–56
  ageism and ableism as barriers to participation 149–52
  arts and culture sector 140–45
  continuum of services 139
  COVID-19 pandemic 145, 148–51
  examples of programs 141, 142b, 153b
  health and well-being outcomes 145–49
  organizations 141
  questions for arts programs 156b
  resource availability 138–45
  rural locations 139
  transformative learning 131–32
competencies, transformative learning 133, 134b
compression of mortality 6
Congdon, K. 140
Connor, S. R. 189
continuing care retirement community 178–79
Convergence Center for Policy Resolution report 167
COVID-19 pandemic 3–4, 34, 43, 145, 148–51, 167, 209
Cranton, P. 124, 126, 133
creating art 84–85
creative aging 1, 29
  arts in health 29–33
  folklore 113–14
  institutional infrastructure 207–12, 213f
  interdisciplinary fields 20–24
  policy 62–69
  see also arts in healthy aging
Creative Aging Innovation Forums 210–12
Creative Aging Institute 67–68
Creative Aging Mid-South 153b
creative arts therapies 30–31
creative participation 84–85, 97–99
creative sector 18–20
creativity 105–6
Creativity and Aging Study: The Impact of Professionally Conducted Cultural Programs on Older Adults (Cohen/NEA) 59, 64, 85
Creativity Matters: Arts and Aging in America (NCCA) 64–65

Creativity Matters: The Arts and Aging Toolkit (Boyer) 64–65
critical gerontology 33–34, 110
critical reflection 116
cultural context 71–72
cultural engagement 39
cultural mapping 157
cultural policy, *see* policy
cultural value 40
cultural well-being 92
culture
  arts and 13
  broad concept 38–39
  creativity and 106
  definition 13, 106
  expressive culture 108, 114
  folklore 106–7
  needs and motivations 76–77
  transformative learning 127–28
Culture Matters: Using a Cultural Contexts of Health Approach to Enhance Policy-Making (WHO) 71–72
cumulative disadvantage 112
curative care 192*t*
curatorial participation 43

Dance for PD 142*b*
death and dying, *see* end-of-life care
Death with Dignity law 188–89
dementia 9, 68, 81, 172, 180
demographics of older adults 2–6
Designing and Delivering Arts Programs for Older Adult Learners (NCCA) 82
developmental intelligence 74
Dewey, J. 115, 131
dignity 188
disability 151–52
Dissanayake, E. 107
diversity 37

E.A. Michelson Philanthropy 66–68, 144–45, 214–15
Ecker, D. 131
ecological model, age-friendly communities 154–55
economic well-being 4
educational attainment 4, 7, 139
education-focused programs 22, 63, 94–97, 114–16
Edwards, L. 146
8Ps Framework for Arts in Healthy Aging 45–47, 219–22
  Participation 103–5
  Partnerships 207
  People 198
  person-centered 168–72
  place 56–62
  policy 51
  program design 100
  purpose 43–45
eldercare 159–60
Elders Share the Arts (ESTA) 65
emotional health 80–81
Encore Creativity 142*b*
end-of-life care
  anticipatory grief 188
  autonomy 186–87
  dignity 188
  examples of arts programs 199*b*
  "good death" 184–89
  hospice care 182, 189–93, 194, 196
  landmarks and task work 187*t*
  legacy 198
  meaning-making 188, 196–97
  pain control 193
  physician-assisted death 188–89
  psychosocial support 198*b*
  reminiscence 197
  ritual 198–200
  spiritual care 194–96
  types of care in end-of-life settings 192*t*
  "What Matters" 186
engaging in arts and culture 38–39
Erikson's eight stages of life development 73–74, 77
eudemonic well-being 91
evaluative well-being 91
existential quality of life 90
expressive arts therapy 24, 30–31, 218
expressive culture 108, 114
extrarational transformative learning 128–31

falls 9
Fancourt, D. 84–85, 86, 147
Fareed, C. G. 127–28
federal agencies 14–15
Federal Interagency Forum on Aging-Related Statistics (FIFARS) 7, 9
Findsen, B. 121, 125
Finn, S. 84–85, 86
focusing event 57, 61, 62, 208
folk groups 107
folklore/folk arts 102, 103, 106–7, 112, 113–16, 119–20
Foner, J. W. 111
Formosa, M. 121, 125
forums 210–12
4Ms Framework of an Age-Friendly Health System (Institute for Healthcare Improvement) 168–69

Friedan, Betty 112
functional ability 7–9, 35–37, 205, 221–22
    healthy aging 81–83
    program design 93–94
    subjective well-being 91
    WHO definition 7–8, 81–82
functional age 109–10
functional assessment 175
functional limitations 7, 9, 132–33, 153

Gawande, A. 185, 186–87
generation X 5
Geriatric Education Centers 68
Gerontologist, The, editorial on age-friendly communities 155–56
gerontology 33–34, 109–10
Gifts of Art 183*b*
Gifts of the Muse 41
Gillis, M. 151
Global Age-Friendly Cities: A Guide (WHO) 153–54
"good death" 184–89
"good life" 90
grantmakers, action steps 217*b*
Greene, M. 114–15
grief 188, 195–96
Gullette, M. M. 150–51

Hamer, L. 115
Hanna, G. 64–65
happiness 90
Hartley, N. 197
health and well-being outcomes 1, 13–14, 20, 25, 29–30, 33, 45–46, 71, 95, 145–46, 159, 167–68, 169, 202, 205, 221, 223
health, broad understanding of 23
healthcare
    age-friendly system 168–72
    consumerism 162–64
    continuum 95
    person-centered care 168–72
    quadruple aim 164
    quality 162–64
    scope of practice of healthcare staff 182–83
    supporting healthcare staff through the arts 164
    system 159–60
    triple aim 164
health inequality 37–38
Health Resources Services Administration 68
healthspan 6, 36
healthy aging 6–11
    arts participation 84–89
    in natural aging process 77–83
    societal trends 204–5

healthy life expectancy 6
hedonic well-being 92
helping professionals 124
hierarchy of needs 75–76
Hoggan, H. 133
holistic healthcare 163
home health aides 176–77
home healthcare 176–77
hook rug making 103–4
hospice care 182, 189–93, 194, 196
hospitals 31, 181–82, 183*b*
hospital arts 182–83
House Select Committee on Aging 53
How Art Works (NEA) 44–45, 143–44
How to Care for Aging Parents (Morris) 166
human development 72–75
human rights 38
Hurston, Zora Neale 112

"I Know a Thing or Two" program 135
immersion 129–31
income levels 4
independent living 173–78
    see also aging in place
inequality 37–38, 112
informal caregivers 176–77
Institute for Healthcare Improvement
    4Ms Framework of an Age-Friendly Health System 168–69
    triple aim 162–63
Institute of Medicine, healthcare quality 162
Institute of Museum and Library Services (IMLS) 214–15
institutional infrastructure 207–12, 213*f*
instrumental activities of daily living 175
instrumental benefits 94–95
integrated healthcare 163
interdisciplinary model 148
interpretive participation 42
interprofessional care teams 182–83
inventive participation 42

Jarvis, P. 121
John F. Kennedy Center for the Performing Arts
    action steps 217*b*
    activating the arts in healthy aging ecosystem 215
    field convener 67
    National Council on Aging (NCOA) 54
Johnson, Perry 101–2, 137
Jordan Schnitzer Museum of Art (JSMA)
    Reflections and Connections Program 141
Jost, L. 135

Katz, S. 110, 111–12
Kay, John 103, 112–13
Kirshenblatt-Gimblett, B. 113–14
Kroth, M. 124, 126

Lambert, P.
LaPlaca Cohen 66–67
LaPorte, L. M. 123, 124
Laros, A. 116
late adulthood 5–6
Lawrence, R. L. 128
Lawton, P. H. 123, 124
Learning for Justice program 106
legacy 198
leisure activities 9–10, 23–24, 146–48
LGBT community 119
life care centers 178–79
life course 108–13
life expectancy 2, 3–4
lifelong learning 22, 121–23, 208–9
  program examples 135*b*
life plan communities 178–79
life satisfaction 90–91
life-story objects 112–13
LifeTime Arts 67–68, 135*b*, 217*b*
"Living History" approach 63
Lloyd, T. 113
logic models 44, 86–89, 219–22, 220*f*
Longevity and the New Journey of Retirement
  report 34–35, 36
longevity economy 4
longevity revolution 11, 36–37
long-term care 164–68, 179, 179*b*

MacArthur Research Network on Successful
  Aging 207
"making special" 107
mapping process 206–7
Martinson, M. 151–52
Maslow's hierarchy of needs 75–76
Mature Mind, The (Cohen) 74–75
Maze, Collete 104–5
McGarth, V. 115–16
meaning making 188, 196–97
Medicaid 164–68
medical tourism 162–63
Medicare 4–5, 54, 60, 164–68
Meeks, S. 155–56
Meet Me at MoMA 142*b*
memories 103–4, 109
memory care facilities 180
Menec, V. H. 154–55
Mezirow, J. 123, 124–25, 126, 129
Miller, J. B. 116, 128–29

Moody, H. R. 55
Morris, V. 166
motivations for arts participation 75–77, 79*f*, 95, 103–5
multigenerational living 174
museum-based program 135–36
music-making 104–5
Music Thanatology 199*b*

Naropa Community Arts Studio 142*b*
National Academies of Science, health inequality
  report 37
National Arts Service Organizations, action
  steps 217*b*
National Assembly of State Arts Agencies
  (NASAA) 65, 67–68
  action steps 217*b*
  activating the arts in healthy aging
    ecosystem 214–15
  Creative Aging Institute 67–68
National Association of Music Merchants
  (NAMM) 59
National Center for Creative Aging (NCCA) 59,
  60, 62–65
  *Creativity Matters: Arts and Aging in
    America* 64–65
  *Designing and Delivering Arts Programs for
    Older Adult Learners* 82
  dissolution 65, 212–14
  *National Leadership and Exchange Conference
    on Creative Aging* 65
National Center on Arts and the Aging 54
National Council of Senior Citizens 57
National Council on Aging (NCOA)
  action steps 217*b*
  activating the arts in healthy aging
    ecosystem 215
  Aging Mastery Program 10–11, 93, 94*f*
  policy activity 51, 54–56, 57–58
National Endowment for the Arts (NEA)
  action steps 217*b*
  activating the arts in healthy aging
    ecosystem 212, 214–15
  communities of practice 65
  *Creativity and Aging Study: The Impact of
    Professionally Conducted Cultural Programs
    on Older Adults* (Cohen) 59, 64, 85
  definition of "the arts" 14*b*
  How Art Works 44–45, 143–44
  Office of AccessAbility 55–56
  Office of Special Constituencies 52–53, 54–56
  policy activity 14–15, 50, 51, 52, 53–56,
    57–58, 59, 60, 61–63
  reports and publications 65, 84

National Endowment for the Arts (NEA) (cont.)
  Staying Engaged: Health Patterns of Older Americans Who Participate in the Arts 84
  Summit on Creativity and Aging in America 60–61, 210, 211b
  Survey of Public Participation in the Arts 40, 84
National Endowment for the Humanities (NEH) 55–56, 57–58
National Guild for Community Arts Education
  action steps 217b
  Catalyzing Creative Aging initiative 67
  Creativity Matters: The Arts and Aging Toolkit (Boyer) 64–65
  see also National Guild of Community Schools of the Arts 63
National Leadership and Exchange Conference on Creative Aging (NCCA) 65
National Organization for Arts in Health (NOAH)
  action steps 217b
  activating the arts in healthy aging ecosystem 215
  arenas of activity 31
National Research Center of the Arts poll 52
natural aging process 77–83
needs
  engaging in arts as a basic human need 38–39
  of older adults 33–38
  see also motivations for arts participation
New Jersey Performing Arts Center 64–65
Next Wave in Creative Aging: Creative Aging Innovation Forums Cross-Industry Report (Saunders) 148
nursing homes 4, 180–81

Obama presidency 60, 61
objective quality of life 90
observational participation 43
Office of AccessAbility 55–56
older adults
  care settings 173–83
  demographics 2–6
  perceptions of in arts policy community 52–53
  social isolation of women 4
  understanding the needs of 33–38
Older Americans 2020: Key Indicators of Well-Being (FIFARS) 9
Older Americans Act, 2020 amendment 68–69
Older Americans and the Arts: A Human Equation (Sunderland) 54
Opening Minds through Arts 179b
O'Rand, A. 112

Osher Lifelong Learning Institutes 135b
O'Sullivan, E. 126–27
outcomes
  arts-based programs 86–88
  community arts 145–49
  healthcare context 162
Owen-Booth, B. 146

Pabst Steinmetz Foundation 68
palliative care 182, 192t
paraprofessional caregivers 176–77
participation, see arts participation
partnerships 46
patient- and family-centered care 163
patient-centered care 163, 172
Payne, M. 197
people 46–47
Perlstein, S. 59, 63, 65
person-centered approach 47, 168–72
physical health 80
physician-assisted death 188–89
place 46–47
policy 49–70
  aging as a special constituency 51–56
  arts aiming for a place on the aging policy agenda 56–62
  challenges 207–12
  coordinated policy community 208–9
  Creative Aging 62–69
  cultural policy 15–18
  decentralizing Creative Aging policy 53
  diffusing arts in healthy aging 66–69
  8Ps Framework 46
  National Council on Aging (NCOA) 51, 54–56, 57–58
  National Endowment for the Arts (NEA) 14–15, 50, 51, 52, 53–56, 57–58, 59, 60, 61–63
  policy actors 49
  policy making 49–50
  second-generation approaches 207
  social structures of aging 111
  subsystems 215–16
  wicked policy problems 207
  window of opportunity 56–57, 68–69, 216
post-acute care 181–82
President's Committee on the Arts and the Humanities (PCAH)
  action steps 217b
  activating the arts in healthy aging ecosystem 215
problem-solving 131
professional associations, action steps 217b

professional development 65
program design
  basic elements 93–99
  considerations for learner-centered programs 97–99, 117–18
  education-focused programs 22, 63, 94–97, 114–16
  in 8Ps Framework 46–47
  goals 97, 98f
  logic models 44, 86–89, 219, 220f
  representative types 96f
  societal trends 205
  therapy-focused programs 30–31, 94–97
Program of All-Inclusive Care for the Elderly (PACE) 177–78
psychobiological view of art 107
psychosocial support 198b
public awareness campaigns 64–65
purpose 46–47

qualitative problem-solving 131
quality of life 90, 196–97, 204–5

Rabheru, K. 151
"rag on" 109
Rajan, K. B. 84, 85
Rajan, R. S 84, 85
Reagan presidency 57–58
receptive arts participation 84–85, 97–99
reflection 116, 129–31
reminiscence 197
respite care 181
Rethinking Care for Older Adults (Convergence Center for Policy Resolution) 167
retirement 5, 34–35
Riley, J. W. 111
Riley, M. W. 111
ritual 198–200
Roberto, K. A. 139
Robinson, Aminah Brenda Lynn 108–13

scholarship, gaps in 205–7
scope of practice 182–83
second-generation approaches 207
selective optimization and compensation (SOC) model 148–49
senior centers 178
senior housing 173, 180, 182–83
sensory loss 80
silent generation 5
Skevington, S. M. 90
skilled nursing facilities 180–81
Slover Linett 66–67

Smithsonian Institute, action steps 217
social connectivity 154–55
social determinants of health 8–9, 71
social gerontology 33–34, 109–10
social health 80–81
social prescribing 148
social theories of aging 111
societal trends 204–5
sociocultural context 71–72, 83f, 89–90
Sonke, J. 30, 32
spiritual care 194–96
Stagebridge 142b
Staying Engaged: Health Patterns of Older Americans Who Participate in the Arts (NEA) 84
StoryCorps 142b
storytelling 63, 103–4, 135
subacute care 181–82
subjective age 109–10
subjective well-being 89–93
Summit on Creativity and Aging in America (NEA) 60–61, 210, 211b
Survey of Public Participation in the Arts (NEA) 40, 84
Sykes, Marion 103–4

Tam, M. 122
Taylor, E. 116, 125–26
Teaching Artists Guild, action steps 217b
technological proficiency 149
Terry, P. 54–55
theater programs 119
therapy-focused programs 30–31, 94–97
Tighe, M.A. 53
TimeSlips 63, 179b
training 65, 67, 115, 164
transformative learning 116, 120, 123–28
  aims in the transformative learning environment 132b
  arts educator 131–33
  assessment strategies 133
  community setting 131–32
  competencies 133, 134b
  extrarational and the arts 128–31
  phases 125b, 130f
transitional care 181
Trump presidency 150–51

United Nations General Assembly, "Decade of Healthy Aging" 7
universal design (for learning) 132–33
Untapped Opportunity: Older Americans and the Arts (Culture Track) 66–67, 144–45, 210–12

values 89–90
Village Movement 174
virtual forums 210–12

Wacker, R. R. 139
well-being 23
  subjective 89–93
"What Matters" 168–69, 186
White House Conferences on Aging
  (WHCoAs) 55–61, 62, 64–65, 208
Whole person
  body 77
  mind 77
  spirit 77
  whole-person healthcare 77, 78f, 163

wicked policy problems 207
Wolf, M. A. 122–23
Wonock, C. 148
World Health Organization (WHO)
  Agenda for Sustainable Development 71–72
  Culture Matters: Using a Cultural Contexts of Health Approach to Enhance Policy-Making 71–72
  functional ability 7–8, 81–82
  Global Age-Friendly Cities: A Guide 153–54
  healthy aging 7–8, 81–82
  quality of life 90
  What is the evidence on the role of the arts in improving health and well-being? 84–85
Wyszomirski, M 58